Put Your Best FACE Forward

Put Your Best FACE Forward

The Ultimate Guide to Skincare from Acne to Anti-Aging

SANDRA LEE, MD

Board-Certified Cosmetic and Surgical Dermatologist

Star of TLC's *Dr. Pimple Popper*

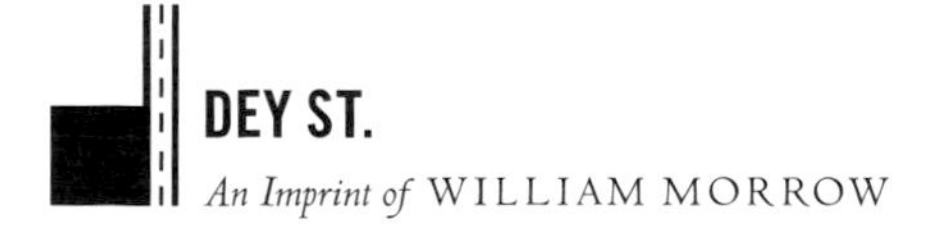

All photographs are courtesy of the author.

All illustrations are courtesy of SkinPhysicians and Surgeons.

This book contains advice and information relating to health care. It should be used to supplement rather than replace the advice of your doctor or another trained health professional. If you know or suspect you have a health problem, it is recommended that you seek your physician's advice before embarking on any medical program or treatment. All efforts have been made to assure the accuracy of the information contained in this book as of the date of publication. This publisher and the author disclaim liability for any medical outcomes that may occur as a result of applying the methods suggested in this book.

HarperCollins books may be purchased for educational, business, or sales promotional use. For information, please email the Special Markets Department at SPsales@harpercollins.com.

FIRST EDITION

Designed by Paula Russell Szafranski

Library of Congress Cataloging-in-Publication Data has been applied for.

ISBN 978-0-06-287229-6

18 19 20 21 22 LSC 10 9 8 7 6 5 4 3 2 1

This book is dedicated to those I'm most dedicated to:

my two boys, Chance and Stratton,

and my husband, Jeff.

Love you three to the moon and back.

CONTENTS

INTRODUCTION: GIRL MEETS PIMPLE 1

CHAPTER 1

Dr. Pimple Popper 101 19

CHAPTER 2

Thanks for Popping In! 39

CHAPTER 3

Acne: An Issue for the Ages 133

CHAPTER 4

Time Won't Tell 165

CHAPTER 5

Prescription for Beauty 181

CHAPTER 6

Sack the Lies, Hack the Truth 227

CONCLUSION: I'M NOT HURTING YOU, RIGHT? 253

ACKNOWLEDGMENTS 257

BDD AND BFRB RESOURCES 259

NOTES 261

INDEX 267

Put Your Best FACE Forward

INTRODUCTION

Girl Meets Pimple

YOU KNOW THOSE TIMES WHEN—*BING!*—YOUR EYES JUST POP OPEN WITH some profound realization you had overlooked before? For me, it was just past three o'clock in the morning when I felt a wave of anxiety wash over me. "What did I *do* yesterday?" I thought to myself. Did I *really* just start a GoFundMe page for one of my patients, whom I affectionately call Pops, without asking his permission? The day before, I had posted a video on my YouTube channel, Dr. Sandra Lee (also known as Dr. Pimple Popper), of some amazing blackhead extractions I had done on Pops. Blackheads, which are open comedones, are like snowflakes: each one is an individual; they are so satisfyingly unpredictable. Sometimes you squeeze one and get the most amazing pop: you never know if it will sputter out with a little light pressure from my comedone extractor or if it will slide out smoothly. Pops's blackheads were no different, and removing them had been an ongoing journey for us, since he had so many of them.

I have to back up a bit here for those of you who are not avid "popaholics," as I like to call them. The story of how I came to be Dr. Pimple Popper was unexpected—kind of a happy accident that I noticed and seized upon, and Pops has a lot to do with it. I have been a board-certified dermatologist in private practice for more than a decade, specializing in skin cancer and cosmetic surgery and reconstruction and laser surgery. You may wonder, aren't extractions something a dermatologist does regularly? Isn't this what a dermatologist *is supposed to do*? It's not that dermatologists aren't capable of "pimple popping"—that is, extracting blackheads, whiteheads, and milia, and surgically excising cysts. It's that this is such a small part of what our profession is about. We are experts who deal with all medical conditions of the skin, hair, and nails. And believe you me, there are *so* many!

In 2014 I had started an Instagram account, @DrSandraLee, intending to showcase my life as a dermatologist—to educate people on the many facets of my profession. Instagram is flush with gorgeous filtered images: mouthwatering pictures of food, exotic places traveled, and beautiful do-it-yourself makeup, hair coloring, and styling tutorials. I saw a quickly increasing popularity among makeup and hair gurus, as well as a growing interest in spa treatments and cosmetic treatments. Would these same people, and others, be interested to see what I do day-to-day, as well? Hmm . . .

One day Pops came in for a regular appointment, but something was different. For years, I had seen him as one half of a whole, or what I lovingly call a "package deal," meaning that he and his wife came together. Always. Except this time, his wife wasn't with him. I knew she had been ill; recently, she had taken to waiting in the car during his appointments, not feeling up to coming into the office. I couldn't help but ask how she was doing, and instantly regretted doing so.

"She's gone." Pops choked back tears and looked down at his hands. She'd been his whole life. She ran the show. And now he was lost without her. I noticed that his clothes weren't as neatly pressed as they usually were, he had a stain on his slacks, and his hair appeared a little more disheveled. Nothing I do can take away a person's emotional anguish, but I wish I could have waved a magic wand and made some of that pain and sadness disappear. Opening a GoFundMe page in his name was an impulse move—a result of my learning about his economic hardships and overwhelming grief since his wife had passed away. People who watched my videos from around the world sent the kindest messages of hope and love to Pops and donated money to help someone whose face they'd never seen! They'd just heard his story and knew every blackhead extracted from him by heart! My popaholic fans are amazing: we ended up exceeding the $5,000 goal and raised more than $14,000 for Pops!

Pops and his wife had been my patients for many years, but in all that time, I was examining his skin and mainly treating and controlling his precancerous skin lesions and skin cancers (non-life-threatening but locally destructive squamous cell carcinomas and basal cell carcinomas). It actually took the unfortunate passing of his dear wife for me to bring up the fact that those bumps on his nose were benign blackheads and whiteheads. It wasn't until this point that he confided that he knew they weren't dangerous, but he absolutely detested them. Not because he could see them; his eyesight was failing and he couldn't. But because he could feel them, and he couldn't get rid of them himself, and they made him feel ugly and ashamed.

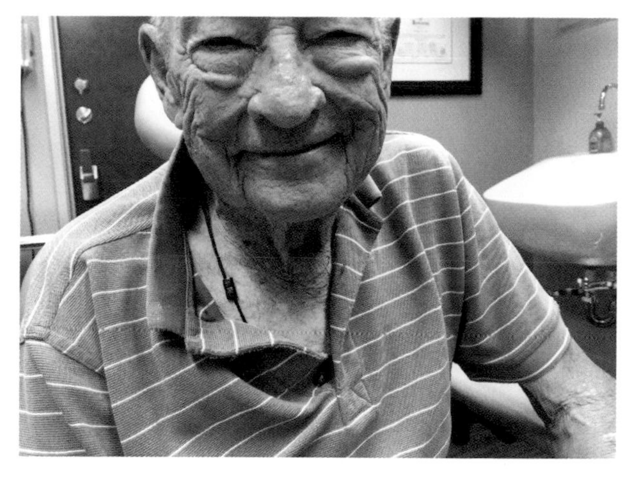

Pops after he was surprised with more than $14,000 from his fans around the world.

So I asked him, "Would you like me to extract as many of these as I can? This is a procedure I can't bill to insurance, but if you allow me to film the procedure for others to watch, I won't charge you." He immediately agreed, very happy that I was going to take care of them. This surprised me. I had never offered this service to my patients in the past because, as a dermatologist, I avoid extractions that aren't medically necessary, as health insurance doesn't cover them. Patients normally have to pay out of pocket for these "cosmetic" procedures, and they can be very expensive because they are time consuming.

Just a couple of months prior to this, I had posted a video on Instagram of me extracting a blackhead on the back. To my surprise and curiosity, there was a noticeable increase in "likes" on this post and, subsequently, on any posts involving "pimple popping." In fact, my most popular Instagram posts were simple blackhead extractions. Would followers be interested in other things that I pop out of people's skin? Yes! People were mildly interested in what it looked like to administer Botox or treat a wart, or even to see what psoriasis looked like. People seemed to get really excited, though, when I posted a milia extraction or a blackhead squeeze. Once they saw that, they were hooked. I am talking about unbridled enthusiasm. People who liked it loved and obsessed about it. People who hated it detested it. Either way, they tagged their friends because they just *had* to share. I had happened upon the discovery of a pretty substantial demographic of popaholics.

No longer wanting to limit myself to fifteen-second clips on Instagram (today the app lets you post one-minute clips, but back in the olden days—a couple of years ago—fifteen seconds was its limit), I posted a full-length pimple-popping video to my YouTube channel, a platform I had created and originally used for TV appearances, and which was meant to appeal to a much smaller fan base. What should I call this Instagram page and YouTube channel that I would devote mainly to sharing things that I'm able to pop from the skin? Well, I gave myself the moniker Dr. Pimple Popper, and things really *erupted* from there.

People were demonstrating a substantial interest in an area of medicine that usually doesn't get much attention. My YouTube videos of Pops, his blackheads, and his emotional progress after losing his wife have been viewed—get this—more than sixty million times! As I write this, I have exceeded 2.5 billion total views on my YouTube channel, with the vast majority of them coming since 2015. Because of this social media exposure, which I created in a very DIY fashion, I went from being a private-practice physician to an international social media personality and influencer, with beauty magazines and TV talk shows seeking my expert opinion, and my social media pimple popping being featured in the *Wall Street Journal,* the *Washington Post,* and *New York* magazine.

I've come to realize that it's a shame most dermatologists don't treat these benign cosmetic conditions, because it's very obvious to me that these "ugly" bumps and embarrassing spots on our faces and bodies have so much to do with how we feel about ourselves, and this, of course, affects every aspect of our lives.

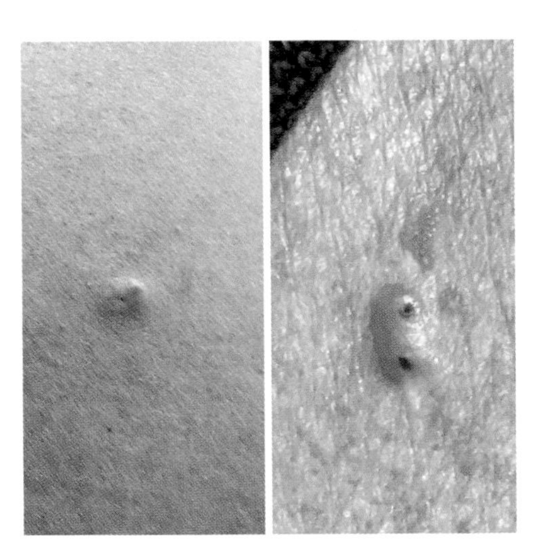

Blackheads on the back.

Now if I notice that one of my acne or skin cancer patients has a blackhead or milium, I like to offer to extract it for free in exchange for permission to videotape the procedure so I can post it on my social media. Happily, very few people decline this offer. I've been pleasantly surprised to learn that they are extremely grateful that I suggest it, making for win-win-win situations. My patient gets rid of something that has been bothering them for some time, and at no cost. Viewers of my YouTube channel, Instagram, Snapchat, Twitter, and Facebook page get to witness the glory and satisfaction of a good blackhead extraction. Finally, for me it's been an unexpected win, as I hadn't realized how very appreciative many of my

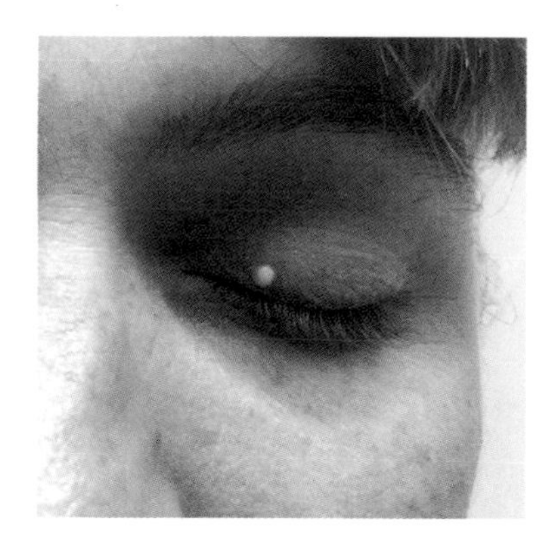

Milium on left upper eyelid.

patients would be after I removed a growth that had been a source of embarrassment, shame, and even depression because other physicians may have refused to remove it.

I really have no simple clear concrete idea why people like to watch pimple popping, but I certainly have some theories. For many, it's akin to slowing down and staring when driving past a car wreck, while for others, there is this feeling of fright followed by euphoria and exhilaration, similar to riding a roller coaster or watching a scary movie. And for those who keep coming back, there is something hypnotic about watching a pop or a squeeze or even an incision; it's satisfying on a deep psychological level, perhaps because eliminating a blemish of any kind offers a sense of closure, resolution, and accomplishment. Ultimately, the reason I continue to do this, and why my viewership continues to grow, is that watching pimple popping seems to make people *happy*. Can you believe that? It's fascinating to me and mind boggling at the same time.

How my life has changed since I started posting my work on social media. I would have thought the private practice I share with my dermatologist husband, Jeff Rebish, in a quiet suburb of Los Angeles would continue to grow gradually over time and that my workdays would be filled with surgical and cosmetic procedures: Mohs micrographic surgery (a technique to remove skin cancers), Botox and fillers, acne treatment, eyelifts, liposuction, and lasers to treat brown spots, red spots, and fine lines and wrinkles. A few years ago, I never would have believed that I would be extracting thousands of blackheads, cysts, lipomas—anything that pops from the skin. I have removed more blackheads, excised more cysts, and popped out more lipomas in the last few years than I have during my whole dermatology career before then—times a hundred!

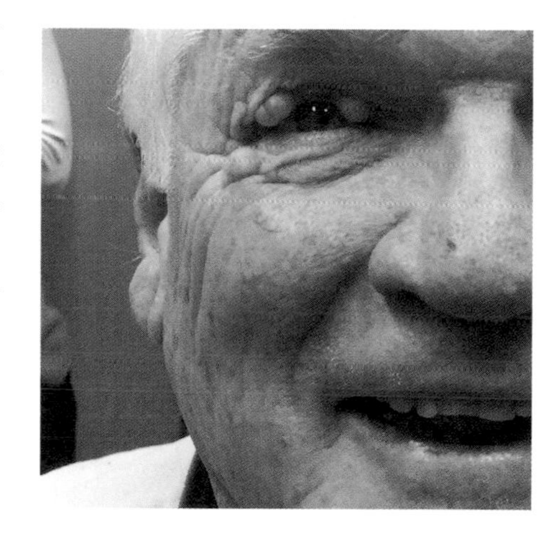

Patient with benign cysts called hidrocystomas around the eyes. You can see why he would want these removed even though it's not medically necessary.

I still do all the things a dermatologist does in private practice, but the other day, before my first patient arrived, I filmed a segment with a British TV talk show about how celebrities with acne get red-carpet ready.

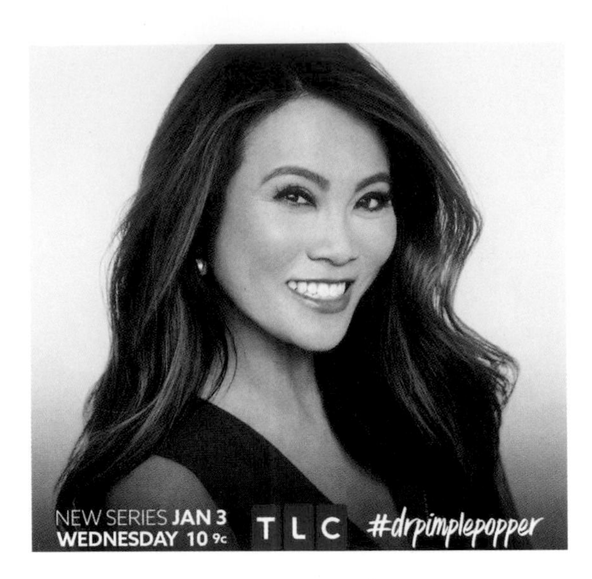

My new show on TLC is called Dr. Pimple Popper.

The next day, I talked to an Australian morning radio show about what makes people obsessed with popping pimples. A few days later, I answered questions about skin on Facebook Live with a well-known American magazine. After that, I collaborated on a video with a famous YouTube star from Amsterdam. And now I have a television series on the TLC channel, named, appropriately, *Dr. Pimple Popper.*

Fame has its moments too—good and bad. My least favorite experience was when I just had my first child via C-section and I was in the hospital recovering. The nurse came in the day after delivery, woke me by opening the drapes to bring light into my room, and announced I needed to get up and use the bathroom. One of the first major steps you have to take to get a hospital discharge is to be able to use the bathroom on your own. Man, that was tough! I hobbled slowly, completely stooped over, making my way to the bathroom while almost overcome with waves of nausea and light-headedness—I thought I was going to pass out! I left the bathroom door open so the nurse could get to me in case I hit the floor. As I was sitting on the toilet trying to catch my breath, I'm sure with no color in my face, the secretary at the labor and delivery desk darkened my bathroom doorway. "Hi, remember me?" she said excitedly. "You saw me for the spots on my back a few months ago, and I have more and was wondering if you could take a look and tell me how I can get rid of them?" Please don't do that to *anyone.*

Another instance was when a patient's daughter approached me on the golf course. I was in midswing when I heard a golf cart approach me from behind. Her father had instructed her to cross over two golf fairways to ask me to look at the mole on her back and tell her it was okay! Please don't do this to your dermatologist. It's difficult to assess your moles or give you any skin advice when we are away from our office and don't have your personal history in your chart or our instruments to properly assess your skin growth. Needless to say, I took a mulligan on that hole!

It's not that I don't want you to say hello when you see me, but try to save the medical questions for the office setting, please. Okay, well, I do secretly have a favorite time when a patient of mine approached me. In the grocery store, this happens every now and again: A sweet patient will come up to me and say "Hi, Dr. Lee, it's So-and-So. Remember me? You did surgery on me last month!" My favorite response: "Oh, hi! Sorry, I didn't recognize you with your clothes on!" I love doing that. Makes my day, haha.

Putting my work life on display on social media was eye-opening to me, because it validated to me that the hard work I put into making sure my patients are comfortable and relaxed in my office is truly one of my best attributes as a physician. And I really learned this from my father. I still recall the words he told me in the first few weeks I began work as a dermatologist myself. He said to me: "Always remember, Sandra, that the physician that graduates at the very top of his medical school class, who receives the most respected accolades and awards in medical school and residency, who is considered one of the most intelligent physicians around, can have a crappy bedside manner—be cold and curt, impolite and condescending, and will quickly be regarded as a terrible doctor. Conversely, the physician who had mediocre grades and accomplishments during her training but who has a wonderful bedside manner—who is open, warm, inviting, confident, and inspiring—will easily be touted as an excellent physician in intellect and skill." Obviously, we all ideally want to be smart and accomplished *and* have a great bedside manner, but this advice was meant to explain to me that how we treat our patients emotionally is just as important as how we treat them physically. This is one of the very best (but certainly not the only) pieces of advice my father has given me.

LET'S REWIND

I should explain how and why I became a dermatologist, which was much more complicated than a standard résumé can express. The most obvious reason that dermatology was on my radar at all was because my father was a dermatologist (now retired). My father grew up very poor in Singapore, one of ten kids. As a child, he loved to read and was obsessed with books. He would stare longingly into the windows of bookstores. All the money he could scrounge up by doing odd jobs was used to buy books. Needless to say, the house that I grew up in was *full* of books, with stacks of volumes on every conceivable subject to be found on every table, bedroom nightstand, and even available counter space.

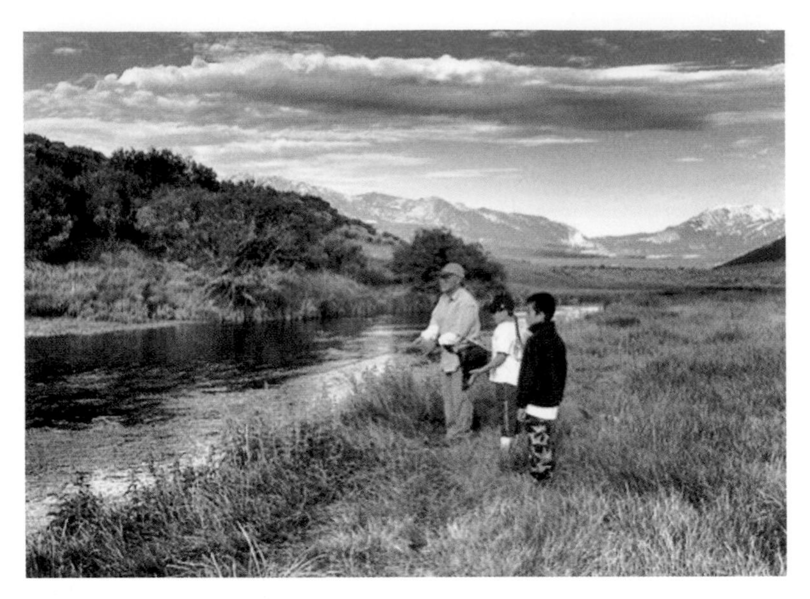

My father teaching my two boys how to fly-fish in nearby Mammoth Lakes, California.

If my dad didn't know the answer to a question or was just curious about a particular subject, what would he do? He'd buy a book! I knew the aisles of our local bookstore intimately. Nearly every weekend, we used to spend a couple of hours at the shop, where I would wander off to discover the wonderful titles lined up neatly on the store shelves. I'd listen for the comforting sounds of my dad's keys jingling in his pockets and his whistling familiar tunes—reminders that he was close by. I think my father bought every dermatology textbook ever published!

As a result, I grew up unfazed by photographs of, say, a person with psoriasis, a maddening chronic skin disease characterized by bright red plaques with a thick layer of overlying silvery scales sometimes covering 80 percent of the body. I didn't have any qualms about eating dinner next to my dad while he read a medical journal that included pictures of a patient with a fungating, oozing baseball-sized mass growing from the side of his head. Only one image ever really bothered me and I have to admit it is still ingrained in my memory: that of a young child, about my age, afflicted with tapeworms that emerged like long strands of linguine from his backside. That image turned me off noodles for a while! I couldn't stop staring at it, and to this day, I avoid any pork that looks slightly undercooked, as tapeworm infestations can be caused by eating undercooked meat from an infected animal.

My parents didn't behave like the typical Chinese immigrants who moved to the United States—you know, the so-called tiger parents who demand their offspring learn to play the violin and piano, study hard, and attain only As. They were not parents who dictated no sleepovers. No joke! I like to say we're a hybrid, and I admire that my parents recognized and took advantage of all the positives of being immigrants and left many of the negatives behind. Okay, so my brother and I did learn to play the piano, but instead of the violin, we tried to master different musical instruments, such as the flute (me) and the double bass (my brother). We both played classical guitar quite seriously, competing at young ages nationally.

My father is self-taught on piano and ukulele, so in addition to books, our home was always filled with music, too. My parents expected us to do well in school, but they were not helicopter parents. In fact, I'm embarrassed to admit that I got a D in physics in college and this went unbeknownst to my mother and father until after I graduated. (And I *still* got into medical school and became a dermatologist, so there is hope for us all!) My brother and I participated in plenty of extracurricular activities, but they were a little "off the grid": we didn't just play soccer or basketball, and I didn't just attend gymnastics or tap-dancing class. I threw myself into ice skating, baton twirling, and fly-fishing. I was lucky that my parents could and wanted to provide me with so many opportunities and rich experiences.

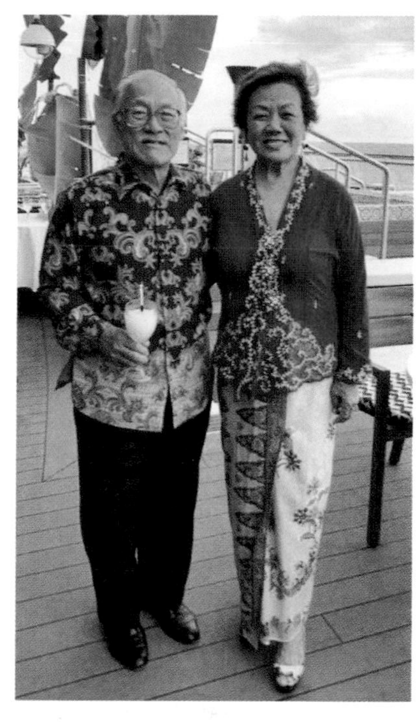

My parents.

My mom temporarily stopped working as a nurse to raise my brother and me, taking us to and from our many activities. Despite being a busy physician, my father made it a priority to be home every night for dinner and to listen to us practice our music. I always believed that I take mainly after my father. After all, I did follow him in his profession, and I've really listened to and incorporated all the advice he's given me through the years. But more recently, I've realized that I am also like my mother. She has a vibrant, inviting personality, always smiling, always happy, always intent on pleasing others and making them feel good. My mother is a fantastic cook who whips up incredible multicourse meals with no prior preparation, and with no distress. I am in awe of that.

Okay, I digress. Where was I?

I studied biology at the University of California, Los Angeles. Nearing the end of my four-plus years at UCLA, I still wasn't entirely sure what I wanted to do in my life. I'd always been strong in math and science, but did I really want to go to medical school? Sure, I wanted to follow in my father's footsteps, but I knew that getting into a dermatology program would be extremely competitive and difficult. To be honest, I applied halfheartedly to medical school, primarily to delay entering the "real world" for a few more years. I was so lucky to be accepted to Hahnemann University School of Medicine (now the Drexel University College of Medicine). I packed up and moved clear across the country to Philadelphia.

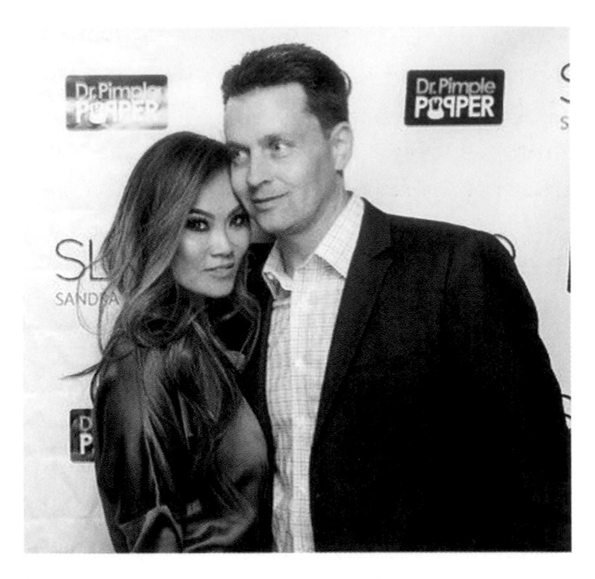

Me and my husband, Jeff Rebish, MD.

The City of Brotherly Love is where I met *my* love, my husband, who attended medical school along with me! Jeff may adamantly dispute the methods he went through to court me, but this is my book, and I'm sticking with my story! So here we go:

All first-year medical students must complete a course in gross anatomy. It's common practice to form small groups and slowly but meticulously take apart a human cadaver. Now, a medical cadaver was once a person who consciously made the decision to allow future physicians to study his or her remains in order to understand the difference between the large and small intestine, to identify the pancreas versus the spleen, to observe how a ball-and-socket joint truly moves, to dissect the facial nerve and all its tributaries along the face, and so on, as an introduction to what we may do to humans in the future . . . who are still alive.

During the course, I befriended five fellow medical students over a delicately thin, small-boned cadaver of a woman, probably in her nineties, with long silver hair and pink painted nails. Jeff would find time during the hourlong course to wander over to my cadaver table. He would be intensely curious about what we were doing. "Oh, you found the cecum [pronounced *see*-cum]?" he'd ask. "Yes," I'd reply. "We had a little trouble finding it, but we just did." I'll show you our amygdala if you show me yours. Ha!

Yes, he courted me over my cadaver in gross anatomy. I'm not ashamed to say that it worked. I love telling this story, but seriously, in hindsight, it should have been an indication to me of how romantic he would be as a life partner. Let's just say . . . not very romantic, but neither am I, so we're even!

In every medical school in the United States, third-year students do rotations in various medical specialties. It's when you apply classroom knowledge to clinical experience, usually in a hospital setting. You are required to rotate among the major general specialties to give you a broad range of exposure, since it is during this time that students determine the area of medicine in which they will specialize. Med students are required to spend time in obstetrics and gynecology (ob-gyn), surgery, pediatrics, internal medicine, and psychiatry. They also get to choose two or three *sub*specialties such as radiology, anesthesiology, emergency medicine, orthopedic surgery, ophthalmology, and dermatology. It's helpful to have prior interest in a specialty so that you know it's right for you. However, I imagine there are just as many students who decide that a specialty is *not* for them during this time. For example, Jeff discovered that he didn't enjoy orthopedic surgery; instead, he wanted to also apply for a dermatology residency position.

The beginning of the fourth year of medical school is when you must decide which medical specialty you wish to pursue and begin scheduling interviews with various programs around the country. Did you know that dermatology is one of the most competitive specialties? Do you think it's because everyone wants to be a pimple popper? (Actually, popping pimples is a small part of a dermatologist's day.) According to the National Resident Matching Program, of the more than thirty thousand residencies in the United States in 2015, just over a hundred were in dermatology. Consequently, you have many people competing to fill a much smaller pool of positions. The primary reason why it's so competitive is that we deal with very few dermatology emergencies or life threatening conditions that are really complicated multisystem diseases. Unlike a general surgeon or obstetrician, dermatologists aren't often beckoned by the hospital in the dead of night or during weekends.

In general, we interact with healthy, happy patients of all sexes and all ages, from the neonate to the octogenarian, and with all races and ethnicities. Sometimes I joke that I'm a glorified hairdresser in the way that I develop relationships with my patients. They may look forward to visiting me, and often recruit their family and friends as well. We get a lot of hands-on work—skin biopsies, tissue cultures, fungal preparations, surgical excisions—which keep the days moving quickly and easily. We can avoid getting too caught up in the intricacies and difficulties of health insurance, since many of the procedures and treatments we perform are cosmetic and therefore on a fee-for-service basis. I like to say we don't live to work but work to live. Basically, the kind of dermatology I do is a low-stress, high-satisfaction, exclusive, potentially highly lucrative medical specialty, and for these reasons, it is *really* hard to snag a dermatology residency position.

Many dermatology residents are smarty-pants—at the top of their medical school classes. Yet I was determined. I really wanted to specialize in dermatology, and I'm pretty intense when I get my mind set on something. I applied to every program I could and wound up invited on about thirty interviews, more than anyone else I knew applying for a dermatology residency position. I thought I was sitting pretty at that point.

I was confident—perhaps too confident—because my dad was a dermatologist, and I had grown up in that world. However, this certainty may have been my biggest mistake. Jeff also applied for a dermatology residency position, and at many of the same programs as I did, in an attempt to "couples match"—if not in the same dermatology program, then at least in the same area of the country. While we weren't yet married, we were linked together, and programs knew that we wished to be a package deal. Well, this was my second mistake because most programs have maybe one, two, or three dermatology positions available per year. This greatly decreased our stock. No program wants to feel forced to take two people when it may want only one of them.

It's a pretty crazy process in the United States, if you don't know how this whole find-a-residency-position-after-medical-school thing works. Students interview and create a prioritized list of where they would like to train and in what specialty. Similarly, residency training programs interview medical school applicants and compile lists of who *they* wish to see in their program. This is all fed into one secretive computer program, and everyone's priority lists are tabulated there to create the most matches between student and program. Then there's one day in March, called Match Day, when all around the nation, all fourth-year medical students receive notice simultaneously telling them which program has accepted them.

Essentially, all fourth-year medical students find out on the same day what they will potentially be doing for the rest of their lives, and where they will be training. Well, I never got to experience this exhilaration, this excitement. I didn't get into *any* program at all.

What was I going to do? How did this happen? I was devastated and so embarrassed and ashamed. Everyone else was popping open the champagne, excitedly discussing and sharing where in the country they would be spending the next few years, relieved that this entirely stressful process was over. Not me. I felt numb and wanted to just disappear. I had failed at the most important thing in my life and, apparently, had wasted all this time and effort.

But life goes on, and with the support of Jeff (who, by the way, *did* match into a dermatology program in his home state of New York), I moved on and fulfilled my first-year residency requirement, which is to do a transitional medicine internship year. I was fortunate to have an extremely helpful and encouraging program director at my internship at Pittsburgh's Allegheny General Hospital. He generously allowed me a month to rotate at a dermatology program at Southern Illinois University, six hundred miles away. I rented an apartment next to a cornfield in Springfield, Illinois. I had to show SIU how much I wanted to be a dermatologist and how great I would be to work with. I had to win them over and make sure they wanted to spend the next few years working with me on almost a daily basis. I never gave up, and although I felt like I had a huge mountain to climb, I wanted to try one more time. What other choice did I have? Give up medicine after having spent so many years slowly but surely trudging toward this goal? Go into another specialty and learn to love it like I already knew I loved dermatology? I faced some dark days.

Long, stressful story short: against *many* odds, the next year I matched in dermatology at SIU. I went from feeling like the unluckiest person on earth to feeling like the most fortunate. I had been swimming upstream against a strong and uncertain current but had made it. And I could not waste the opportunity that was finally granted to me. I will always be grateful for these people who gave me a chance and for the people who supported me in this highly stressful journey. I had done it. In retrospect, I see that my most satisfying successes were usually preceded by giant failures.

The next year, I knew I had to marry this wonderful man who had stood by my side and helped me through this difficult time. There were still sacrifices to be made, as we trained in separate dermatology programs in different states—heck, in different time zones!—for the next few years. However, these are the concessions you often have to make in order to do what you love, what you feel like you should be doing, what you know you will be the happiest doing.

In another important stroke of luck, I matched into a truly wonderful, nurturing program. Although I was married, I lived alone, without any relatives or friends in the area. But the staff, nurses, and dermatologists at the SIU Division of

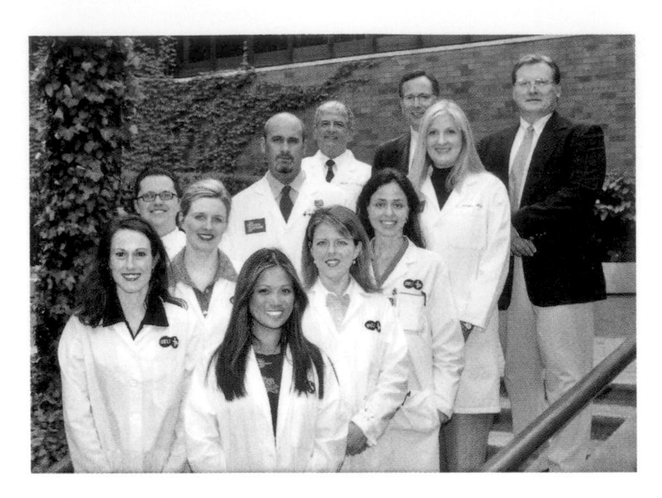

SIU dermatology program.

Dermatology invited me into their homes and included me in their lives. Perhaps this is the Midwestern mentality—it was certainly a welcome one for me, and one I won't ever forget.

I wasn't training in a fancy, fast-paced city with bosses who cared more about their celebrity patients than about their residents. I didn't have the distractions of trendy dance clubs or bars to go to (or of waking up the next morning with a hangover). It was dermatology 24/7. I knew that I loved to work with my hands, and I was lucky to train with a top-notch physician skilled in Mohs micrographic surgery, the most effective and advanced treatment for skin cancer today. The female dermatologist who served as program director had the most amazing bedside manner, which I observed closely and still try to emulate. They let me be my goofy self and didn't treat us unfairly or take advantage of us, as some other dermatology programs can do. They cared about us, our opinions, and, most important, were dedicated to helping mold excellent dermatologists.

It's a big deal and stressful to me to tell this story, because I have never spoken these words before. I have never told my staff or my colleagues or my close friends about the run-up to my career. Of course, I can't bring myself to say that if I had the chance to do it all over again, I would do it differently. The fact that everything didn't fit into place easily, and that I reached a point where I felt all my future goals had been washed away, was extremely humbling—but also highly motivating. I likely wouldn't be the dermatologist that I'm proud to say I am today if I hadn't had to truly examine how badly I wanted it and then tried again to make it happen. I'm pretty convinced that I certainly would not have become Dr. Pimple Popper if I hadn't gone through these dark, stressful, seemingly fruitless times. These experiences made me into a much better doctor. I'm lucky to be a dermatologist, and I don't *ever* take it for granted.

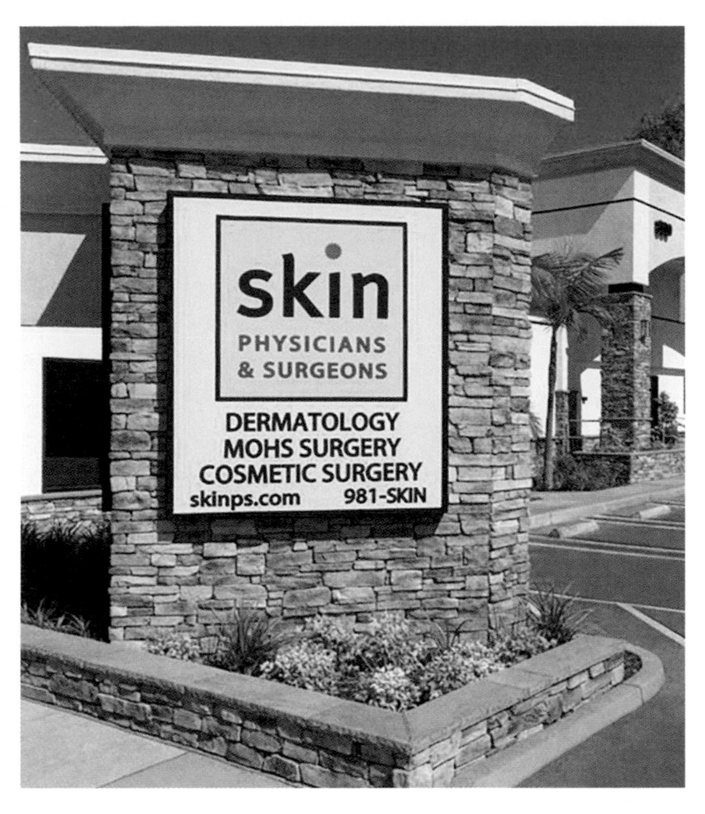

My office in Upland, California.

After a couple of years, my husband and I were able to make it back to California and start our own practice together. Remember, though, that I'm pretty type A: when I reach for the stars, I try to grab the farthest, brightest star out there. Not surprisingly, I decided to complete an extra year of training in a laser and cosmetic surgery fellowship in San Diego with a world-renowned dermatologist and laser surgeon, Richard Fitzpatrick, MD. Many famous dermatologists are pompous, self-absorbed, and just plain mean, but Dr. Fitzpatrick is not only extremely intelligent but also very down-to-earth and just a pleasure to be around. Everyone loves him! I had excellent surgical training in Illinois during my residency, but it is during this fellowship that I used my surgical skills to explore more cosmetic treatments, including hair transplants, lower face facelifts, aggressive laser resurfacing, eyelifts, and tumescent liposuction.

Finally, after four-plus years of undergraduate school, four years of medical school, four years of dermatology residency training, plus that extra year in between, and a final fellowship training year, at thirty-three years old, I was ready to be a dermatologist on my own! Phew, that took awhile! In 2004, Jeff and I took over my father's dermatology practice in Upland, renaming it Skin Physicians & Surgeons. It would have been amazing to work alongside my dad, but the day I started working was the day he retired. Deservedly so, since he had worked many years beyond what he would have chosen for himself to keep his practice afloat so that we could take the helm easily. Now he was free to strum his ukulele and plan his many fly-fishing adventures around the world.

My dad has always been an excellent source for honest advice, and I will readily admit that the first couple of times I performed surgery on my own, I asked him to be available in the office while I worked. It's nerve-racking to do that first surgery on your own, without the umbrella of someone else over you protecting you. I could hear him strumming his ukulele and singing while I whittled away at someone's nose, removing a skin cancer and reconstructing the area so that it was barely visible. Yup, the good ol' days. Here I am now, more than a decade later. My dad doesn't need to watch over me anymore, haha. We have two sons and a thriving practice that we love.

Here I am, working in a suburb of Los Angeles, and people travel from Northern California, Texas, New York, Canada, London, Malaysia, Saudi Arabia, and even Nigeria to see me. Why do people travel from far distances to see me when there are thousands of dermatologists to choose from? It boggles my mind. Strangers stop me at the store or the gas station with adoration in their eyes, and they tell me that I have been a positive influence in their lives. Adults have actually trembled and cried when they shook my hand to say hello. I joke that I've attained rock-star status in the world of dermatology. What the heck happened here?

I enjoy what I do, and get to know such interesting people, treat fascinating skin diseases, and perform many cosmetic procedures that I felt people would find interesting and like to learn about and follow. My gut told me that people would be interested in seeing how Botox treatments are administered, witness what liposuction under local anesthesia looks like, or understand the skin diseases I see and diagnose. And, yes, see what kinds of growths I pop out of perfectly normal people. As a result, with the permission of my patients, I made the decision to post my work.

In *Put Your Best Face Forward,* I expand on the excitement created by my videos and take the opportunity to give in-depth answers to questions about skin conditions and skincare. You will meet some of my most special patients in the pages that follow, including Pops, Mr. Wilson, Mr. Gold, the Masked Man, and Momma Squishy—a wonderful lady who had been dealing with large, embarrassing bumps on her body for twenty years until I was able to remove most of them.

You'll also learn a lot about your skin and how to best take care of it. This is not a medical textbook, but I have included everything that I think is important for you to know to improve your skincare at home, at your doctor's office, and beyond: from identifying your skin type, to learning how to safely remove blackheads, to understanding how to protect your skin from aging and from environmental and other factors. *Put Your Best Face Forward* is a fun, accessible, yet scientific and informative guide. It's a book I hope you turn to again and again—for there is nothing in here that I do not stand behind. I share with you only the ideas and treatments I believe in, and I am clear in my warnings when I don't think you should do something, especially in terms of at-home treatments. Know when to pop and when to stop!

I have been so blessed with fans and followers, and I am so excited to share even more knowledge with you. The more you know, the better and more glowing your skin can and will be!

Chapter 1

Dr. Pimple Popper 101

IF YOU ARE A REGULAR VIEWER OF MY YOUTUBE CHANNEL, YOU WATCH ME address all kinds of skin-related topics, using specific medical terms. I tend to stick with what works, the tried and true, but, of course, I have learned many things along the way. Here I'm going to give you a crash course in Dr. Pimple Popper and some skin basics. This will set you up for what follows in the rest of the book and give you a chance to think about your own skin. It's important when you read *Put Your Best Face Forward* that you don't think I'm speaking a foreign language! Just as people use the metric system to talk about measurements, dermatologists use their own special terms to understand and communicate skincare concerns and concepts. These important terms and techniques help you understand the different conditions and treatments I refer to in the book and on my social media. This guide can even help you to understand your own skin better, and to discuss questions and concerns with your dermatologist. (They'll be impressed by your new vocabulary!)

A PRIMER ON DERMATOLOGIC LESIONS

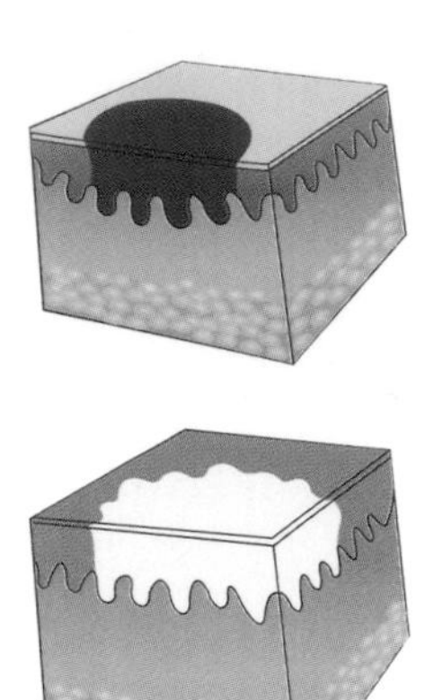

Top: Macule. Bottom: Patch.

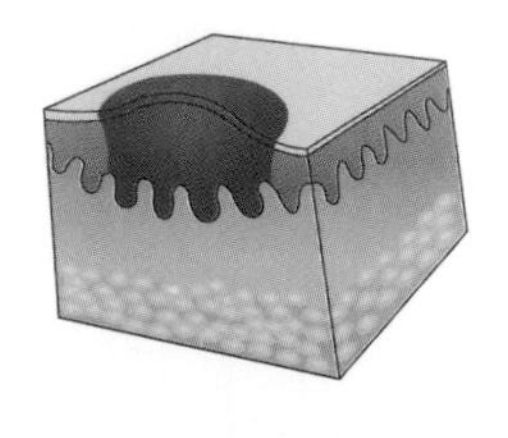

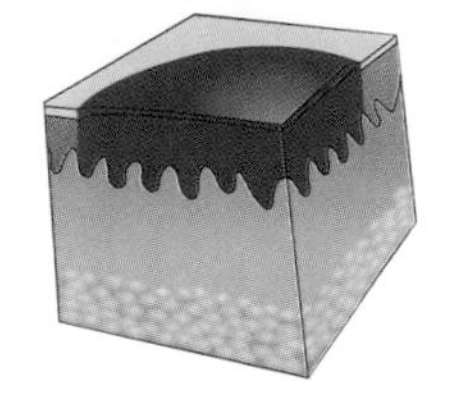

Top: Papule. Bottom: Plaque.

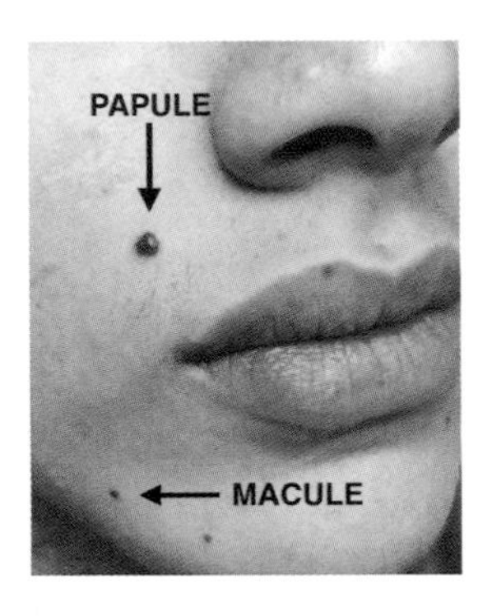

Macule versus papule.

MACULE This completely flat lesion on the skin measures less than 1 centimeter in diameter and can be any color of the rainbow. A good example is a freckle or a flat mole. When you run your finger over it, you don't feel any change in the surface of the skin.

PATCH A patch is flat just like a macule, only larger (greater than 1 centimeter in diameter). Examples include vitiligo (white patches where pigment cells have been destroyed), melasma (see page 55), and a large, flat birthmark.

PAPULE An elevated, raised, well-rounded growth projecting from the skin's surface that is less than 1 centimeter in diameter. This is different from a blister, a vesicle, or a pustule. Good examples are a raised mole, a cherry angioma, a seborrheic keratosis, and a wart.

PLAQUE This is what we call a papule that is greater than 1 centimeter in diameter. Again, it's elevated and well circumscribed. Psoriasis is commonly described as plaque-like growths, but many other dermatologic conditions appear as plaques.

NODULE A raised growth under the skin, but it is deeper seated and not as superficial as a papule. You popaholics

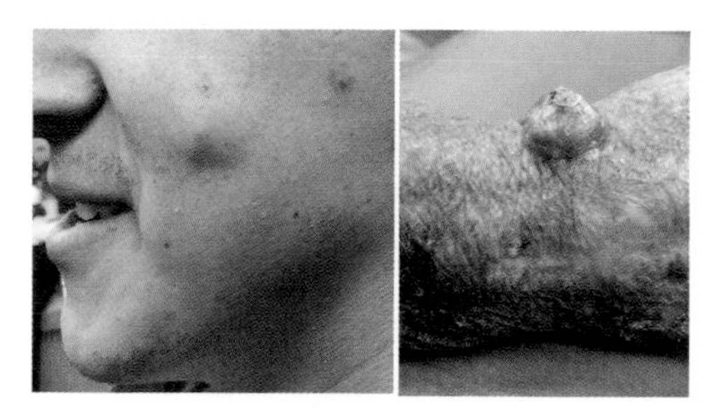

Left: Nodule (cyst) on the cheek. Right: Nodule (squamous cell carcinoma) on the wrist.

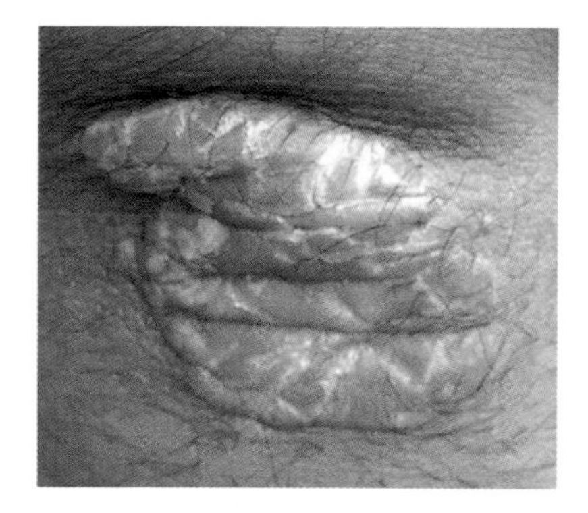

Example of a plaque: psoriasis on the elbow.

know this well. A nodule is often at least 2 centimeters in diameter, or about the size of a penny. We use this term to describe lesions such as cysts, lipomas, keloids, and two common skin cancers, basal cell carcinoma and squamous cell

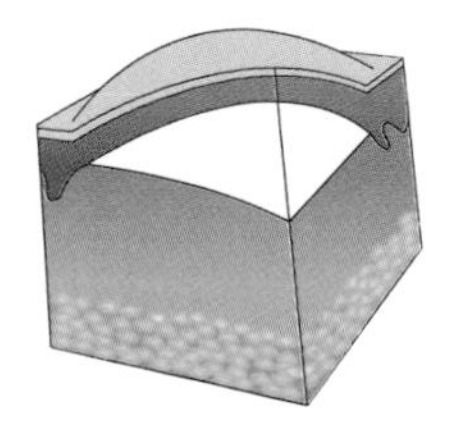

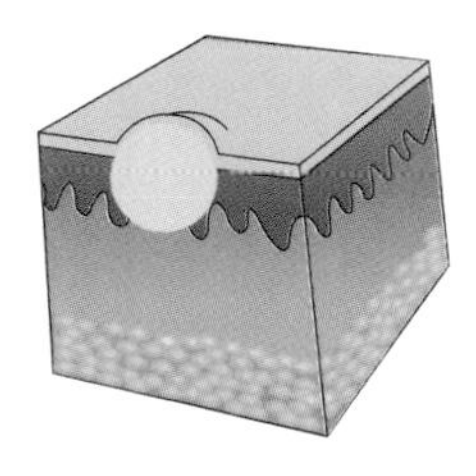

Top: Bulla. Bottom: Pustule.

carcinoma. See, I taught you something without your even knowing it!

VESICLE A raised, well-circumscribed growth, less than 1 centimeter in diameter, but primarily filled with a clear liquid. This is what we see in cold sores (herpesvirus), chicken pox, and shingles.

BULLA This is something many of you popaholics would get excited to see, because it's essentially a big blister; a large, water-filled vesicle greater than 1 centimeter in diameter. This is how we

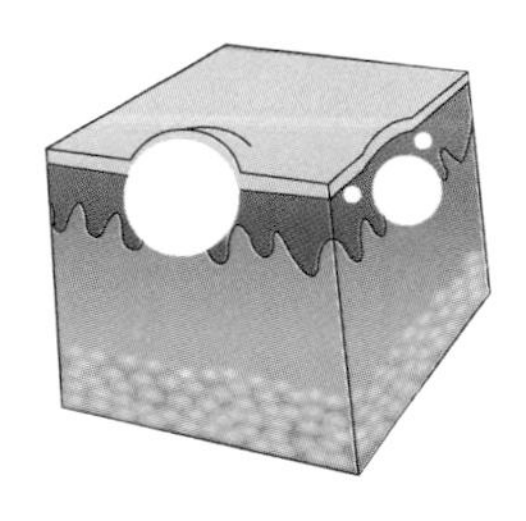

Nodule.

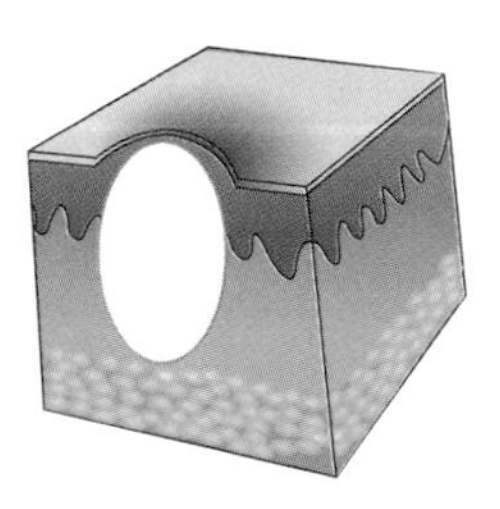

Vesicle.

describe a friction blister (the type of blister we get from ill-fitting shoes), and also, we see it in many blistering disorders of the skin.

PUSTULE An elevated, circumscribed growth that is much like a vesicle, but instead of being filled with a clear liquid, it is filled with a purulent fluid, pus. This is seen in acne.

CRUST A layer of dried sebum (an oily substance secreted by the sebaceous glands located in the skin and often attached to hair follicles), pus, or blood mixed with epithelial (tissue) or bacterial debris.

SCALE An excess buildup and/or shedding of stratum corneum, the outermost layer of the skin.

FISSURE A linear crack in the skin, which can often be quite painful. You may get one or more of these on the heel of your foot or even on your tips of your fingers when the areas are irritated.

EROSION A superficial open wound with loss of skin.

ULCERATION A deep open wound with a partial or sometimes complete loss of skin and even deeper structures.

EXCORIATION: Loss of skin due to picking or scratching.

ATROPHY: A thinning of the epidermal or dermal tissue.

LICHENIFICATION: An increase in skin lines and creases as a result of chronic rubbing.

If you want to know more specific morphological terms we use in dermatology, go to my website, at www.drpimplepopper.com.

The Truth About Tumors

When many people hear the word *tumor,* they automatically think of something malignant (cancerous) and life threatening. I think of that scene in the movie *Kindergarten Cop* where Arnold Schwarzenegger yells to the kids, "It's *not* a *too-mahhhhh!!*" Actually, *tumor* is a generic term, simply meaning a growth on the skin or on an organ within the body. We refer to nonmalignant tumors as benign. So don't let the word *tumor* frighten you!

THE TECHNIQUES AND INSTRUMENTS I USE AS DR. PIMPLE POPPER

NUMBING MEDICATION AND 30-GAUGE NEEDLE

I probably get the most complaints about posting video footage of numbing procedures, including videotape of my administering anesthesia with a needle and syringe. It gives many people more heebie-jeebies than the purulence, or pus, that emits from an abscess does! But it's important you see what I do here.

I would certainly argue that dermatologists are the best compared with any other medical specialty when it comes to administering local anesthesia with the least amount of pain and discomfort possible, since we do this on a daily basis. I actually perform many maneuvers at the same time when I stick someone with a needle. I know that this is one of the main reasons why some people avoid going to the doctor: they are afraid of needles. My ultimate goal is to anesthetize patients painlessly—in fact, to numb them before they even realize I'm doing anything at all to their skin—because it instills trust between patient and dermatologist. Here are several of my favorite techniques:

1. HIDE THE SYRINGE: Needles are not on display in my office. They are hidden in my pocket or held close to my side, passed to me on the sly by my assistant—certainly not waved in front of patients to increase their anxiety.
2. I'M "BASIC": Numbing medication such as lidocaine is acidic, which is why it burns when we inject it under the skin. We temper this burning sensation by adding sodium bicarbonate to the mix. $NaHCO_3$ raises the pH of the liquid, reducing the acidity and thus making the injection more comfortable.
3. 30-GAUGE NEEDLE ONLY: I don't use any needle thicker than a 30-gauge, which is very thin: not much wider than the size of a single hair. Because the smaller the needle, the smaller the pinch; the smaller the pain, the smaller the hate.
4. SHAKE OR PINCH THE SKIN WITH MY NONDOMINANT HAND: This is an important one, and one that draws a lot of attention on my videos. People watching sometimes think I'm nervous or have a tremor. I don't. I'm actually doing this purposefully.
5. INJECT SLOWLY AND TAKE ADVANTAGE OF FIELD EFFECT: This is actually something I don't think a lot of physicians realize if they don't inject as often as we dermatologists do all day, every day.

6. TALK-ESTHESIA: An important one. I don't think I'm actually a chatterbox in real life. (I'll bet that many of you who've watched my videos find this hard to believe.) But I ask open-ended questions, or just chatter on about current events or even about myself, to distract the patient from the task at hand, including the sounds that the scalpel makes as it cuts the skin and the "sliding" sound of the suture (stitch) that passes through the skin. Also, if a patient is formulating an answer to one of my questions, his or her focus is no longer on the surgery. It's all about distraction, and it works.

11 BLADE VERSUS 15 BLADE

These are the two main types of surgical blades I use. The 11 blade is what I rely on instead of lancets (small, short pins), because it comes to a very sharp point and allows me to nick the skin very superficially to cause as little damage as possible before I extract a whitehead or milium. I use a 15 blade in surgeries to excise tissue before I place sutures, or to shave off a layer of skin to send for a biopsy.

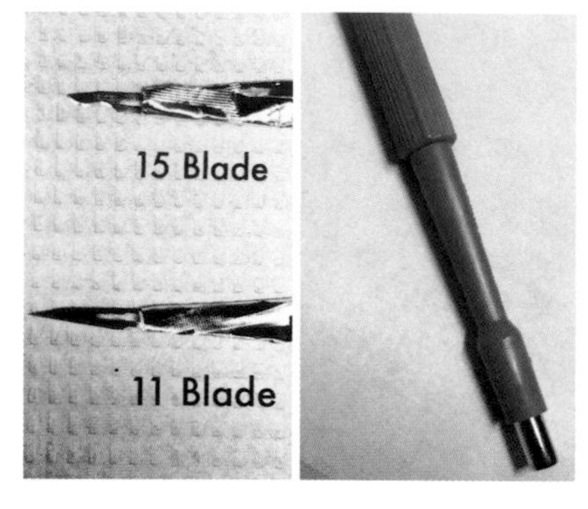

Left: 15 blade and 11 blade. Right: A punch biopsy tool.

COMEDONE EXTRACTOR AND TWEEZER

There are so many different types of comedone extractors, but the Schamberg-type tool is really my jam. It avoids excess trauma to the skin and allows controlled, even pressure around blackheads or milia in order to best extract them efficiently.

The comedone tweezer is something I've discovered myself because of—guess what?—social media! I, too, was transfixed by videos that I saw on Facebook and Instagram of a physician using a curved tweezer to push against the skin and then

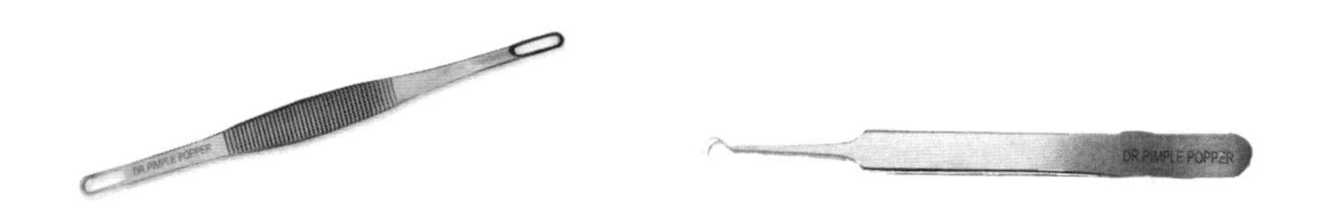

Left to right: The official Dr. Pimple Popper comedone extractor and blackhead tweezers.

to pull out completely the extruded blackhead. I've tried it out, and I like it, but it doesn't replace my original comedone extractor. It's also particularly satisfying to pull out sebaceous filaments using these funky-shaped tweezers designed specifically to get into tight spaces and pull gently from the skin stuff that shouldn't be there.

THE PUNCH VERSUS EXCISION

Many of you ask me how I decide which approach to use in removing a cyst: whether to excise the area or to pull out the "punch" biopsy tool that so many of you are enamored of. Well, it has everything to do with the size of the cyst, its location, and my mood that day. In other words, there are many instances when I can do either a punch or a standard elliptical excision, but let me explain my criteria for choosing one option over the other.

In all instances, I could perform a standard elliptical excision, but sometimes the punch excision is quicker, which is partly why I may choose it. First, you should understand that this circular cookie-cutter-type tool is traditionally used to take a skin sample (biopsy) when the goal is to obtain a deeper component of skin, as opposed to a shave biopsy, where we merely take off the superficial layer. We also use the shaving technique to take off a mole sitting up on the skin, so that the area is left flat and flush with the regular skin.

The punch biopsy tool takes a core of tissue so that we can assess the dermal and subcutaneous tissues, the deeper components of the skin. In the case of cyst removal specifically, I use the punch tool to create a larger opening in the cyst so that I can squeeze out its contents and keep the surgical repair line short. Punches come in many different sizes, from as small as 1 millimeter to probably as big as 2 centimeters or so. There are even elliptical-shaped punches (which I don't use because you can't cut through the skin with a twist, as the tool is not circular). It's important to understand that the larger the circular punch, the more difficult it is to close the resulting wound from side to side without creating "dog ears" or "Burow's flaps"—that is, pooching up of the outer edges of the surgical wound.

This is actually why excisions are elliptical or diamond shaped. Seamstresses understand this concept, as they know that a circle cannot be sewn together without getting bumpy, but "darts" have to be created on the outer edges so that the clothing will lie flat. This is why I perform punch excisions of cysts only if the sacs are on the smaller side. I really use only punches that range in size from 2 millimeters to 5 millimeters; any larger than, say, 6 millimeters, and the dermatologist will need to convert to a more elliptical excision, so I might as well do that in the first place!

Location is also important when determining punch versus standard excision. Areas with thinner and more mobile skin and areas that are generally covered by clothing would be possibly punchworthy. You really won't see me doing a punch on the face unless the skin is really loose and movable, as in the case of an older gentleman with thin cheek skin. Elliptical excisions are more elegant and cosmetically superior. I don't use a large punch excision on the thick and stiff skin of the back in a large person because a slit excision may be preferable: any wideness to an excision has to be pulled together, and the more tension that is created, the wider the excision, with increased risk of the scar spreading and an inferior cosmetic result.

AND THE CURETTE RAN AWAY FROM THE SPOON

Before I "became" Dr. Pimple Popper, I was handling maybe ten cyst excisions a year; now I probably do about that much in a week. Needless to say, I've gotten better at preparing and predicting cyst behavior, improving the final result, and decreasing the incidence of recurrences. There's actually a video on my YouTube channel that shows the moment I realized that the curette would be pretty useful when ensuring the complete removal of cysts. The curette is a standard instrument used by medical dermatologists, but most commonly, it's for scratching or scraping off lesions that grow atop the skin—particularly seborrheic keratosis (see page 48). I also use a curette to clean out the "hole" at the excision site, to ensure that the entire cyst and cyst wall have been eliminated. Leaving behind any tissue from the cyst wall heightens the risk of a recurrence.

MESSY VERSUS CLEAN CYST EXTRACTION

As with politics, this is a divisive topic. Some people prefer watching messy cyst extractions; others prefer watching a cyst excised completely cleanly and intact. I just wonder if one group is composed more of Democrats and the other of Republicans. But as a physician, I always stay away from the topic of politics! Personally and professionally, I prefer a clean extraction, mainly because this reduces the odds of the cyst recurring. Also, as you have seen from my videos, the contents of a cyst sac can be all colors of the rainbow, chunky like cottage cheese or egg salad, creamy like mashed potatoes, or thick and sticky like oatmeal or wet newspaper.

I know you're not grossed out if you're a popaholic! In addition, I have learned that the larger the cyst size and the longer it's been around, the more likely the contents have liquefied somewhat, so if this cyst is opened rather than removed intact, it can create quite a mess. And you guys don't have smell-o-vision, but you often comment on this; you both want to know and *don't* want to know what the contents of the cyst smell like. Well, in general, we in the room don't want to know, so if we avoid opening up the cyst, we minimize any odor detected.

What do these pops smell like? Not all of these growths I pop out from the skin smell, but like I say all the time, I don't really try to smell them! We all wear masks, and I would say that smell is not my dominant sense. (Thank goodness in this case.) However, I know that so many of you people are curious about this, so let me give you the best idea, and maybe one of these days I can create a scratch-and-sniff that you guys can get and see for yourself! First of all, it's mainly epidermoid cysts and infected cysts that have a strong odor. But not all epidermoid cysts have a strong smell. Lipomas don't smell; they look like raw chicken breast, so I'm guessing if I stuck my nose real close and took a whiff, they would smell like that?

But trust me, I'm not trying this anytime soon. Pilar cysts often don't give off an odor. However, noninflamed epidermoid cysts can certainly emit a pungent odor that often stays with you hours later, and I'm always reminded that the reason we smell things is because tiny microparticles actually escape into the air and get caught in our nasal passages and nasal hairs, so we are actually inhaling and ingesting odors in order to "smell" them. Gross, huh? Thought I would share that with you. Since I have to deal with that unnecessary and regrettable knowledge, so should you!

I'll tell you what I think, but let's ask my staff their opinions. Kristi, one of my medical assistants, says: "Spoiled Progresso soup. I know that's weird; it's only because I worked in claims at Sam's Club, so I know how awful that stuff smells when it's gone bad."

Me: "A certain kind of soup, would you say? Like, cream of mushroom, maybe?"

Kristi: "Whatever they sell in bulk there, haha!"

Sorry, Progresso, I love your soup (when it's not spoiled), so don't sue me! Valeria, another one of my medical assistants, says: "It smells like toe jam or one of those really expensive superstinky soft cheeses."

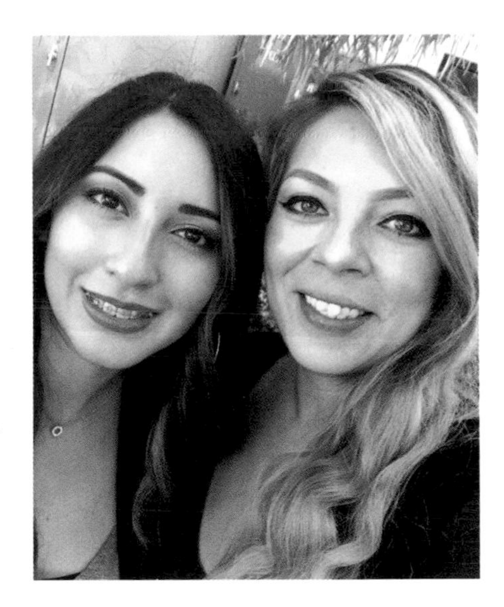

Valeria (left) and Kristi (right), my two medical assistants.

Cyst Superstar: Mrs. Gold

Mr. and Mrs. Gold represent why I love dermatology so much. They are couple goals. They are why I would never want to just see young acne patients or limit my dermatology practice to only cosmetic procedures. Then I would never get to meet people like them! I love the couples who have been married for decades, who are ornery and sassy and witty, who know each other so well that they can easily push each other's buttons but choose to do so in a loving and teasing way.

Mr. Gold is really the one we focused on, and the main reason they came to see me in the first place. But Mrs. Gold has an inflamed cyst on her upper back, one that many popaholics were salivating over and pleading with me to remove, which we did as well. Mr. Gold has rhinophyma, which causes disfiguring enlargement of his nose. He is a proud and witty man, and doesn't really like to express how much it bothered him and how embarrassed he felt when interacting with others. Imagine that with every single person you speak to, you feel self-conscious that they are not really listening to you or looking you in the eyes. They are instead looking at your nose and noticing that it looks like you have three nostrils instead of two. I did something called electrosurgery, using a device that can cut through the oily, thickened skin of the nose like a hot knife through butter, essentially resculpting the nose. I'm quite proud of the outcome. How impressive that such a relatively simple procedure conducted under local anesthesia can have such a resoundingly positive impact on someone. It's why I'm proud to be a dermatologic surgeon and really what makes my job so enjoyable. I get to be creative and meet wonderful people who will touch my life as I have touched theirs.

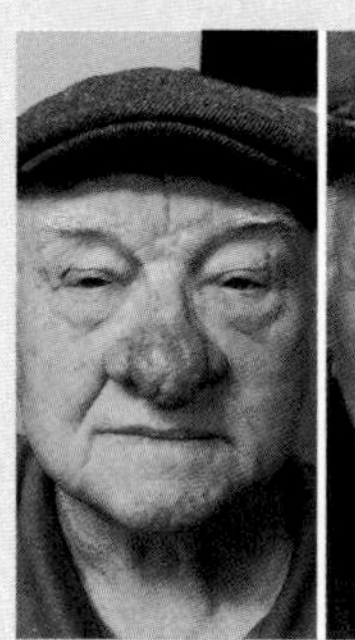

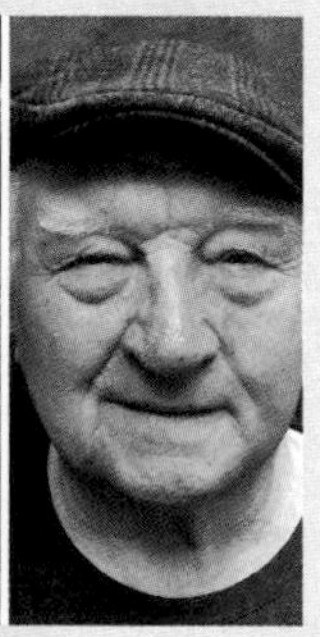

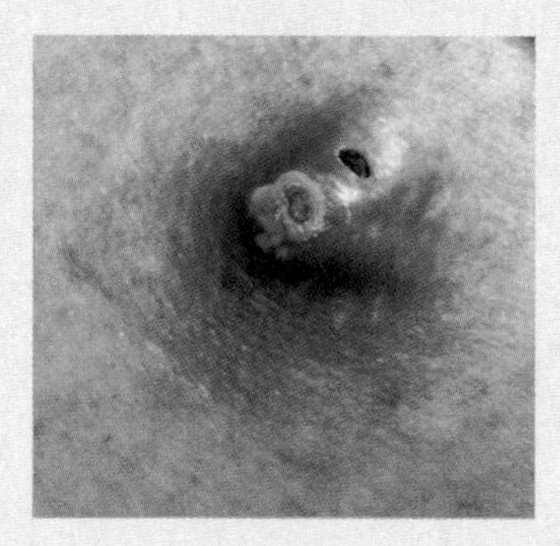

Left: Mr. Gold before and after rhinophyma surgery.

Right: Mrs. Gold's inflamed cyst.

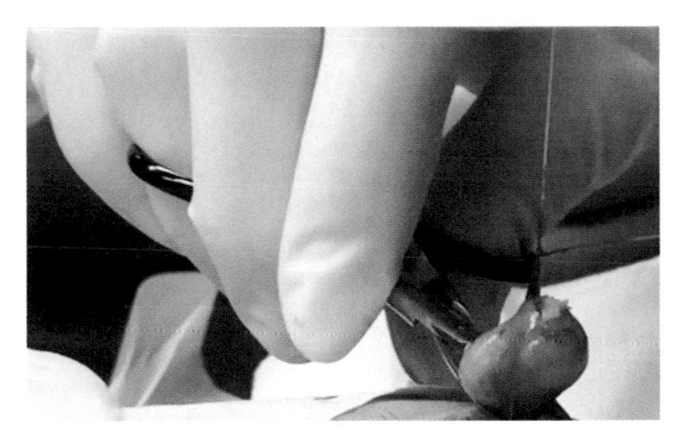

What I call a suspension stitch.

SUSPENSION STITCH

Suspension stitch is my name for this method. This is a temporary stitch that I place in the cyst or growth itself, and I use it to help provide traction, so that I can pull this growth out from under the skin—especially when I'm trying to not disrupt the cyst or growth and want to take it out intact.

BURIED VERTICAL MATTRESS STITCH

This is the type of stitch I place first in almost all my excisions. I most commonly use Vicryl, an absorbable suture, so that in about six to eight weeks, the stitch should dissolve or break down. (Sometimes your skin "spits" out this partially digested suture at this time.) It is a very important stitch to use because it's actually the "muscle" stitch, providing longer-lasting strength during that critical healing time in the first one or two months after surgery. Don't let anyone stitch you up anywhere on the body without putting in deep stitches like this if the wound edges gape open "at rest." In other words, if there is *any* tension on the wound edges, a deep buried vertical mattress stitch is essential for keeping the resulting scar line a small, thin straight line and not a widened, ugly scar that resembles a stretch mark.

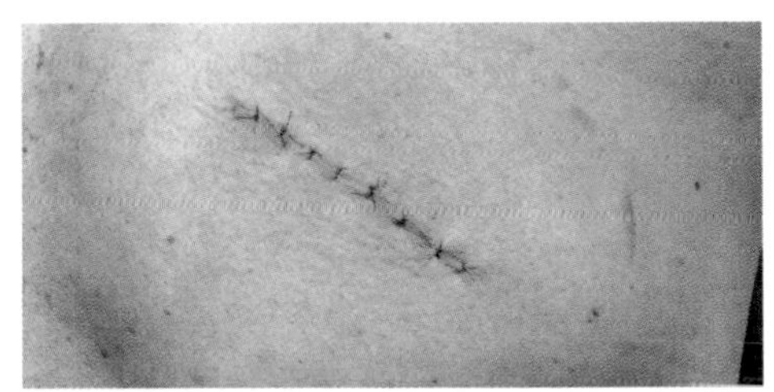

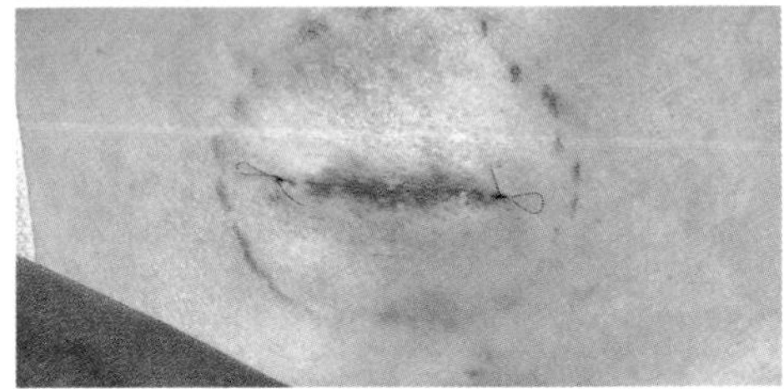

Top: Interrupted stitch. Bottom: Running subcuticular stitch.

INTERRUPTED STITCH VERSUS RUNNING SUBCUTICULAR STITCH

Top stitches are placed after the wound is fully closed. Many people ask me why I don't just use skin glue. Well, I guess I could, but I suppose I like the extra insurance that individual sutures placed on the wound gives me, in case a deeper stitch were to unravel or snap. If I place sutures on the face, they are usually removed within five to seven days, but on the body, I often keep sutures in ten to fourteen days, depending on the type of suture placed. I use individual interrupted sutures on the face almost exclusively because I remove them so soon; if we take out these sutures between five and seven days, we avoid the appearance of "railroad tracks" or the "Frankenstein" look of the hash lines that go perpendicular to the surgical wound line.

For a sutured closure on the body, if I put interrupted sutures in place, I often leave these in a little longer—about seven to ten days—because there is usually more tension on the wound; as we move about, we often stretch and pull the thicker skin on our body (more than on our face), and wounds are more likely to pull apart, or dehisce. If a suture line is straight, and there is likely less stress on the wound edges, I will then opt for the running subcuticular stitch, which I describe as the "cosmetic or plastic surgery type" stitch. This is a single stitch placed completely under the skin, which won't leave any track marks whatsoever. However, it is only one stitch: if it snaps, you have no stitch at all. It is used to precisely and carefully oppose the wound edges, hopefully with a slight turning out (i.e., eversion) of the wound edges, which, as the wound heals and contracts, will settle down and look great. It's a cool stitch to perform, it is also pretty quick to do, and when it all works out perfectly, it can leave an imperceptible scar.

WHAT ABOUT SKIN TYPE?

Just the other day, I was meeting with a group of ladies in their late twenties. One of the women, who is struggling with adult acne, asked me a question that I kind of dread: "What is the *one single thing* we all can do that can get rid of our pimples?" If I could give her a simple one-size-fits-all answer, I wouldn't have to work another day in my life and would be living on my own private island!

As with most skincare-related questions, the answer is complicated. I need to know important information before I can give a correct answer that is specific to the person asking a question. *You* are unique, and so is your skin! Is your skin oily or dry? How old are you? Is your skin sensitive and/or red, or do you have family members with severe acne or other chronic skin conditions? It's helpful to know your occupation, your hobbies, your interests. In other words, a variety of skin types, genetic factors, and environmental conditions play a role in the kinds of skin issues that plague us. That's why there are so many treatment options for acne and other conditions. A successful acne treatment plan—or any skincare treatment plan—must be tailored to you personally. And it must be based on your specific skin type.

The Fitzpatrick test is a well-known and dependable skin classification system that was developed in 1975 by Harvard Medical School professor Thomas Fitzpatrick, MD. It's pretty straightforward, and an excellent and fun way to figure out what kind of skin you have. Remember, our skin changes as we age: your skin at nineteen is not the same as it will be at thirty, forty, or beyond. So even if you think you know your skin type, if you haven't taken this or another similar skin quiz in a while, you might be due for a redo. Skin type quizzes like the Fitzpatrick Skin Type measure two factors: genetic disposition and your skin's reaction to sun exposure. Skin type quizzes are available online—and they even do the calculations for you!

MAKE THE RIGHT CHOICES

Different kinds of skin types are determined by genetics. We are born with a certain kind of skin, and we have to make the best of whatever gifts we've been given. Such skin types vary and depend on several factors that can include:

- water content, related to your skin's firmness and comfort;
- lipid or oil content, related to your skin's texture and nutrition; and
- sensitivity, or the degree to which your skin tolerates topical and ingested substances.

Once you know the kind of skin you have, you can make the appropriate choices to take care of it. What follows are some general guidelines for taking care of your skin according to type.

NORMAL

The majority of people have normal skin—a balance of water and lipids in your skin. You don't have many imperfections or harsh sensitivities to external stimuli. Your pores are small, and your complexion is clear. Normal skin usually has good circulation, little trace of oil, and a soft, smooth, even tone.

Basic Care for Normal Skin

- Wash your face two times a day using a mild cleanser and lukewarm water.
- Use sunscreen during the day.
- At night, apply a light moisturizer.

Did You Know

Soaps, in general, have gotten a bad rap, and now most people prefer to wash their faces with cleansers or washes. Soaps definitely clean our skin, but they contain harsher ingredients such as sodium lauryl sulfate, which is a surfactant, using foam and bubbles to help remove the oil, dirt, sweat, and debris. However, this can strip the protective layer of natural oils and proteins on the surface of our skin that helps to maintain the moisture barrier. Antibacterial soaps contain triclosan, which helps to destroy bacteria on the skin; however, this ingredient irritates some people's skin. I'll admit it's nice to use a soap that leaves your skin smelling fragrant, but soaps with a strong scent actually work against you, drying you out more.

All this being said, not all soaps are bad! Those bar soaps that you can see through contain glycerin, which helps keep the moisture in your skin. Also, there are superfatted soaps impregnated with extra lipids such as stearic acid, lanolin, or triglycerides to form a protective barrier on the skin's surface, minimizing the loss of moisture. Cleansers and washes were created to be less harsh on the skin, and more moisturizing and hydrating, which is why many dermatologists recommend them over soaps.

DRY

Dry skin often has visible pores and sometimes a visibly dull, rough complexion. Red patches are sometimes evident. As you age, your skin loses its elasticity, and lines are visible. When dry skin is exposed to conditions such as wind, sun, dry air, cold air, dry indoor heat, long, hot showers and baths, and certain ingredients in soaps and cosmetics, it can become flaky, or it can crack and peel, itch, and even become inflamed. Very dry skin can develop a scaly appearance, especially on the hands, arms, and legs. Severely dry skin can become itchy and painful and lead to eczema (inflamed and irritated skin). Menopause can also contribute to dry skin, and more women begin to experience drier skin as they age.

I have very dry skin. In fact, I have a skin condition called atopic dermatitis, meaning my skin's moisture barrier is not that great. I keep a tub of moisturizer in my shower and by my bedside. If I don't have moisturizer close at hand, I'm usually in trouble after twenty-four hours. If I start to itch a little, I know I've got to get up from my (probably comfortable) position and put on some moisturizer stat, because the more I scratch, the more I'll itch. Sometimes, when I'm particularly dry, I'll put petroleum jelly such as Aquaphor or Vaseline on my skin. Some of you with oily skin probably recoil in horror imagining zit central after doing the same, but those of us with dry skin sometimes need to slather on a heavy ointment in order to keep our skin hydrated.

Did You Know

Drinking water does nothing to hydrate dry skin! I mean, if you're dehydrated, yes, your skin can look more sallow. But the more you drink, the more you'll . . . pee, and your skin won't look amazingly improved.

Basic Care for Dry Skin

- Switch out long, hot showers and baths in favor of warm, short showers. Go for the coolest temperature that you can. Avoid long Jacuzzi soaks. Personally, I hate cool showers, so I compromise and take very quick hot showers, with minimal soap or cleanser.
- Instead of soap, use a gentle, unscented, soap-free cleanser. You don't need an expensive brand, either. Cetaphil, CeraVe, and Dove have great, inexpensive mild cleansers.
- After washing, pat skin dry gently with a soft towel.
- Moisturize while your skin is still damp. I keep a tub of moisturizing cream in the shower so that when I'm just towel dry and still damp, I slather on the moisturizer. This keeps water from evaporating from your skin and drying you out more.
- When outdoors, use sunscreen and wear sunglasses rated for blocking 99 to 100 percent of UVB and UVA to protect both your eyes and the skin around your eyes.
- Avoid putting direct heat on your face from blow-dryers, portable heaters, and other similar implements.

SENSITIVE

Sensitive skin reacts to environmental elements more severely than other skin types. You may be more prone to allergies or to contact dermatitis, which is when your skin reacts after having come in contact with an irritant such as makeup, certain plants, or even something that blows in from a breeze, like pollen. If you have sensitive skin, understand what external factors cause it to react, leading to rashes, dryness, or bumps. Common irritants include perfumes, bath soaps, laundry detergents, cosmetics, household cleaners, dryer sheets, certain fabrics, latex, plants, certain foods, nickel (which can be found in watches, zippers, and jewelry), and even some moisturizers. People with sensitive skin can often develop allergic contact dermatitis. Interestingly, although this is often seen as a rash around the eyes, the condition is *not* usually caused by eye shadow or moisturizer or anything else applied *on* the eye area. See page 236 for more information.

Did You Know

You can use the same exact cosmetic product daily for decades and then suddenly, out of the blue, develop a sensitivity to one of its ingredients. So don't immediately eliminate a product that you have been using for years as the possible culprit for your red, irritated, bumpy, itchy skin. If you don't know the cause of your rash but suspect it's something you are coming into contact with, try to eliminate everything that you apply to your skin. Then stick with only a mild cleanser such as Cetaphil, and slowly add products back into your regimen, one at a time, to see if you can isolate the source of the irritation.

Basic Care for Sensitive Skin

- Use scent-free products.
- Avoid products with dyes, such as laundry detergents.
- Don't use topical products that are acidic or that contain alcohols.
- Stick to fibers or fabrics that are nonirritating. (For example, some people are sensitive to wool, which is a natural fiber. "Natural" doesn't guarantee a product or fiber won't be irritating to your skin.)
- Use fragrance-free sunscreen.

I have dry *and* sensitive skin. And the older I get, the more sensitive and drier it seems. The key is knowing what type of skin you have, because then you can head off problems at the pass before you are deeply involved in a relationship with redness, irritation, flaking, and bumpiness.

COMBINATION

Combination skin has an imbalance of lipids and water. It can be dry or normal in some areas and oily in others, especially around the so-called T-zone, commonly defined as the forehead, nose, and chin. Combination skin is common, and requires that different areas of the face and body must be treated accordingly. Combination skin can sometimes show itself through enlarged pores on some areas of the face, blackheads on the nose or the T-zone in general, and shiny skin on the forehead or chin.

What about if you're unsure which type of skin you have? You're not alone; some people just aren't sure. Sometimes I'll ask a patient if they are dry or oily, and they'll reply, "I just don't know." So I'll ask them about two situations: (1) When they wash their face, does the skin feel a little tighter a few minutes later? This is a sign of dry skin. (2) When their photo is taken, do they notice a conspicuous shine on the forehead, cheeks, or chin? Well, they likely have an oily complexion.

Basic Care for Combination Skin

- Use a soap-free cleanser.
- Treat oily sections with a light moisturizer and dry sections with an oil-based moisturizer.
- Use a gentle exfoliation product.
- Use sunscreen during the day.

Did You Know

Pore size is largely genetic. There are many products and devices out there devoted to the promise of shrinking the size of these "holes" we hate in our face, but this is largely temporary. We're all really born this way, and we pore this way. So, in general, don't expect these products or treatments to make pores disappear for good.

OILY

The technical term for oily skin is excess sebum on the face. Oily skin peaks in younger people, who are going through hormonal changes that happen during puberty, adolescence, and even into the twenties and sometimes into the thirties. As with other skin types, a tendency toward oily skin is genetic. So no, the pizza you ate last night does not cause oily skin! It happens when glands in the skin secrete too much oil. If you have oily skin, you might notice that your pores are large, your skin often has a sheen that is not caused by perspiration, and you have a propensity for blackheads and other blemishes. But remember the positive side of having oily skin:

you have your own built-in moisturizer! One of my dear friends, also a dermatologist, has oily skin. One day during our dermatology residency training in Illinois, I mentioned to her that my skin was so terribly dry. She looked at me with subtle contempt, rubbed her nose and cheek with her finger, and said, "Here," as she presented me with her own human-made moisturizer. We still laugh about this. People like my oily friend will stay younger looking for longer, unlike us dry skin types!

Did You Know

You may detest your oily skin, but you are actually lucky! Your built-in moisturizer will keep your skin more youthful, and the fact is that you will likely get a little drier as you age. So don't detest it. Embrace it while it lasts.

Basic Care for Oily Skin

- Wash twice a day with a mild cleanser.
- Use a light moisturizer at night that is labeled "noncomedogenic" and "oil free." The same holds true for sunscreens.
- Avoid cosmetics and lotions that contain ingredients such as lanolin, mineral oil, and cocoa and shea butters.
- Use spot acne treatments as needed.
- Blot oily skin with a skin blotting paper.

Chapter 2

Thanks for Popping In!

WHAT FOLLOWS IS AN EXPLANATION OF SOME OF THE VARIOUS TYPES OF benign bumps you can see on the face, neck, and body. I include not only your favorites, such as blackheads, skin tags, and cysts, but also those common skin ailments that I get asked about most often. This is certainly not all skin conditions you can find—not even *close*: there are thousands of skin conditions, and probably more that have yet to be recognized. As we age, we grow a literal garden of stuff on our skin. In this chapter, I cover some basics, and also discuss the most common noncancerous and malignant growths.

If you are able to recognize all of the following, congratulations! You're gaining the knowledge of a first-year dermatology resident in training. And if it's interesting to you, there is so much more. It's all about experience, though, and seeing and recognizing the same thing over and over again, in all its shapes and forms and presentations on the skin. Sometimes it may seem easy, but often it is not.

BUMPS AND SPOTS COMMONLY FOUND ON THE FACE

FRECKLES

Most of us can identify freckles. They are small (usually less than 0.5 centimeters), harmless brown spots that show up on the face, neck, shoulders, chest, arms, and backs of hands. Fair-skinned people and people of Celtic origin with light or red hair and blue eyes often have freckles. Freckles develop due to a combination of genetics and sun exposure. Your skin contains cells called melanocytes, which manufacture the pigment melanin. After exposure to ultraviolet (UV) rays, the melanocytes accelerate production and deposit the pigment in one spot in the skin.[1] The spots fade or disappear when you stay out of the sun but then reappear with sun exposure. That's the key difference between these brown spots and others that occur on our skin. They are neither moles (nevi) nor skin cancers, because those don't come and go but, rather, barely change or continue to grow.

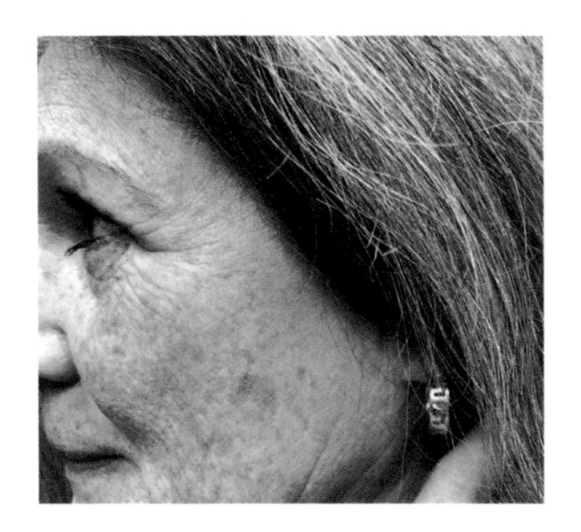

Freckles and a solar lentigo.

How to Prevent Them (If Possible)

While the freckles themselves do not pose a health risk, people with a proclivity to freckles are also candidates for skin cancer. Therefore, those who easily develop freckles should avoid the sun and certainly tanning beds, and use a broad-spectrum sunscreen of at least SPF 30. The National Weather Service and the Environmental Protection Agency (EPA) developed a zip-code-based UV index to forecast the risk of excessive exposure to UV rays. You can access the index, which tells you how cautious you should be when outdoors in your area, on the EPA's website: www.epa.gov/sunsafety/uv-index-1.

Treatment Options

Freckles are generally harmless. However, if you don't like your freckles for cosmetic reasons, try covering them up with makeup, or better yet, stay out of the sun, to minimize their appearance and decrease your risk for premature aging and skin cancer, too! There are treatment options to lighten many of your freckles and maybe even eliminate some of them, but in general, the results are temporary. Sunlight is the main instigator, so if you protect yourself from UV rays, you may be able to slow the return of your freckles, but don't be surprised if they reappear. Embrace them! Many people consider freckles a sign of cuteness or youthfulness. Smile and be proud of your freckles!

1. SKIN-LIGHTENING CREAMS, also known as bleaching creams, containing kojic acid and up to 2 percent of a depigmenting agent called hydroquinone can be purchased over the counter. You'll have to get a prescription for products containing higher concentrations of hydroquinone. You must apply these creams consistently over several months to see lightening. The best results come by combining regular use with sun avoidance.

   Dermatologists in the United States typically prescribe topical hydroquinone cream in higher strengths—usually 4 percent and sometimes as high as 8 percent or more—but this is not without some controversy: in 2006 the US Food and Drug Administration (FDA) proposed banning hydroquinone because studies testing the medication in rodents showed that it heightened the risk of cancer if administered to the animals in very high doses via a feeding tube. Keep in mind that the results of animal studies are not always replicated in humans. There remains no ban on the topical use of hydroquinone; in fact, no evidence of increased carcinogenic risk in human beings has ever been reported. But due to this history and information, some people fear using this product on their skin. Personally, I don't know a dermatologist anywhere in the world who refuses to prescribe topical hydroquinone in the strengths we favor. However, hydroquinone needs to be prescribed responsibly—not because of any risk of cancer but rather the risk of developing a skin condition called ochronosis.

   It is ironic, given that patients may use hydroquinone to lighten their skin, that long-term use of the agent in high concentrations may actually darken the skin, causing a blue-gray pigmentation. Ochronosis may or may not fade after the person discontinues hydroquinone. Because of this, many dermatologists will not prescribe it in strengths above 4 percent. But I have seen prescriptions as high as 16 percent written by other physicians.

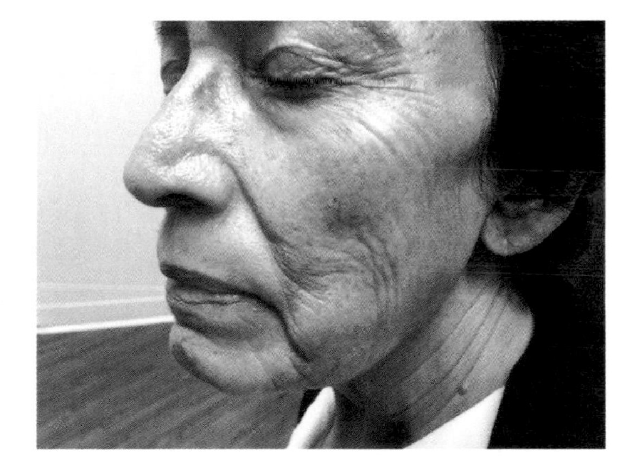

Ochronosis in a patient who had been using hydroquinone 8 percent topically for a long duration.

I advise caution with the use of such high strengths, especially for a long duration. You don't want your skin to turn even darker when you're just trying to lighten and brighten it a little!

2. THE RETINOIDS TRETINOIN (RETIN-A), TAZAROTENE (TAZORAC), AND ADAPALENE (DIFFERIN) are often combined with topical skin-lightening creams to help lighten freckles over several months when applied regularly.

3. IN CRYOSURGERY, LIQUID NITROGEN is applied lightly to the skin, essentially creating a superficial frostbite. Most freckles respond to this safe, simple procedure. Liquid nitrogen treatment can potentially leave a permanent white spot by inadvertently destroying the pigment-producing cells at the treatment site if treatment is too aggressive. Accordingly, your doctor may start slow and small to see how your skin responds.

4. SEVERAL TYPES OF LASER TREATMENTS have demonstrated a high success rate in fading and removing freckles. These are safe procedures with a low risk of discoloration or scarring. Neodymium:YAG and alexandrite lasers, the most common ones used, release small bursts of a specific wavelength to destroy the colored pigment that the freckles absorb.

5. INTENSE PULSED LIGHT (IPL) TREATMENTS also lighten and remove freckles successfully. The pulsed light device distributes a broad wavelength of light, and that energy is also absorbed by the pigment of the freckle, destroying it.

6. CHEMICAL PEELS can provide great results in removing freckles. Peels cause the outermost layers of your skin, which contain much of the pigment that makes up a freckle, to desquamate, or peel off.

Healing Time/Results, or "What to Expect"

The aforementioned treatments are generally successful, but everyone's skin is different, and results will vary. Oftentimes multiple treatments or a combination of treatments are required to achieve optimal results. Even if your freckles are removed completely, it's important to know that the spots can reappear with repetitive UV exposure. Think of it as a maintenance treatment: you will need to return regularly—maybe on a yearly basis—for touch-up visits, depending on the number of freckles you have and the level of improvement you want.

What You Can Do at Home, Where Applicable

Wear your sunscreen daily and reapply it every two hours if you have been actively perspiring or have gotten wet. At home, daily bleaching creams also do not require a visit to the doctor.

Okay, I don't want to freak you out, but what you may think is a freckle could be something dangerous, like a skin cancer. The $10 million question is: How do you know? Well, there is a simple way to remember the potential signs of melanoma, which we commonly call the ABCDEs of melanoma:

- **A** stands for asymmetry. If you drew a line down the middle of a freckle, are the two sides near mirror images of each other? Or does the spot have an irregular shape, with the two parts looking very different? That's a characteristic of melanoma.
- **B** stands for border. Look for a jagged or otherwise irregular border.
- **C** is for color. Does the color look mottled?
- **D** is for diameter. Is the "freckle" larger than a green pea?
- **E** is for evolution. Has it changed noticeably in size, shape, or color over a few weeks or months?

Always see your doctor if you notice changes in your skin, including any of the ABCDEs of melanoma.

When to See a Doctor

Your dermatologist is trained to evaluate you for skin cancer. Make an appointment right away if you notice a freckle, mole, spot, or growth that is new, changing, irritating, bleeding, asymmetric, has irregular borders, is variably colored, or is otherwise bothering you. If you can't see a dermatologist, consult your primary health care professional, and if necessary, they will refer you to a dermatologist.

DERMATOSIS PAPULOSA NIGRA

These dark-brown flat bumps are seen most often on the face, neck, and chest of people with more skin pigmentation, such as those of Asian, African, and Middle Eastern ancestry. If you're not sure what I'm talking about, both President Barack Obama and actor Morgan Freeman have this condition. Dermatosis papulosa nigra (DPN) is not worrisome in terms of health and well-being, but most people who get it remember an older relative who has maybe hundreds of bumps, and these bumps can make us feel self-conscious and old. They're sometimes referred to as age spots, but I prefer "wisdom spots." We get a lot of different kinds of spots the wiser we get, and that's just life.

How to Prevent Them (If Possible)

Unfortunately, it is not possible to prevent dermatosis papulosa nigra. Like many benign skin conditions, they just . . . happen. The longer we live, the more opportunities our skin has to grow various things.

Treatment Options

Treating DPN is not a DIY project. They need to be treated by a professional. Luckily, there are several methods that are very successful:

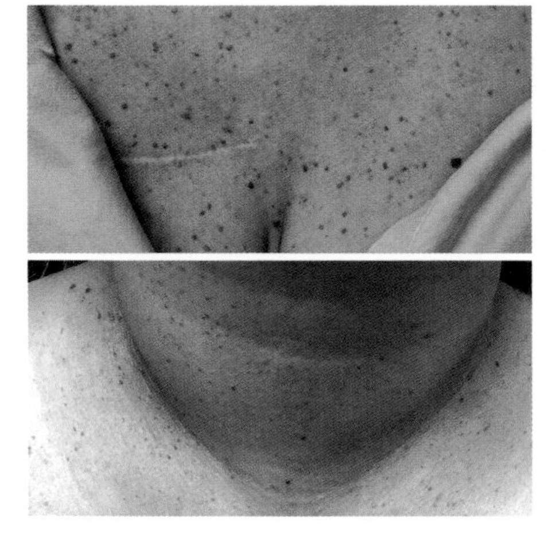

Two different examples of dermatosis papulosa nigra on the neck and chest.

- An electrocautery tool can be used on a very low setting, causing these growths to crust up and fall off. It feels like a very minor electric shock—more annoying than anything else. However, it can be tough to sit still when very sensitive areas around the eyes, nose, and lips are being treated. We can apply a topical numbing cream beforehand to minimize discomfort. The procedure turns them darker, and then they fall off in about a week.
- Certain lasers can also be used to treat these bumps. The one I use in my office is a KTP (potassium-titanyl-phosphate) 532 nanometer laser. It's a very interesting method for treating this condition, because the laser essentially "implodes" the bumps, creating a true popping sound. It can also feel like a hot pen pressed to the skin, so it's a little uncomfortable, but again, numbing cream can be applied beforehand. Like the electrocautery tool, the laser turns the bumps darker, and they fall off in about a week. Never pick them after a procedure—let

the bumps fall off naturally. And apply sunscreen and keep the healing areas out of the sun because otherwise it will take longer for them to fade.

- Another option is to have liquid nitrogen applied to the areas. This essentially treats the bumps with frostbite. As with the other treatments, liquid nitrogen turns the bumps darker, and they fall off in about a week. It's important here to also keep the healing area out of the sun, or else it will take it longer to disappear completely.

Screen It!

It's so important to wear sunscreen, especially right after a DPN falls off. Following the procedure, the newly treated skin is more susceptible to turning dark with ultraviolet exposure. This is called postinflammatory hyperpigmentation, and it essentially replaces the original dark spot with a different kind of dark spot, albeit one that should fade over the course of a few months.

What You Can Do at Home, Where Applicable

Sorry! This is just one of those conditions that will require a trip to the dermatologist if you want them removed.

SOLAR LENTIGOS (AKA AGE SPOTS, LIVER SPOTS, SUN SPOTS)

People may also call these liver spots or age spots, but I never utter such terrible words! I prefer to reassure my patients that they are "wisdom spots" because we get more of them as we acquire more "wisdom." And wow, do some of us get them! Tan, brown, or black spots on the skin appear in areas that get the most exposure to the sun or to direct ultraviolet rays, such as the face, arms, backs of the hands, and shoulders, but they can occur virtually anywhere. It's fascinating to me, and I certainly get a chuckle from my seventy- and eighty-year-old patients when I announce that they have the tush of an eighteen-year-old. The skin there often does not have a single blemish, and has a beautiful, even tone and texture. When you compare this to their forearms, where the skin is now sun damaged, peppered with brown spots, red spots, purple spots, yellow spots, and white spots, you can truly see the difference that the sun can make on your skin.

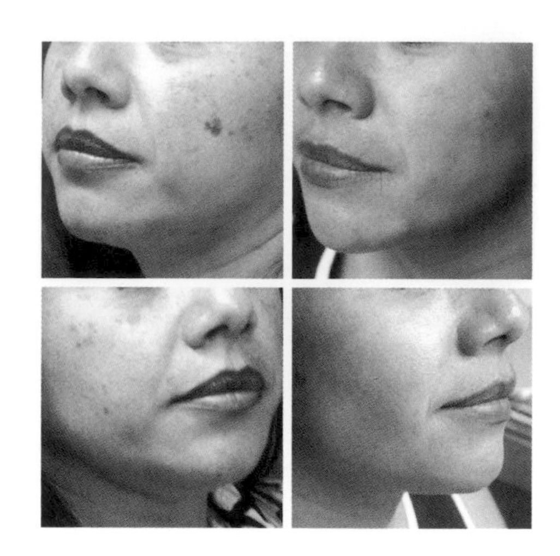

Solar lentigo before and after treatment with chemical peels and topical hydroquinone.

Lentigos make people feel *older.* I mean . . . *wiser*! The surface of a solar lentigo is usually flat, but it can be slightly depressed or slightly raised. Their size can vary from no bigger than 5 millimeters to, less frequently, a couple of centimeters wide. Sometimes they are just slightly pink or flesh color or tan, and there is a slightly defined texture change in the surface of the skin. People most susceptible to this condition include those with a history of sunbathing, those with fair skin but who tan somewhat easily, and older adults in general. We see these dark spots in 90 percent of sixty-plus Caucasians and 20 percent of light-complected people younger than thirty-five; far fewer cases occur in dark-skinned individuals, who have a greater amount of protective natural pigmentation. Sometimes lentigos can't be distinguished completely from seborrheic keratosis—in other words, a very thin seborrheic keratosis can resemble a solar lentigo, or freckles, or even benign moles. These spots are also different from the visually similar melasma.

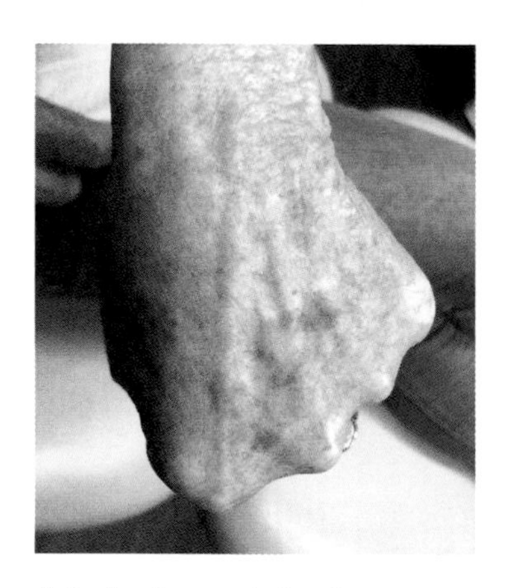

Solar lentigos on the hand.

How to Prevent Them (If Possible)

Sunblock of SPF 15 or higher can help stave off the appearance of these spots, but let me tell ya, for many of us, it can be too late, because lentigos typically don't show up until decades after your sun exposure. As mentioned before, sun obviously plays a huge role; I don't see many of these spots on the derriere, whereas I have seen hundreds on arms, legs, and even the chest. I joke that this confirms my patient doesn't have a history as a nudist. I like to use humor to drive home the fact that sun plays a huge role. It's important to stay out of the sun as much as possible. I know, you say you already stay out of the sun. Well, a lot of what shows up is from sun exposure you had as a teenager or young adult. Young people out there, be forewarned! Look at the arms and legs of your older family members. If you don't want brown spots like they have, I'm giving you notice.

Treatment Options

Rubbing certain natural items on your sunspots may help slightly to exfoliate and lighten them. Tomato, for example, contains enzymes that help repair damage, and so rubbing a slice of tomato on the affected area of your skin could help; the citric acid in lemon juice and other fruits may improve matters, but if they irritate your skin, then please stop. Luckily, lentigos are harmless and don't call for treatment. To make them less noticeable, your health professional might prescribe lightening and sun-protection creams. We can also use cryotherapy, chemical peels, light devices, and lasers to lighten and eliminate them, since they are very superficial on the skin. There are many options, so speak to your dermatologist about the best one for you.

Healing Time/Results, or "What to Expect"

Procedures are very effective, but there can be downtime involved. (Plus, these are often considered cosmetic treatments and therefore are not covered by health insurance.) Laser resurfacing and intense pulsed light treatments require a recovery of one to two weeks. You feel fine, and you are not in any pain, but if you don't want people to know that you "had something done," it's very difficult to hide. A chemical peel might cause redness and peeling for several days after treatment. Cryotherapy results in darkening of the spots; then over the course of a week, they slowly lift up and peel or flake off. In other words, if you look at the treatment options for freckles, beginning on page 40, the same treatment options are used here, but the difference is that the result for solar lentigos is more likely to be permanent.

Spray It!

"Tan in a can" can be a great way to help disguise sun spots, but it can darken these rough bumps, making them stand out more, because the spray tan color gets "stuck" and more concentrated on these growths. Here's a tip: before you spray, take your finger or a Q-tip and dab a little bit of lotion on each of your spots, to prevent the spray tan from collecting within these spots.

What You Should Not Do at Home

You may be very tempted to pick off these spots. Some solar lentigos are raised slightly, as they reside on the very superficial surface of the skin. However, doing so can irritate them and possibly lead to scarring; this in turn brings about darker and lighter spots, which can make your skin pigmentation even more uneven.

When to See a Doctor

See a dermatologist if you've exhausted more conservative measures and still aren't satisfied with the results. And, of course, remember those ABCDEs of melanoma: if a spot doesn't seem right, trust your instinct and get it evaluated by your dermatologist.

SEBORRHEIC KERATOSES

Dermatologists see these kinds of bumps on our patients *every single day*. I'm betting that if you are in your midforties, you have at least one of these, and you may not even know it! Seborrheic keratoses (SK) can be annoying, unsightly, or not bother you at all. What's most important about having a doctor properly identify these benign, harmless growths is that we can reassure patients for certain that they do *not* have melanoma—which is a common worry when you notice one of these on your body. Seborrheic keratoses *can* look pretty ugly; some docs even call them "barnacles"!

Seborrheic is defined as "greasy," and *keratosis* is defined as "thickening of the skin." If that doesn't present an ugly image, I don't know what does! The bumps appear in all shapes, sizes, and colors but turn up mostly as very small, raised, wart-like, and oval shaped, and they can grow to the size of a silver dollar. Some people have literally thousands of them, normally on their chest and back. They are also commonly found on the face, neck, arms, legs, and scalp and, rarely, on the genitals.

Their appearance can change, often starting out as a light tan color that darkens to brown and sometimes almost black. The signature appearance of seborrheic keratoses is their waxy, pasted-on look, kind of like if you dripped brown candle wax onto your skin. Their surface often appears crumbly, like a pastry crust; because of their resemblance to dried-up scabs, patients are often tempted to try picking them off.

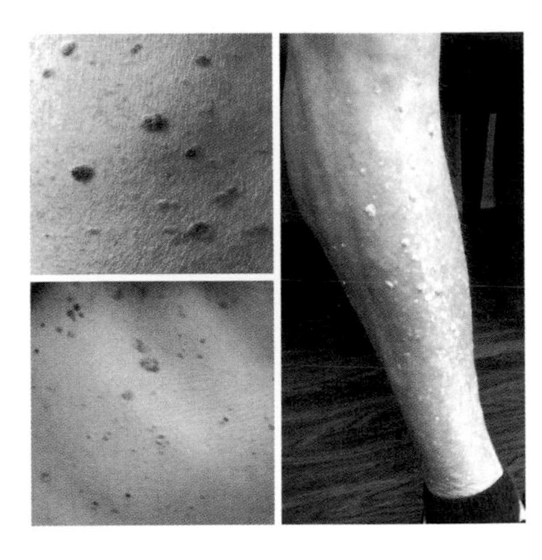

Seborrheic keratoses can present in many different ways. On the right, we call these "stucco keratoses" on the legs because it looks like stucco paint was flicked at the legs with a paintbrush.

Dermatosis papulosa nigra, discussed earlier, is considered a variant on the face, seen usually in African Americans and dark-skinned Asians. SKs are the skin growths that I most frequently call wisdom spots.

How to Prevent Them (If Possible)

Unfortunately, there is not much that can be done to prevent them. I'd like to say that seborrheic keratoses occur only on sun-exposed areas, and therefore you should avoid the sun. That said, they *do* show up on parts of the body where the sun doesn't shine, such as under women's breasts, so we know that ultraviolet rays do *not* play a major role in their development.

Treatment Options

These growths can be removed easily by cryotherapy, using liquid nitrogen, but when they are quite large, it may be easier to anesthetize the area and scrape them off the surface using an instrument called a curette and a process called *curettage*. However, often times we just reassure our patients that SKs don't need to be removed. There's also a new

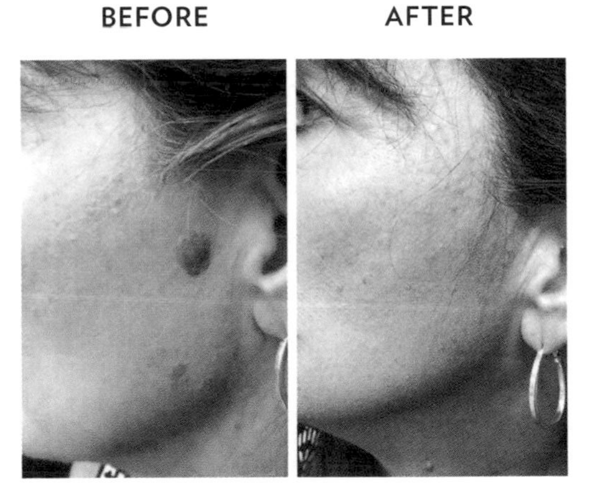

Before and after treatment of a seborrheic keratosis using a curette.

product available at dermatologists' offices for clearing your body of these barnacles. It's called Eskata: a topical liquid that the doctor applies directly to your seborrheic keratoses, causing them to flake and drop off over the following week.

What You Can Do at Home, Where Applicable

Lotions or creams containing an acid such as alpha or beta hydroxy acid or urea can help promote exfoliation. If the keratoses itch or get irritated by clothing, you may consider seeing your doctor, because this is a valid reason for removal.

What You Should Not Do at Home

Avoid scratching these growths or picking them off. Not only will they likely bleed a little but also, and more seriously, you risk infection or scarring, as well as a recurrence.

When to See a Doctor

See a health professional if the growth gets very itchy or irritated, bleeds easily, changes in appearance, shows up without an obvious cause, or is an irregular color with ragged borders. If a seborrheic keratosis blackens it can be challenging to distinguish it from skin cancer without performing a biopsy. Removing the growth or taking a sample and looking at it under the microscope can confirm the diagnosis. Of all noncancerous skin growths, keratoses are most likely to be mistaken for melanoma. Remember your ABCDEs, and when in doubt, see your dermatologist.

Healing Time/Results, or "What to Expect"

A shave removal is a simple five-minute office procedure that requires only local anesthesia. However, you can expect a short recovery time, since the skin will look like something was scraped off—which is essentially what was done. Removing the growths using cryotherapy (liquid nitrogen) is simple and, when done correctly, usually does not cause scars. Overfreezing, though, can produce permanent scarring and hypopigmentation, or a permanently lightened spot on the skin. For seborrheic keratoses on the torso, you might see patches of lighter skin where the growths were removed. Once treated, the lesions rarely return, although, of course, a new one can always form.

FIBROUS PAPULES

If you have a bump on your face that you thought was a whitehead or a pimple and tried to pop it but can't, it could be a fibrous papule. These benign growths, also known as angiofibromas, appear most often on the nose but can also show up on the chin, cheeks, neck, lip, and forehead. They range in size from 1 to 5 millimeters. This common condition affects women and men ages thirty to fifty equally, regardless of race or ethnicity.

The flesh-colored papules are shiny, firm, and dome shaped. While most people will have only one or two, occasionally several will show up, particularly if you're born with a genetic propensity to develop them. Two congenital conditions, tuberous sclerosis and Birt-Hogg-Dube syndrome, can run in families—producing hundreds or even thousands of fibrous papules—and may be accompanied by other skin conditions and even internal/systemic tumors or other issues.[2]

How to Prevent Them (If Possible)

There is no way to prevent angiofibromas. They're just part of life. Seeing a pattern here?

Treatment Options

The harmless fibrous papule doesn't require any treatment. If you want it removed for cosmetic reasons, talk to a doctor about performing a minor surgical procedure such as shave removal, electrosurgery, or ablative laser resurfacing. There is, however, a risk of recurrence.

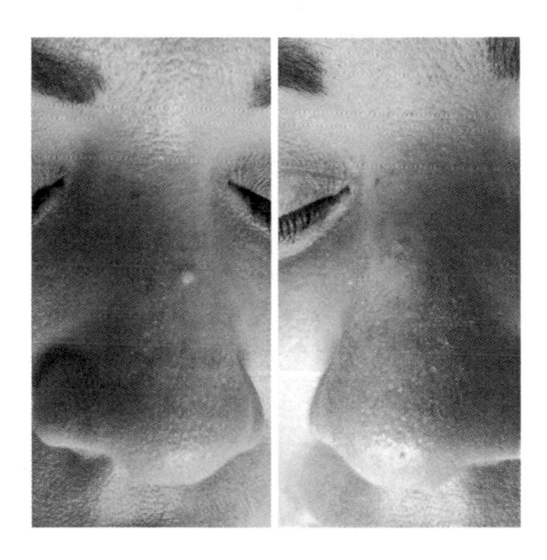

Fibrous papule on the nose before and after shave removal.

What You Can Do at Home, Where Applicable

While there's nothing you can do to prevent fibrous papules, certainly if you have a growth that is of concern, bring it to the attention of your dermatologist. If you have many bumps, you should be evaluated by a dermatologist to see if you have a heritable, congenital condition.

What You Should Not Do at Home

It might be tempting to pick, prod, shave, or otherwise torture this poor fellow at home, but it's best to avoid doing so. You won't be able to pick off the lesion without significant discomfort, and you certainly increase your risk of scarring, infection, and recurrence.

When to See a Doctor

Seek professional help if you're suspicious of *any* growth. Fibrous papules can closely resemble skin cancers such as basal cell carcinomas and melanomas. A dermatologist can often differentiate an angiofibroma from other bumps by examining your skin closely, but sometimes we need to take a tissue biopsy to confirm the diagnosis. See a dermatologist right away if a fibrous papule, or any growth, for that matter, bleeds, forms a scab, or changes in any way. If you have multiple lesions, and this type of bump affects other family members, you may want to bring this to the attention of your doctor.

Healing Time/Results, or "What to Expect"

Even though fibrous papules are benign and asymptomatic, some people might want to remove them for peace of mind or for cosmetic reasons. Surgical means include shave removal or curettage. Some lasers have been used successfully to treat angiofibromas, but there is a risk of recurrence as well as developing new growths.

XANTHELASMA

These sharply demarcated yellowish bumps/papules form just underneath the skin, usually on the inside corners of your eyelids. They aren't harmful, but people who have them often dislike them because they are noticeable. Xanthelasma is a perfect example of how internal conditions can be diagnosed based on a particular eruption in the skin. The condition is a cutaneous manifestation of lipidosis—in other words, a sign that you may have elevated levels of cholesterol and triglycerides, which can increase your chances for heart disease. If you're diagnosed with this uncommon disorder, ask your physician to order a blood test to check your cholesterol and triglycerides. But don't freak out: we do see xanthelasma in people with perfectly normal lipid levels. Most people who get it are middle-aged or older and are of Asian or Mediterranean heritage; women are more at risk than men.

How to Prevent Them (If Possible)

Xanthelasma won't go away on their own, but you should keep your cholesterol levels within a healthy range for you. If it is a hereditary condition, there is even less you can do to prevent them.

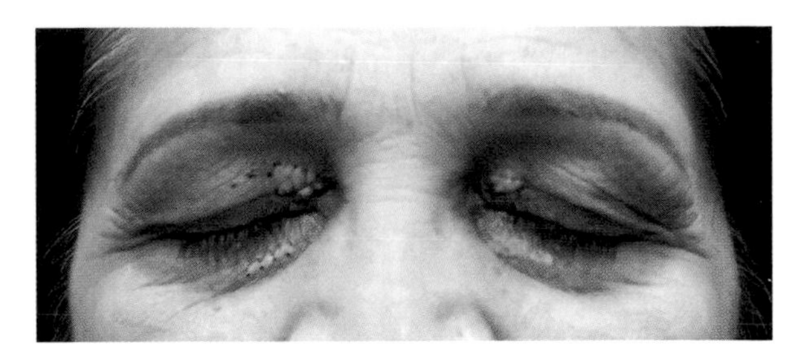

Xanthelasma on the medial upper eyelids.

Treatment Options

Your doctor has a couple of options to remove these growths from your face, including using an electric needle or surgical excision, or destroying them with a strong acid or CO_2 laser. This treatment can be effective, but remember that you can develop a recurrence or brand-new growths, particularly if it is an inherited or genetic condition.

What You Can Do at Home, Where Applicable

There is no home treatment for this condition.

What You Should Not Do at Home

Don't pick or poke!

When to See a Doctor

If you want treatment, you should seek professional help. You should also get your blood cholesterol checked to make sure it is within a healthy range, and if not, discuss with your physician steps you can take to bring down the level.

Healing Time/Results, or "What to Expect"

Healing time can take from one to four weeks, depending on how extensive the condition is and the method used to remove the bumps.

SYRINGOMA

These noncancerous bumps, caused by an overgrowth of cells in your sweat glands (eccrine glands), are harmless but annoying. Syringomas typically appear as small (1 to

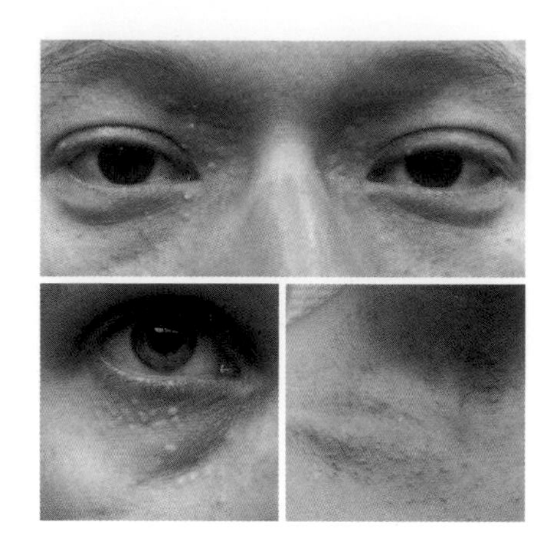

Top and bottom left: Syringomas around the eyes. Bottom right: Eruptive syringomas on the neck and chest.

3 millimeters) growths that range in color from flesh toned to yellowish. They can show up at any age and in people of any ethnic background, though they are seen most frequently in young adults, and primarily females. They occur in clusters in a symmetrical fashion on the upper cheeks and lower eyelids of young adults. We also see them in the armpits and on the chest, abdomen, forehead, and genitalia. The condition can sometimes run in families, and about 18 percent of people with Down syndrome have them.[3] People with diabetes mellitus are more likely to have a type known as clear cell syringomas. A less common variation, eruptive syringoma, is seen more commonly in people with darker skin, presenting as multiple lesions that all surface at the same time, usually on the chest and abdomen.

How to Prevent Them (If Possible)

There is no way to prevent syringomas at this time.

Treatment Options

Because so many people find syringomas disturbing cosmetically, they can be removed, although there is some scarring risk. The destruction of syringomas is simple, and treatments can include burning or cauterization using an electric needle; excising it using a scalpel, scissors, or flexible razor blade; carbon dioxide (CO^2) laser treatment; a procedure to sand down the lesion (dermabrasion); and freezing (cryosurgery) with liquid nitrogen.[4] Because some of these bumps are buried deep in the dermal layer of the skin, they tend to come back. Some patients may wonder why they can't be shaved off, leaving them flush with the surrounding skin and, ta-da, no more syringomas! Well, the problem lies in the fact that even if you do shave off the top, the syringoma is still underneath and will likely grow back.

What You Can Do at Home, Where Applicable

Many people are desperate to find a cure, as is evidenced by many treatment suggestions online, most commonly including the application of lemon juice or apple cider vinegar. Now, both items are acidic and, therefore, exfoliators of the skin. However, there is no way that you can peel the skin deep enough to remove a syringoma without potentially causing hypopigmentation, hyperpigmentation, or scarring. See right for a photo of a patient whose sister told her to apply apple cider vinegar to remove a cyst. As you can see, the vinegar peeled the superficial skin to such a degree as to change its appearance and texture.

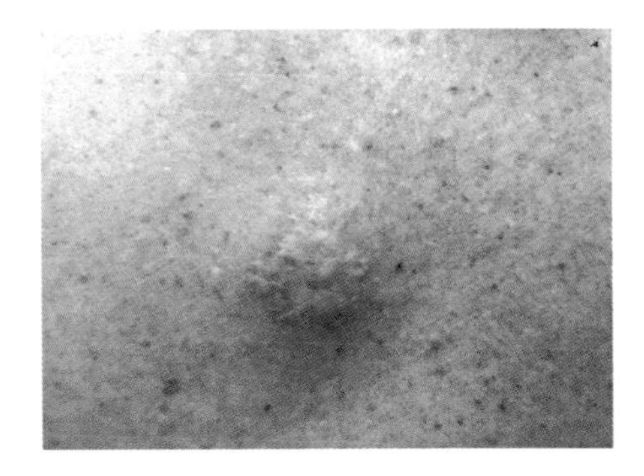

Scarring overlying a cyst because of apple cider vinegar application.

What You Should Not Do at Home

Don't pick at these bumps or try to remove them on your own, as you can damage your skin, including getting an infection or scars!

When to See a Doctor

If these bumps become numerous and unpleasant, you should seek cosmetic removal.

Healing Time/Results, or "What to Expect"

Medical treatment usually takes a few sessions to complete, with visible results in two to three weeks.

MELASMA

This common patchy, brown, tan, or blue-gray skin discoloration on the face is seen most frequently in women with darker complexions, in their reproductive years, twenty to fifty years old. The spots usually appear on the upper cheeks, upper lip, forehead, and chin. The condition can happen in men, but it's fairly uncommon. Melasma is most common among pregnant women; when it affects mothers-to-be, it is called *chloasma,* or the "mask of pregnancy."

How to Prevent Them (If Possible)

I tell my patients how not to develop melasma: live in a cave and never show their skin to the sun. Of course, this creates a host of other, bigger problems, so I don't

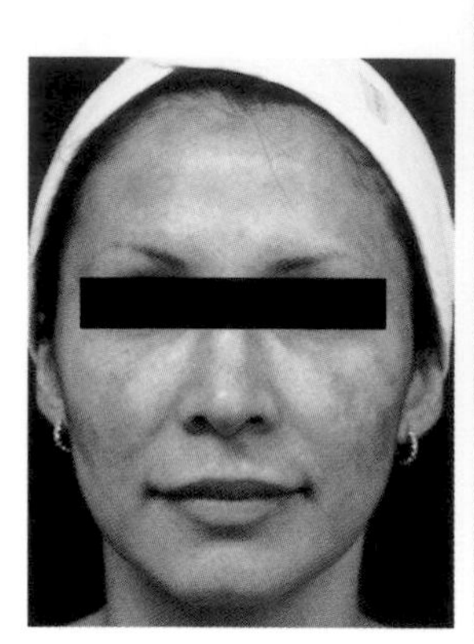
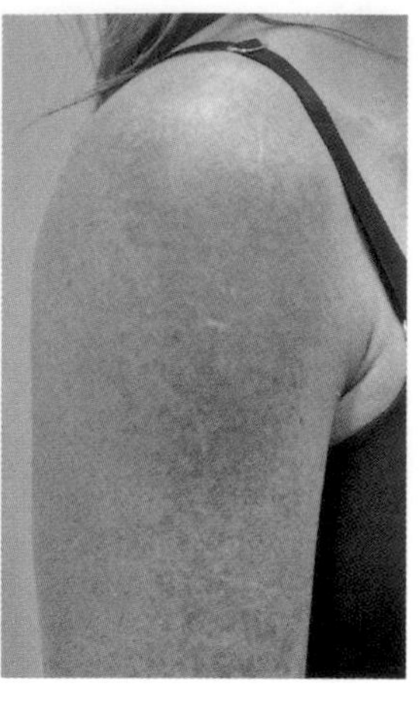

Melasma is seen most commonly on the face but can show up on other sun-exposed areas, such as the shoulders and upper arms.

really advise cave living for anyone. The point I'm trying to make is that the primary culprit is sun exposure and heat. Melasma can also be triggered by birth control pill use and hormonal changes such as those associated with pregnancy.

Treatment Options

Therapies include over-the-counter creams containing up to 2 percent hydroquinone and prescription-strength 4 percent and higher hydroquinone creams. A twice-daily application to the affected areas, morning and night, is generally the accepted treatment. You can add sunscreen on top of the hydroquinone cream every morning. Melasma has the best chance of clearing spontaneously without treatment if it's chloasma, meaning that it developed during pregnancy. You may want to stop taking birth control pills or other kinds of hormone therapy if possible (always consult your doctor before changing or stopping a prescription medication), if this seems to be a causative factor for you. However, please don't be too discouraged and frustrated, for melasma is extremely stubborn and difficult to treat.

Chemical peels, light-assisted devices, and laser treatments, including resurfacing, are tools we dermatologists use to try to clear your melasma. The main issue is that this is not always completely treatable. It has much to do with *where* the pigment discoloration is located in the skin. There are two types of melasma: epidermal and dermal. Epidermal melasma is more superficially placed pigment on the skin and is usually treatable, whereas dermal melasma, which is deeper under the skin, cannot be treated without more risk of scarring or permanent depigmentation of the skin.

What You Can Do at Home, Where Applicable

I tell my patients with melasma that they must become religious fanatics about their sunscreen. Keep your skin out of the sun!

What You Should Not Do at Home

No picking or scratching! You can't scrub it off.

When to See a Doctor

See a doctor when the color darkens or becomes hard to conceal with makeup, or if over-the-counter products aren't working and you want to try to make your melasma less noticeable.

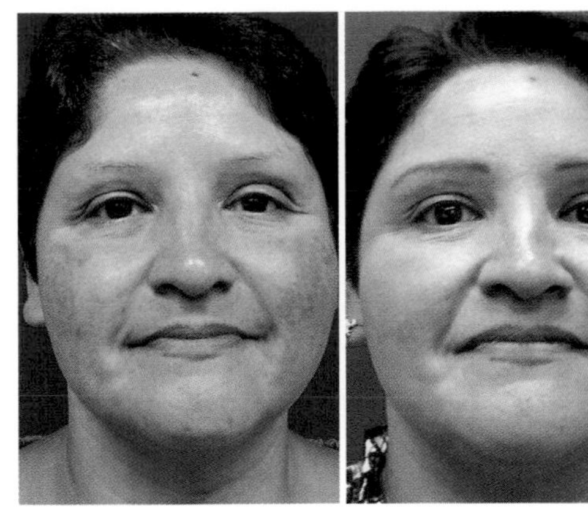

Melasma treated with fractional CO_2 laser.

Healing Time/Results, or "What to Expect"

It may take several weeks or even months for topical creams to make a visible difference in the appearance of spots. And sometimes they don't work at all. Laser treatments and chemical peels usually require some downtime, but it really depends on the type of laser and type of treatment.

REDNESS: THE THREE COMPONENTS OF ROSACEA

Acne is such a big topic, I've given it its own chapter. See pages 133 to 163 for all the deets on acne. However, I will spend some time on rosacea here, since it is so common. It's a chronic skin condition that can look very similar to acne and in fact may be related. It appears primarily on the face and is known for flare-ups and remissions. Rosacea tends to happen often and is more noticeable in people of Celtic descent, but it can occur in any skin type or ethnicity. People with light eyes, hair, and skin tend to be more predisposed, but perhaps this is partly because redness or flushing in the skin is more noticeable in a light-skinned person.

There are essentially three types of rosacea:

1. ERYTHROTELANGIECTATIC: Probably the most common and identifiable form, with red, sometimes purple flushing of the cheeks and nose triggered by and worsened by various stimuli such as sunlight, stress, hot drinks, spicy food, alcohol, exercise, cold or hot temperature, and caffeine.
2. PAPULOPUSTULAR: This type looks very much like acne and is sometimes confused with acne. Luckily, treatment options overlap even if it is misdiagnosed.

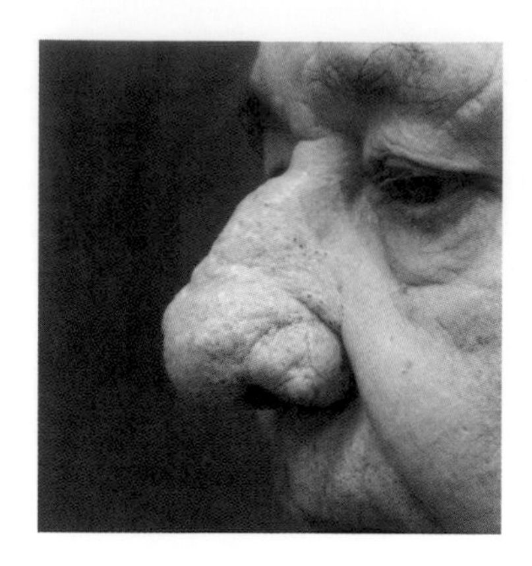

Rhinophyma in Mr. Wilson.

3. GLANDULAR: Probably the least common form, glandular rosacea is associated with a phymatous change, meaning that the skin thickens, especially on the nose. The late actor-director Orson Welles had this condition, and President Bill Clinton has some thickening of his nose from rosacea. This is called rhinophyma.

A common and unfortunate misunderstanding regarding rosacea is that people assume it is tied to alcoholism, and this is simply not true. Alcohol can exacerbate the problem, since it is one of the aforementioned triggers, but it is incorrect and unfair to assume that someone with rosacea suffers also from alcoholism. This condition can present in stages or cycles. Over time the redness becomes more persistent, the color deepens, blood vessels become visible, and when untreated, bumps and pimples can develop.

Generally, rosacea appears after age thirty, although it can show up earlier in life. Symptoms are intermittent redness on the nose, forehead, cheeks, chin, neck, ears, scalp, or chest. Sometime it can affect the eyes, making them irritated and watery or even bloodshot: this is called blepharitis and is usually monitored by an ophthalmologist.

People with fair skin who blush easily are at greatest risk. Women are diagnosed more often than men (maybe because they are more likely to consult a doctor for this condition), but more severe symptoms tend to be seen in men. Recent research tells us that the overabundance of two inflammatory proteins, resulting in abnormally high levels of a third, may cause rosacea's symptoms. Another theory says that the body's response is related to microscopic *Demodex* mites living in hair follicles. How's that for giving you nightmares?!

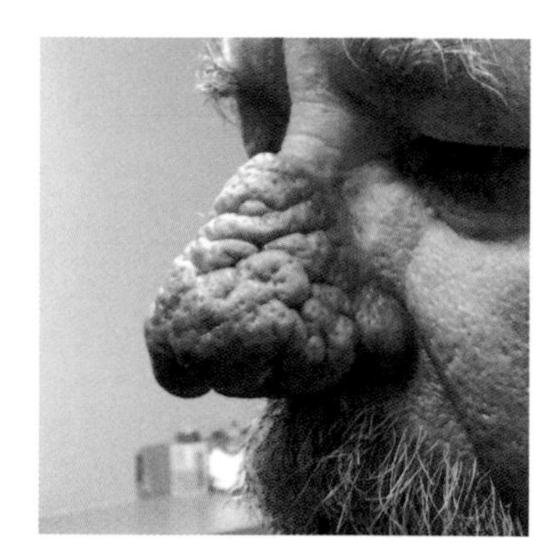

Severe rhinophyma.

Treatment Options

A dermatologist will check out the signs and symptoms of the condition, which is critical to treatment since there is no one-size-fits-all method of managing it: different signs and symptoms require different treatment. The papules and pustules are the most medically treatable feature of rosacea. We can prescribe topical and oral medications that can really improve the red, painful bumps associated with rosacea. However, the flushing and the spidery blood vessels that appear on the face are a little more difficult to treat, and so we focus more on prevention here. We definitely see success with laser treatments, such as the KTP or the pulsed dye laser, which specifically targets the red color in blood and can really improve the redness. But this mainly improves the redness already present and doesn't prevent future redness from forming. Prevent redness by avoiding the triggers that exacerbate your rosacea. Not everyone has the same triggers, though, so learn what aggravates *your* rosacea.

Treatment includes prescription topical and oral medicines, which include crossover treatments with many acne medications and also others such as metronidazole and topical ivermectin. Mirvaso and Rhofade are newer prescription once-daily topical treatments for rosacea. Mirvaso is the first prescription treatment to target the facial redness that many rosacea sufferers experience. The active ingredient, brimonidine, belongs to a class of medicines called alpha-2 adrenergic agonists that cause blood vessels to temporarily constrict or shrink, making redness less apparent. Rhofade contains the active ingredient oxymetazoline, which can be used to fade the persistent facial redness that occurs in many with rosacea. These two topical products use different active ingredients to accomplish the same goal, the temporary improvement of ruddiness and redness that torments many with rosacea.

Sunscreen worn daily can help stop outbreaks. Light treatments including lasers can reduce redness and noticeable blood vessels. There are no topical prescription medications that can temporarily reduce the appearance of redness.

The skin thickening that leads to rhinophyma can be particularly bothersome and a huge source of embarrassment—even depression. Sometimes the growths can be asymmetric and pretty disfiguring, looking like a third nostril is growing. There are ways to improve this, but it requires surgery and is not always covered by medical insurance, and not everyone is a good candidate. Like many dermatologists, I remove the thickening skin on the nose and other parts of the face using a few methods:

- lasers;
- dermabrasion (a procedure that removes skin); and/or
- electrosurgery.

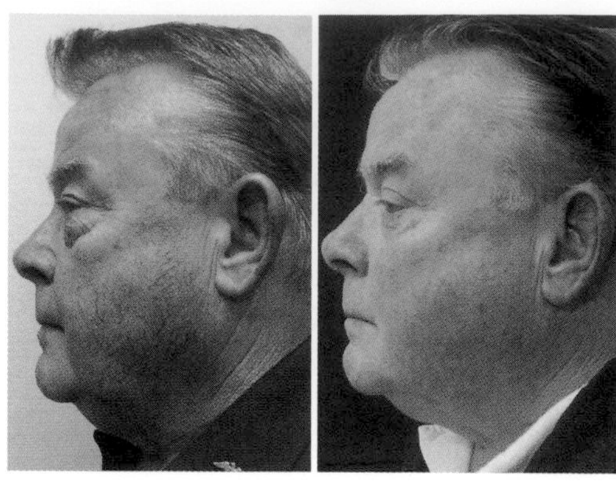

Erythrotelangiectatic rosacea treated with Vbeam and Iriderm lasers.

My preference is usually electrosurgery. It entails using a very hot wire to cut and cauterize tissue similar to a hot knife cutting through butter. This is hard to stomach for some patients and some observers, but it's the best way to describe it, and you can watch the videos on my YouTube channel to see what I'm talking about. This procedure is very gratifying to me because I see the tremendous positive effect it has on my patients. It's rewarding to be able to perform a procedure that can be painless, doesn't require general anesthesia, and yet can transform patients' lives, making them feel like themselves again.

For rosacea that affects the eyes, an ophthalmologist may prescribe an eye medicine along with instructions to wash the eyelids several times a day.

How to Prevent Rosacea (If Possible)

The list of potential rosacea triggers varies in individuals and can seem limitless. Talk with your health professional about creating a diary for you to document your triggers, which will help you to prevent future outbreaks.

What You Can Do at Home, Where Applicable

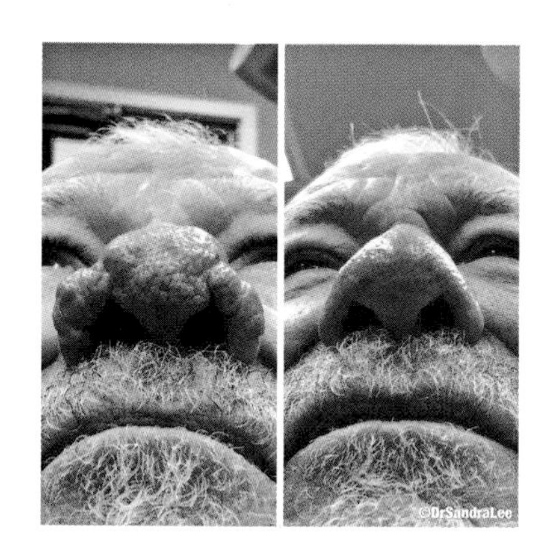

Rhinophyma before and after electrosurgery.

Sunlight is thought to make rosacea symptoms worse. So, here we go again: use sunscreen, and this time it should have a very strong protection factor of 30 or higher, and with both ultraviolet A (UVA) and ultraviolet B (UVB) protection. Use it every day, rain or shine. A hat with a brim and protective sunglasses also help (and add to your mystery!). For those of you with dry skin, I recommend using a hypoallergenic, perfume-free and grease-free moisturizer. Unless your doctor tells you otherwise, I also recommend avoiding steroid creams or abrasive face creams and cleansers. Guys, you may find that an electric razor helps symptoms over a traditional blade razor.

When to See a Doctor

If you suspect you have rosacea, see your dermatologist before the condition worsens. According to the National Rosacea Society, people with any of the following warning signs should see a dermatologist.[5]

Signs That You May Have Rosacea

- Redness and ruddiness on the cheeks, nose, chin, or forehead.
- Small, visible blood vessels on the face. These tiny blood vessels can be reduced or removed with lasers or other forms of light therapy.
- Red bumps on the face. Don't use over-the-counter acne creams without talking to your doctor, because they can make rosacea bumps worse.
- Watery, irritated eyes. This could be a sign of ocular rosacea, most commonly blepharitis. Symptoms include burning and stinging, swollen eyelids and styes. Unfortunately, most people don't think an eye condition can be related to a skin condition, and they may not seek out help. But if you think you have rosacea and your eyes are bothering you, do have it checked out ASAP. Ocular rosacea does have serious risks, including corneal damage.

Healing Time/Results, or "What to Expect"

Some people experience rosacea outbreaks throughout their lives. Some people see a reduction of or no symptoms as they age. While treatments can reduce symptoms, as of this writing there's no cure.

DILATED BLOOD VESSELS (AKA TELANGIECTASIAS, NEVUS ARANEUS, SPIDER ANGIOMA)

Now, it can be difficult to differentiate rosacea from simply dilated vessels that can occur anywhere on the skin, but are usually most noticeable on the face. These little clusters of fine blood vessels on your face are called spider angiomas because they look like little spider webs, except, of course, they are red! If you have a lighter complexion or more translucent skin, these are more visible. They can be caused by trauma—maybe something hitting you on the cheek or nose—which makes a superficial blood vessel weaken and dilate a little so that it is now visible. Even blowing your nose or vomiting often can increase your chances of developing broken blood vessels because such activity increases pressure to the superficial skin. Excessive sun exposure is also definitely a factor since the sun can thin our skin and weaken blood vessels.

Is It Them . . . or Is It You?

I tend to see young children whose parents bring them in to show me a nevus araneus on the face that really bothers the child. The spot tends to really bother the parents too, sometimes more than it bothers the child. I think I see this often in young children not because it is more common in youngsters but because their skin is so pristine, without a zit or a brown spot, and often without any moles, even, that any blemish stands out like a beacon. I reassure the patient and his or her parents that this spot is nothing to be concerned about, but it may not ever fully go away. There are treatment options, but the child must know that they have to sit still for treatment, and I always want to be certain that the young patient, and not just the parents, wants treatment. It's important for young patients to feel in control and to feel *they* are making the decision to treat a lesion.

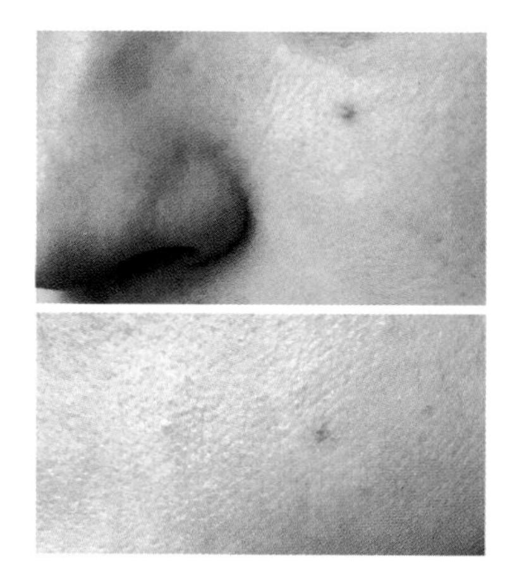

Nevus araneus on the left cheek and left jawline.

How to Prevent Them (If Possible)

Use sunscreen and try to avoid activities that increase the blood pressure to the face. Also avoid certain maneuvers that can increase blood flow to the face such as a forceful exhalation—which is what we do when bearing down—or doing something like clearing your eardrums, which is when you close your mouth and pinch your nose shut while expelling air out your mouth as if blowing up a balloon. Think about it, and you will realize that there are times when you do this and don't even realize it!

Treatment Options

There is no at-home treatment for dilated blood vessels. However, a dermatologist can use a couple of techniques that are pretty effective. Laser treatments can be very good at eradicating these red spider veins. Smaller blood vessels can also be treated successfully with a light electrocautery tool, which essentially closes and seals the vessels. It will feel like a slight electrical shock, but it's quite manageable.

Laser Baloney

When you see a laser advertisement that seems to promise the world, put on your skeptic's hat! So much of what is advertised, especially claims that lasers can erase blemishes or wrinkles easily with no downtime, is more often than not pure baloney!

What You Can Do at Home, Where Applicable

As I said, there is no safe way to treat dilated blood vessels at home. The best advice I can give is that you try avoiding maneuvers that would increase your chance of developing them. Please don't nick or squeeze them. They are blood vessels, and they *will* bleed if nicked, which can be a little scary! They don't gush blood or anything, but they don't stop bleeding that easily. Though trauma to them won't lead to your needing a blood transfusion, they can often scare people because of how much they bleed. If this does happen, apply firm, continuous pressure to the area for ten minutes, and this should stop the bleed.

Healing Time/Results, or "What to Expect"

After a laser or electrocautery treatment at the doctor's office, expect some slight scabbing and maybe some bruising (called ecchymosis), which can take a week or two to subside. Keep your face clean (of course). The light bruising can be masked with a good-quality foundation that matches the color of your skin. Consider a green concealer; since green is the opposite of red on the color wheel, it offsets the redness.

CHERRY ANGIOMAS: RED BUMPS, FLAT AND RAISED, CROPPING UP ALL OVER YOUR BODY!

Cherry angiomas are extremely common, round, slightly raised spots that are 0.5 to 6 millimeters or more in diameter. These bumps derive their usually ruby-red color from the densely packed blood vessels that comprise them, but the color can range from light red to a dark purple. You'll find these most often on the trunk of the body, and sometimes on the face, hands, or feet. Some people have a few of them, while others have literally hundreds. People start noticing these bumps in their twenties and thirties, but if we were to play attention, nearly 100 percent of us would notice at least one on our bodies by eighteen years old. We don't know exactly what causes cherry angiomas, but there may be genetic factors involved. They've also been linked to pregnancy, exposure to chemicals, and climate extremes. They are completely benign, but if they are nicked or scratched, they can bleed like the dickens, causing concern.

How to Prevent Them (If Possible)

We don't know yet how to prevent them.

Treatment Options

This harmless, bright-red or purple bump requires no treatment, but several options exist if you want to remove it for cosmetic reasons or if it's in a location on your body that is bumped easily, resulting in regular bleeding. They can be removed via shave removal, a minor office procedure. They can be lasered off with lasers such as the KTP, pulsed dye laser, or an IPL device. Small flat ones can be eliminated using a light electrocautery device. However, in my experience these procedures are usually considered cosmetic, and as a result, medical insurance doesn't cover the cost of removal. Depending on how many you want treated, treating them can be an expensive proposition. Instead, embrace them and learn to live with them if you can. Remember, we *all* have at least one!

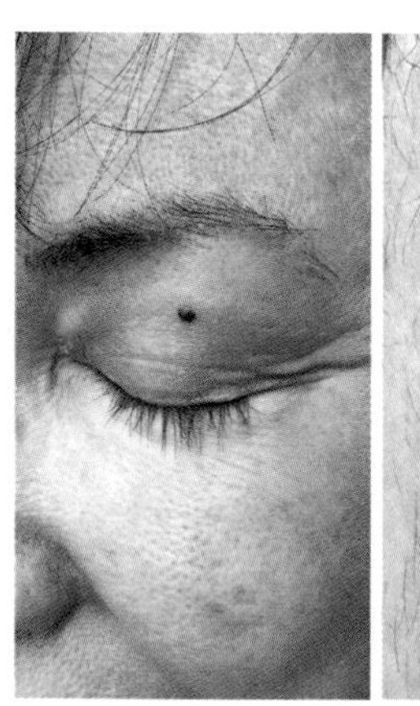
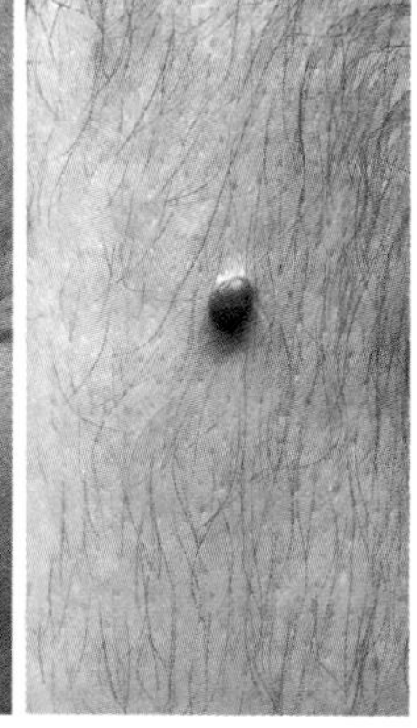

Angiomas.

What You Can Do at Home, Where Applicable

Inspect your angiomas and any bumps on your body closely for any changes in shape, size, or color. As I always say, trust your instincts, because if something looks strange to you or concerns you, get peace of mind and have it checked out by a dermatologist.

What You Should Not Do at Home

If scratched, rubbed, or cut open, cherry angiomas will bleed. It's possible that the bump will bleed if your clothes rub against it as well, so pay extra attention to the location of the bump to manage it well.

When to See a Doctor

A health professional should examine your cherry angioma if it changes in shape, size, or color. If a purplish hue or patches surround the bump, see a doctor to make sure you don't actually have a different condition.

Healing Time/Results, or "What to Expect"

Your health professional will remove the bumps using light electrodesiccation (a technique that uses heat to dry the skin) or ablation with pulsed dye lasers, KTP lasers, and intense pulse light devices. Shave excision can also be used. Again, unless the bumps are causing problems such as irritation, pain, or bleeding, these are considered cosmetic procedures and can be very time consuming and laborious for a dermatologist to do, and all this translates to increased cost!

ENLARGED OIL GLANDS

These are often mistaken for something you can pop. Enlarged oil glands, or sebaceous hyperplasia, is a benign skin condition of sebaceous (oil) glands common in people ages forty and older. People with an oily complexion are particularly prone to these, as their oil glands are more active. Sebaceous hyperplasias are small (from 2 millimeters to 9 millimeters), soft, yellowish or pink-colored or salmon-colored papules that often have a "dell," or depression, in the center, and appear most commonly on the cheeks, nose, and forehead. This condition is basically a harmless overgrowth and clustering of oil glands that can occur anywhere that sebaceous glands are present, but they are mainly noticeable on the face. Typically, papules pop up alone or in a cluster, and although sometimes they may look like a skin cancer, they are benign.

This is a very common complaint for patients at a dermatologist's office: many people have sebaceous hyperplasias, and they don't like them because they make their skin look and feel bumpy. What's more, it's common for them to develop on the rounded curves of our face, our forehead our nose, and our cheeks, and so they make many people highly self-conscious. While patients request removal of these harmless bumps for cosmetic reasons, it's difficult to remove them permanently, and it's possible to develop new ones at any time.

How to Prevent Them (If Possible)

This is another type of skin growth that is *not* your fault but is determined by your genetics. Those with oily skin have a propensity to develop sebaceous hyperplasia.

Treatment Options

Lasers and heat energy may possibly shrink sebaceous glands to some degree, which then decreases their oil production. Goodness knows that this has been touted by many of these laser companies, but I have not been impressed with the results. And it's expensive! Other treatments can include prescription medications and therefore require a doctor's care. Personally, my treatment of choice is to use an electrocautery/electrodesiccation device and a very fine electrocautery "needle" to essentially apply electric current to them and desiccate or dry them up. I explain this to my patients by comparing the treatment to frying bacon on a griddle: the bacon shrivels up and gets smaller.

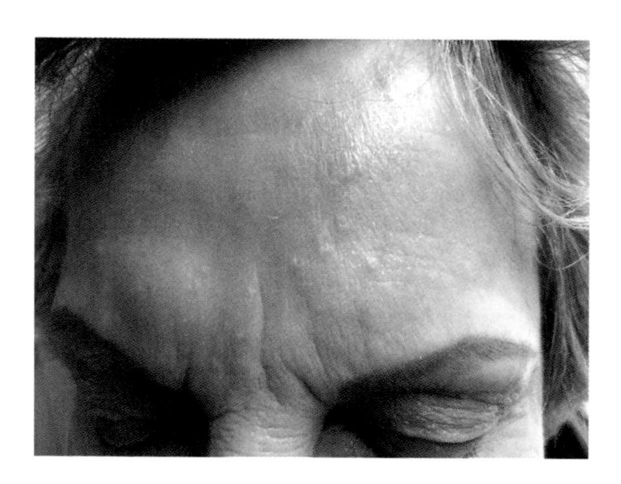

Sebaceous hyperplasias on the forehead.

I always caution my patients not to expect complete elimination of the sebaceous hyperplasia but to hope that this treatment will shrink them somewhat. I can't guarantee they will be eliminated, nor that they won't grow back. Patients may wonder why I can't just laser them or even shave them off with a sharp blade. Well, this is because these growths not only protrude from the surface of the skin but also reside under it and have a deeper component to them—I certainly don't want to "scoop" them out, as doing so would leave a scar.

What You Can Do at Home, Where Applicable

The usual suspects: wear sunscreen to protect your skin and wash your face regularly to avoid the buildup of oil. Look for the over-the-counter anti-aging, anti-acne treatment retinol (vitamin A), which can suppress the growth of skin cells that clog the lining of oil glands and lead to this condition. Better yet, you may be able to get a stronger variant of retinol, but this requires a doctor's prescription and may not be covered by insurance.

What You Should Not Do at Home

Lesions might become irritated or bleed if located where they can be affected by trauma (for instance, from the friction of brushing or combing your hair), after shaving, or from scratching. Don't pick at these bumps and don't try to extract or squeeze them. These are not blackheads or milia; nothing will come out of them. Manipulating sebaceous hyperplasias will only make them red, swollen, and irritated, and certainly increases your risk of infecting the area and leaving a scar behind.

When to See a Doctor

If you are suspicious of any growth on your skin, trust your intuition and make an appointment with your doc. Every dermatologist has seen patients who have found their own skin cancers and brought them to our attention, all because they suspected that a certain inconspicuous bump was just "not right." A benign sebaceous hyperplasia can resemble basal cell carcinoma or life-threatening types of skin cancer such as amelanotic melanoma, so it's important to have a doctor take a look. He or she may perform a biopsy to ensure that the growth is benign. This minor office or hospital outpatient procedure takes just a couple of minutes. If the lesion bleeds, grows, or itches, see a doctor as well. A rule of thumb is to watch your bumps closely and see a doctor if any changes occur.

TRUE POPS

MILIA: SMALL, HARD, WHITE BUMPS

If you have milia, you know they are stubborn little buggers! This is because they are really very superficial, tiny cysts protected from your finger squeezes, tucked just under the skin's surface. They feel like tiny BBs under the skin when you run your fingernail over them, and if you manage to pop one out whole, it looks like your body expelled a tiny, perfect white pearl. It's pretty satisfying to pop out one of these! But it is hard to do this on your own, so I don't advise taking your milia into your own hands.

Milia can often be found in little clusters. If you have just one, the singular term is *milium*—and then I joke that you have *one in a milium,* he-he-he. These white cysts are usually very small, less than 1 millimeter or up to 4 millimeters in diameter, and usually occur around the eyes and the mouth, but they can appear on other parts of your face. Interestingly, milia also occur often in newborns but usually resolve on their own over time. Milia can also be caused by certain cosmetic procedures, such as a chemical peel or laser resurfacing, cropping up during the healing process. Milia apparently occur equally in men and women, but I certainly see more women who bring them to my attention, probably because we look at our facial skin so much more closely, since many of us apply makeup, and certainly makeup and occlusive products we put on our skin can also promote milia.

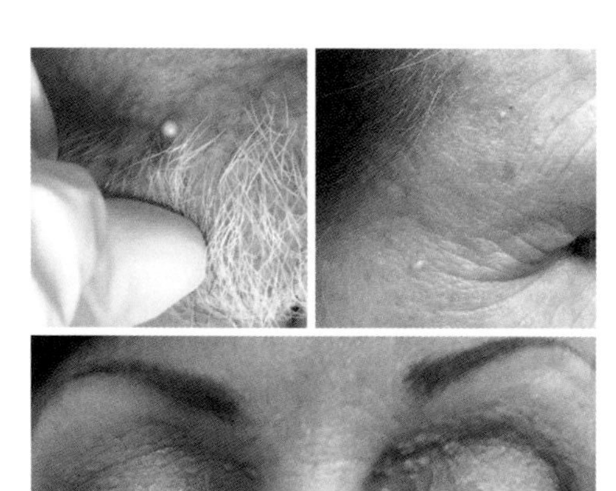

Milia.

How to Prevent Them (If Possible)

Avoid using cleansers that have small beads in them intended to exfoliate the skin, because these beads may actually disrupt your skin's surface too much and promote milia formation. Avoid products around your eyes that are very thick and potentially occlusive, as they can also cause milia to form. Sometimes people are just prone to them, though. Keep your face clean, limit your time in the sun, and exfoliate gently without overdoing it. Use sunscreen with an SPF of 30 or higher as a matter of course. Exfoliating and deep cleansing once or twice weekly can help prevent milia while addressing other cosmetic concerns. Retinol, which is available over the counter, or prescription tretinoin can be used to potentially minimize the appearance of new milia.

Treatment Options

Milia are diagnosed by their appearance and do not usually need any treatment. However, it's hard to stare at them and feel a little ball under the skin day after day. Sometimes they resolve on their own, but this can take a while. A dermatologist will often use a sharp, pointed blade or needle to prick the surface and expose the milium before using a comedone extractor to squeeze it out. Alternatively, when milia are really tiny, I will zap the surface using an electrocautery device at a very low setting. This exposes the milia, and they will often dry up and roll off your skin in a few days. Although anesthesia is not always needed, I believe it is greatly appreciated, and so I almost always use some form of numbing, whether it is topical or local anesthesia.

What You Can Do at Home, Where Applicable

Exfoliation can work somewhat with milia-prone skin. However, the thicker your skin and the deeper the milium, of course, the more unlikely exfoliation is to succeed. Over-the-counter retinol or prescription tretinoin can help to "soften up" the skin and make the milia more easily expressed in the future.

What You Should Not Do at Home

As always, it is not a good idea to squeeze or try to treat milia yourself. They often can't simply be squeezed out because they are under the skin! Squeezing, pinching, and poking will likely be unsuccessful and can lead to scarring and other skin damage or even local skin infection.

When to See a Doctor

Of course, if you are unsure that what you have are milia, see a dermatologist to get confirmation! See a doctor if you want your milia removed, but I caution you, this is considered a cosmetic procedure and therefore is not covered by health insurance. It may be an expensive endeavor!

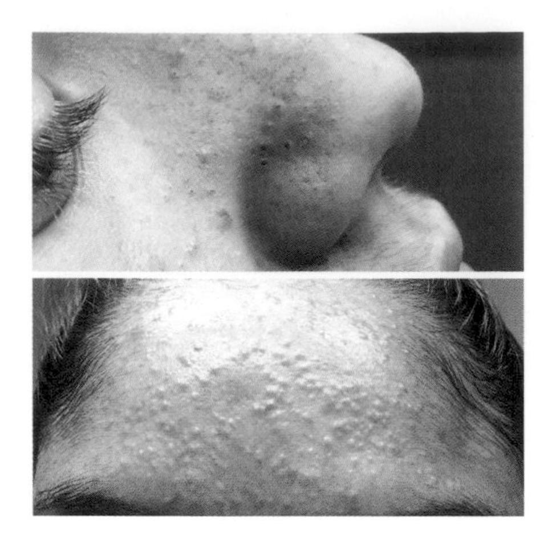

Top: Blackheads. Bottom: Whiteheads.

Healing Time/Results, or "What to Expect"

These simple treatments cause little to no pain and require little to no downtime. After a milium is extracted, you may develop a tiny scab that should fall off within a couple of days. Leave the area alone, and it will heal faster!

BLACKHEADS AND WHITEHEADS (OPEN AND CLOSED COMEDONES)

There is a whole chapter here on acne, but not all comedones come from acne, so let's include information here as well. The medical term for a blackhead or whitehead is *comedone* or *comedo*. (I prefer *comedone*.) Most of us know a blackhead or a whitehead when we see one, because most of us have had one or two, or many more, in our lifetimes. We see them most commonly during puberty, when production of certain hormones peaks, and oil production in our skin is at its highest.

There is another peak in comedones in people in their sixties and beyond into the seventies, eighties, and nineties. I have never seen anyone with such a thick mask of blackheads as my patient known affectionately as the Masked Man. It was as if he were wearing a mask, like Zorro. I suspect he developed such a severe case due to a variety of factors: his oily complexion, his history of smoking and sun exposure, and his occupation working with jet engines (the heat of that working environment essentially baked skin oil into his pores). All this combined created the perfect storm of comedones. And, man, those were *fun* to extract, and it was amazing to see the transformation! Love his sass, love his kindness, love his blackheads!

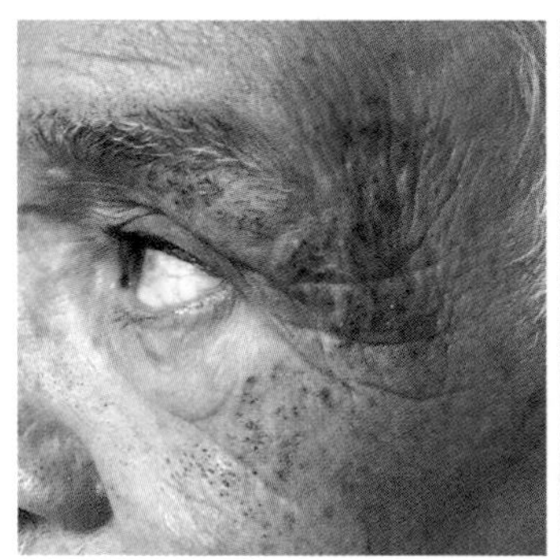

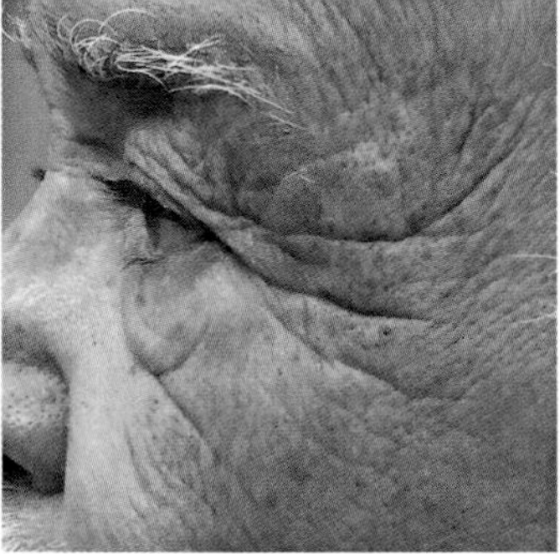

The Masked Man and his comedones before and after treatment.

The type of blackheads the Masked Man had, as well as whiteheads, appear due to years and years of cumulative sun exposure, which is why we call them solar comedones. Clusters of solar comedones, especially those seen commonly around the eyes and the cheeks, are specifically called Favre-Racouchot syndrome. (Thought you'd like to know those names so you can impress your nonpopaholic friends! He-he.)

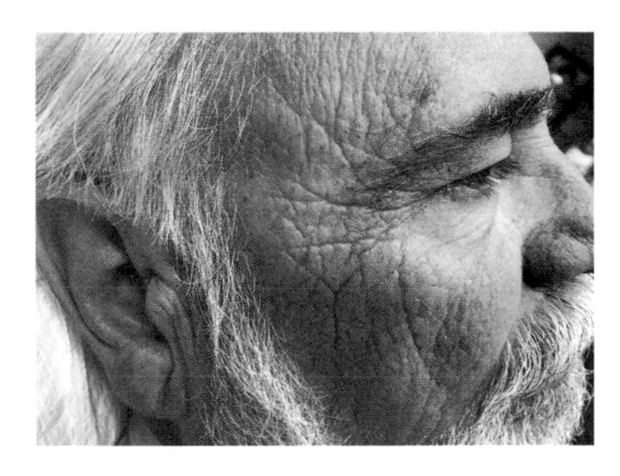

Favre-Racouchot–type blackheads around eyes.

What, Exactly, Are Comedones?

A comedone is a blocked or clogged pore, which leads to a buildup of oil and keratin (dead skin cells), creating a mass effect just below the opening of the pore that we see as a bump. If the bump has a dilated or widened pore, it's called a blackhead. A blackhead is dark in color because the keratin plugging the pore is exposed to air, specifically oxygen, which causes it to oxidize and turn black. Sometimes when you extract an especially deep blackhead, the inner material is lighter in color. If the bump has no dilated pore and no obvious communication to the skin surface, it's called a whitehead. A whitehead is just a "closed" comedone, while a blackhead is an "open" comedone. People often mistakenly believe pustules are whiteheads. But a pustule is an inflamed pimple that has come to a "head" with a porcelain white bubble on the surface of the skin. Most true whiteheads are actually not white in color, but more often flesh-colored bumps/papules on the skin.

How to Prevent Them (If Possible)

If you're a teenager, remember that blackheads and whiteheads are not your fault! Comedones are an inevitable part of adolescence, and the foundation of acne. When the environment is "perfect," they can transform into pustules, pimples, and cysts. So let's try to make the environment less than perfect. Some of the ways we do this are obvious: try to keep your skin as free from oil as you can, but don't go overboard and dry and irritate your skin, either.

Many of you may notice that sun exposure can improve your breakouts, but this is a temporary fix and will increase your chances of developing solar comedones later in life. So sun protection is nonnegotiable.

There are over-the-counter products that can help remove oil efficiently, and there are prescription medications such as tretinoin, which are great at preventing comedones in the first place. Retinol and adapalene, both over-the-counter retinoids, treat blackheads and whiteheads. I discuss this in more detail later.

1. Occlusion: Don't Block the Hole

If you don't keep what you put on your face clean, your skin won't be clean, either. The linings of hats can be grimy, and scarves can carry dirt; your sunglasses can be a repository of grease and dirt; and your cellphone can transfer grossness (bacteria! oil!) onto your chin and cheek area if you don't keep it clean. Holding your chin in your hand puts whatever is on your hands right onto your face. All of this stuff can result in clogged pores, blackheads, whiteheads, and zits. Other culprits in leaving dirt and oil on your face include helmets worn by football players, wrestlers, and motorcyclists; hair that has been treated with heavy products such as gels and pomades ("pomade acne" is an actual diagnosis), and then styled to lie against the skin of the forehead and cheek; and tight, nonbreathable fabrics wrapped, draped, or pulled against the skin. Keep everything that touches your face super clean.

Acne spot treatment medications containing salicylic acid, retinol, or adapalene can also be applied to the skin, which helps remind us to keep our hands off our face, especially if the products are goopy or thick. Of course, something thick and noticeable is probably best applied in the evenings in the privacy of your own home. Just remember that you have spot treatment acne medication on your face before you order food delivery and answer the door!

2. Don't Sweat It!

I love to work up a good sweat. It's actually great for your health, including your skin—but only if you wash it off as soon as your sweat session is over. Not doing so can trap dirt in your pores and, in turn, cause problems, including acne breakouts. If showering isn't possible after exercise or other forms of exertion, use a gentle cleansing wipe (I always have a pack in my tote) to wipe away sweat, pore-clogging oil, and other debris. In a pinch, over-the-counter medicated wipes or sprays that contain salicylic acid or benzoyl peroxide are ideal for acne-prone skin of the neck, back, and chest. I have a great salicylic acid body spray in my acne skincare line, and you can learn more about it at SLMDskincare.com.

3. Avoid Hairy Situations

Oil-based hair products such as serums and scalp treatments have become very popular. Yet they can cause some nasty clogged pores when your hair transfers those oils to your skin. If you're prone to breakouts, skip heavy oil-based products to style your hair, especially those that contain petroleum, silicones, jojoba oil, and shea butter. Consider eliminating bangs and other short layers that tend to sit on or around the face, as the oil from your hair can also cause skin problems. At the very least, when you're relaxing and not "on display," use a headband or hair tie to pull the hair out of your face and away from your skin. Hair conditioners can sometimes cause blackheads or breakouts along your hairline and even on your back. If you suspect your conditioner, try another brand to see if the problem clears up—and wash and rinse off your face and body *after* conditioning your hair.

4. Get a Great Cleanser

As a first line of defense, purchase a good facial cleanser that is formulated to treat and prevent blackheads and whiteheads, such as those that contain salicylic acid or glycolic acid. Just be careful if you have dry skin, because some of these products will dry you out even more. There are many over-the-counter acne cleansers that contain salicylic acid, and my SLMD Salicylic Acid Cleanser is one of the most popular products in my line.

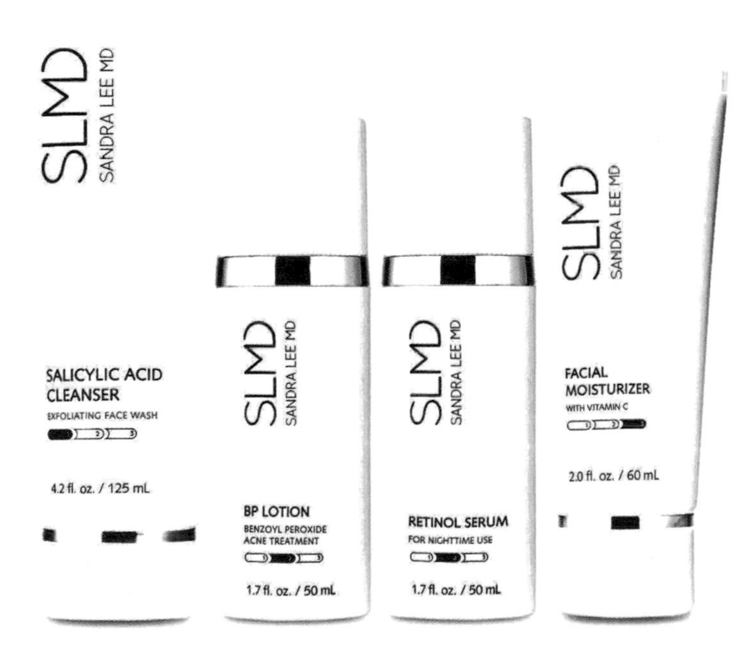

SLMD Acne System, including retinol, salicylic acid, benzoyl peroxide, and sulfur.

5. Steam Gently

Try steaming your face for a few minutes over a pot of water that has been boiled but is off the heat. Hold your face at least twelve inches from the water with a towel over your head to trap the steam so it envelops your face. This softens the contents of the pore, making blackheads easier to extract. One tip I like to recommend: if you're cooking pasta or steaming vegetables, and you're pouring out the excess boiling water into the sink, hold your face above that wonderful steam!

6. Pillow Talk

Make sure you launder your pillowcase and sheets once a week in hot or warm water to keep them clean and to avoid transferring oil and dirt onto your face while you sleep.

7. Sun Protection

Yes, I am a broken record: don't forget the sunscreen, a hat with a brim, and sunglasses when venturing outdoors!

Treatment Options

Should You Squeeze It?

I can tell you not to squeeze your own blackheads, but are you really going to listen to me? It's hard for many of us to keep our hands off our skin, especially when we see a blackhead taunting us. You may try to extract your blackheads; you can give it a good go, but don't force it. *Know when to pop and when to stop!* If nothing gives after a couple of gentle squeezes, it may not be a blackhead, or it may be a blackhead that's really stuck and needs loosening up with steam or topical products first. Patience is key, but persistence is *not.*

Squeezing Blackheads Step by Step

1. Use a mild cleanser to clean your skin.
2. As I mentioned earlier, giving your skin a brief steam bath will open the pores and soften their contents. Placing a very warm, damp washcloth on your face for a few minutes accomplishes the same thing.
3. Set your impeccably clean index fingers on either side of the blackhead and squeeze gently. Some blackheads come out easily at this point.

4. If the gentle squeezing method doesn't work on a stubborn blackhead, do not apply more pressure. Move on to the next one instead.

How to Use a Blackhead Extractor Tool

Comedone extractors are wonderful tools if used properly. Specifically, I use a Schamberg-style comedone extractor that is made from medical-grade steel, with well-honed edges without any hitches, so that it is smooth and glides easily on the skin. You see me use this tool in my videos. (On my website, at drpimplepopper .com/shop, you can purchase the actual comedone extractor that I use.) It allows for precise, targeted pressure, which can extract a blackhead easily, with little or no trauma. You'll either get the blackhead out entirely, or you'll loosen it enough so you can finish up with the squeezing technique described earlier.

My preferred way to use the extractor tool is as follows:

1. Place the loop of the tool on top of the blackhead.
2. Apply pressure in a circular motion, much like when a spinning coin on a table settles down. I put pressure circumferentially around a blackhead, and I avoid dragging the extractor along the skin with heavy pressure, which can produce more damage.
3. Press down firmly on all sides but *don't* press and drag.
4. If a blackhead doesn't budge, regroup and reposition. Change the direction from which you are applying the pressure from the comedone extractor. This often helps to release the blackhead from all sides.

SCRUB SOFTLY: Some people like using a gentle facial scrub—it makes them feel like they are exfoliating and cleaning their skin really well—but I caution against using them too often or too enthusiastically, since scrubs with small beads actually promote milia: tiny, superficial cysts filled with dead skin! An alternative that introduces less risk of developing milia is the rotating skin brush.

BLACKHEAD NOSE STRIPS: What about those nose strips for blackheads? You know, the ones that seem to pull out blackheads and lay them out for all to see like new shoots of grass emerging from a freshly fertilized lawn? Are they useful or just purely for a popaholic's entertainment? Well, these nasal strips can certainly be satisfying to use and make you feel good that you are getting all that junk out of your skin, putting it on display like a comedone trophy. As long as they don't strip healthy skin from your nose, they are not harmful, and they can make your nose look better temporarily.

However, these strips do nothing to prevent future blackheads, and yes, those blackheads will eventually return. If you really like using them on yourself or your significant other and derive great satisfaction from seeing all that debris and oil pulled out of your skin, then go for it. But make sure you do it for good and not for evil! Don't overstrip your skin and remove the natural oils and moisture, and don't irritate your skin. If you're finding redness, irritation, more acne, or even a rash, please take a blackhead break!

Caring for Your Skin After a Blackhead Squeeze Session

After squeezing blackheads, your pores may appear like small holes in your skin. How many times do you see an advertisement or hear someone of authority say "This [product/laser/device] shrinks your pores!" Well, I'm here to give you some bad news: pore size is not really under our control. We are born with what we have. However, you can prevent your pores from dilating excessively by keeping your skin clean and preventing dirt and oil from collecting within the pores and permanently stretching and increasing their size.

It's the type and thickness of our skin that really determines pore size. As we age, our skin loses elasticity; also, gravity gets a stronghold on us, leading to more saggy skin. Just as our bodies get less tight as we age, so do our pores, and since they relax a little, they can open up a little more and become more apparent to us—especially on the more oily parts of our face, which are usually located in the center, right where we can see them when we look in the mirror! Pores can't be "closed," but you *can* minimize their appearance with some simple techniques following blackhead extraction:

- If there are any cuts or abrasions on the skin, avoid using a toner, as it can really sting and inflame already irritated skin.
- Use a mask with soothing properties that has been cooled in the refrigerator to reduce any inflammation.
- A good old-fashioned splash of ice water is great—it will cause some pore shrinkage and can slightly tighten pores.
- Routinely keep your pores clean of oil and debris, which if they collect and harden in the pore can permanently dilate it. And if they also oxidize, this can make the pores more noticeable. I recommend the use of an alpha or beta hydroxy acid such as glycolic acid and especially salicylic acid, which keeps pores clear. When pores are clear, they are less noticeable and less likely to get larger, and you will likely experience fewer acne breakouts.

CLEANSING TIP: My acne skincare line, called SLMD Acne System, contains a salicylic acid cleanser that is great on all skin types. It crystallizes to a small enough size to settle within the pores and encourage exfoliation while cleaning pores of dirt and debris. My tip: if you're looking for a deeper clean, apply the cleanser to your blackhead-prone areas and let it sit for five to ten minutes before you wash it off. Maybe apply it a few minutes before you jump in the shower. Multitasking, to me, is *key*.

Blackhead Superstar: Mr. Wilson

Mr. Wilson starred in the very first blackhead-extraction video series I ever posted. He's the first, and one of the few, whose face is completely recognizable (shown full face) in my videos. If I were to do it again, I would have not shown his entire face because it's unnecessary to get the point across about the technique of extraction and how it can really improve the appearance. Above all, it's my responsibility and my intention to protect my patients, so many of whom are kind enough to allow me to videotape and post publicly something very personal.

The video is how he got his nickname. He could be the doppelgänger of the perpetually cranky, long-suffering elderly neighbor of Dennis the Menace. He's a man of few words, mainly grunts single-word responses to my long-winded and animated questions. He's also the first patient of mine who had truly amazing blackheads—I mean the kind that slide out when you just touch the skin. The unpredictable ones: when you use a comedone extractor and the blackheads seem so eager to escape, they pop out unexpectedly. You squeeze in one area, but they pop out of another. Then, just when you think there are no more blackheads to squeeze, suddenly one curls out like a long streamer.

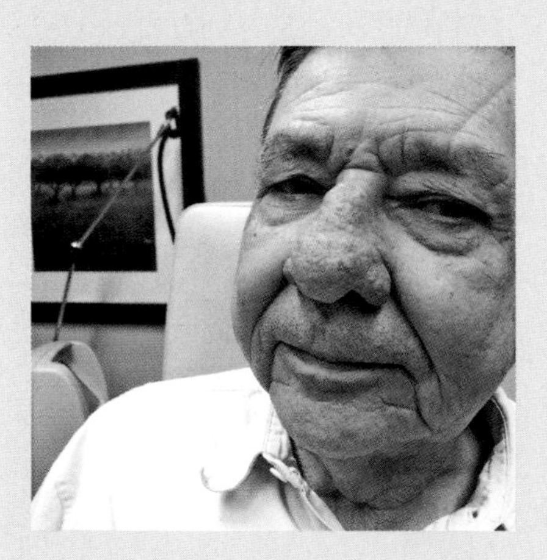

We love Mr. Wilson.

Mr. Wilson is the person who sparked the idea of making a special Fourth of July Pops spectacular and putting these pops to Tchaikovsky's *1812 Overture* so they seem like fireworks that pop out of the skin. I sometimes wonder if people approach him and ask him if he's Mr. Wilson. I mean, he knows we call him this, but I don't think he's a World Wide Web kinda guy. More of a morning-coffee-and-read-the-newspaper-from-start-to-finish-every-day kind of man. Though he is a man of few words, I do know that he appreciated what we did for him, and he wanted it done—he came back for more many times. We subtly reshaped his nose, which was getting thicker and a little amorphous from a condition called rhinophyma, and I was shocked to see clumps of solidified oil like chips of butter emerge from under his skin. Quite amazing. I'm so fortunate that he appeared in my life at the perfect time. Just a few months earlier, had he come to me, I might never have extracted any of his blackheads! And I certainly wouldn't have recorded the experience for tens of millions to see. I feel the gift he has given me, and all you popaholics out there, is greater than the one I have given him. And we all thank him for that!

How to Get Rid of Whiteheads

I'm sure you've figured out that whiteheads are more difficult to remove than blackheads. I don't endorse removing whiteheads manually at home, because they don't have an opening to the surface of the skin (as a blackhead does), so you often have to either squeeze a lot harder or superficially pierce the skin to expel the contents of a whitehead. I caution people about doing this at home, because it can cause scarring when done too aggressively. There is also increased risk of infection when breaking the skin, and if you pierce the skin too deeply and nick a blood vessel, you can certainly bleed excessively. When I remove whiteheads, I use very sharp instruments that are hygienic and sterile.

All this being said . . . do I think people will try to do it on their own? Yes, I do, because it's human nature. It happens all the time, and they are often too darn tempting to ignore! So let me be clear: *don't do it.* But here is how I recommend you proceed, step by step, if you decide to go against my medical advice:

1. Wash your hands with antiseptic soap. Make sure your "work area" and any instruments you use are clean!
2. To remove whiteheads, it's ideal that you soften the skin overlying the whitehead. Apply a warm washcloth to the area for a few minutes, or steam your skin, as discussed previously.
3. If you feel the need to pierce the superficial skin to express the whitehead, make sure you use a sterile lancet, pin, or sharp needle. At home, clean the instrument you use with rubbing alcohol or run it under a flame to sterilize it. Remember, the more deeply you pierce the skin, the greater your risk of scarring, and scarring can be permanent. Always remind yourself of this!

4. Before using the comedone extractor, sanitize it with rubbing alcohol. Position the extractor so the loop is centered over the whitehead and then push downward gently against the skin until the contents are extracted completely. As in blackhead extraction, if the whitehead doesn't want to budge, don't force it. You could end up with an infection or scar.
5. If pressure in one direction doesn't work, lift up the extractor and restart the process in a different, even opposite direction. Sometimes it's nice to take a break and come back to the same whitehead a little later, so that any inflammation and irritation can subside somewhat, but don't do this repeatedly! Remember, patience is key. Also remember to not drag the extractor with excess pressure along the skin, as this promotes more damage to the skin's surface. You may even want to set a timer, so that you know when to stop! Thirty seconds is plenty of time to try to extract a whitehead. Remember, if you can't extract anything, it might not be a whitehead. A milium can look identical to a whitehead, but these are usually situated a little more deeply in the skin and are more difficult to extract. Even a fibrous papule, a sebaceous hyperplasia, or a mole can look deceptively like a whitehead, but no matter how much you squeeze or pinch, nothing can be extracted from such growths. Know when to pop and, soon, please *stop*.
6. After extracting the whitehead, wash your hands and press a cool washcloth or ice wrapped in gauze or a towel on the area. This will act as a skin "tightener" and minimize redness and swelling.

Why Isn't It Working?

Oftentimes you will squeeze, using either your fingers or an extractor, and nothing happens. This is for one of two reasons:

1. What you're squeezing is not "squeezable"! It's not something you can extract! Again, know when to stop, and if you are still really bothered by this bump that won't go away, seek the advice of an expert, who can examine your bumps under magnification and discern what they are. Fibrous papule, mole, sebaceous hyperplasia, and syringoma are the most common whitehead deceivers.

2. This extractable bump is covered by healthy skin, and there is no opening to the skin's surface. This is especially true for whiteheads and milia, and in this case, the very superficial layer of skin needs to be nicked first to allow proper extraction. Milia can be set deeper under the skin, especially on areas of the body where the skin is thicker. Milia are more noticeable around the eyes because the skin there is very thin, but they can lie deep under the comparatively thick skin around the mouth.

PIMPLES

Please see chapter 3, page 133. Acne, including pimples, has its own section!

DILATED PORE OF WINER

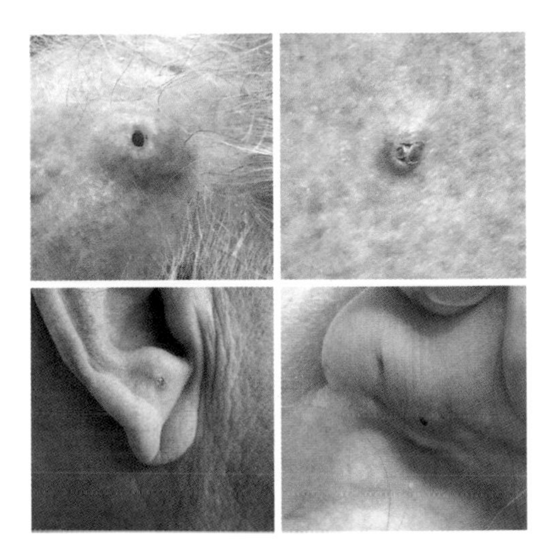

Large blackheads, aka dilated pores of Winer.

This is the king of the comedones, and easily the favorite of all you popaholics. A dilated pore of Winer (DPOW) is a condition that causes the appearance of a single, protruding, open comedone or clogged pore. They usually occur on the face but can afflict other areas of the body, especially the back. We're not really sure what causes a dilated pore of Winer, though it may result from an obstruction or infection of a hair follicle. Hey, pimple popping wouldn't be nearly as exciting or fun if they didn't exist, since they best resemble a giant blackhead (emphasis on *giant*). Pores of Winer are also more predominant in men than in women, and in people forty and over. I usually find really huge ones on the elderly, who may have poor vision and arthritic hands, and on the middle of the back where few people can reach, no matter how young. This is a recipe for a huge DPOW. I would have to say these are *the* most popular types of extractions seen on my YouTube channel and social media. They tend to pop out whole, and cleanly, with no blood or other liquid. This is the best of the soft pops, for sure, and a true crowd-pleaser!

How to Prevent Them (If Possible)

As with many skin conditions, maintaining good skincare habits is your first line of defense. Keep your face and body clean, and don't scratch or pick at affected areas—because they can get worse and, indeed, possibly infected, which can lead to scarring. Don't let one get bigger; have it extracted when it's small. If you allow it to grow to a large size, you risk creating a large permanent dilation of your superficial skin that will just collect debris.

What You Can Do at Home, Where Applicable

Unfortunately, there is no topical remedy for preventing the condition (and popaholics would surely applaud this fact). If you have a DPOW, and if you are persistent, you could likely extract it with a few squeezes—perhaps with no anesthetic and no blood loss or trauma to your skin. However, they usually run on the big side, and you should know that I always anesthetize the area locally for my patients' comfort, and this is not available for you at home.

When to See a Doctor

Of course, you should always talk to your doctor whenever you are concerned about any suspicious changes in your skin. However, if you truly have a DPOW, you don't have to see a doctor unless it's causing you discomfort. Again, this is not something that threatens your well-being, and removing it is unnecessary. Of course, if the pore is very large or looks red and inflamed in any way, seek professional guidance.

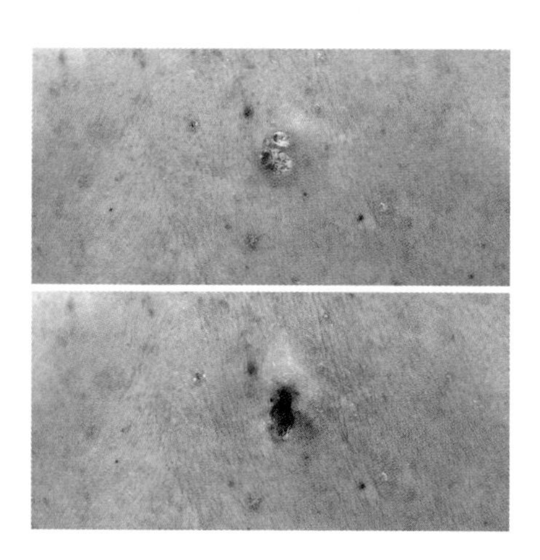

Large DPOW, like a rock, before and after removal.

A dermatologist often uses a local anesthetic, which is injected into the skin around the affected pore. The contents of the pore and its wall will be removed. If the residual dilation of the skin is large and will likely reaccumulate debris, the only option is for the physician to excise that tissue and stitch the edges together, closing the hole. This replaces a dilated pore with a linear scar.

I'm pretty sure that if you have a DPOW yourself, you're not a popaholic. I can't imagine that a popaholic could keep their hands off a DPOW unless it was in a difficult-to-reach place on the body. So if you want to keep that DPOW, please, *don't show it to a popaholic!* Because a popaholic will not leave you alone until you get that taken care of!

Healing Time/Results, or "What to Expect"

If you have a dilated pore excised so that it won't recur, sutures likely stay in place for between seven and fourteen days, depending on the part of the body and the type and pattern of sutures placed.

Pore of Winer Superstar: Like a Rock

A gentleman in his early nineties actually had three large dilated pores of Winer. He came to me because his family was concerned that a quarter-sized lump, with a black core, on his forehead could be something life threatening, such as a melanoma. Thankfully, it was not. It was a large epidermoid cyst with a dilated pore of Winer at its entrance. Then I went to examine his back and found two of the biggest DPOWs I've seen to date—like small rocks wedged under his skin. I locally anesthetized the area and, using my forceps, easily slipped them out. What was most amazing was that I rapped the blackhead on the table, and it was rock hard. It's common to see such benign growths on the elderly, especially on their backs where few of us can reach, but these were particularly huge!

EPIDERMOID CYSTS (EPIDERMAL INCLUSION CYSTS, INFUNDIBULAR CYSTS)

I've never met a person who loved his or her cyst. What's to love about it? It's a bump that protrudes from the skin and makes people self-conscious about having others touch them, for fear they will feel the cyst and be grossed out. But cysts could coexist happily with us if they didn't have to go get inflamed. This is a risk from any cyst, but of course the risk increases if they are located in areas that are easily traumatized

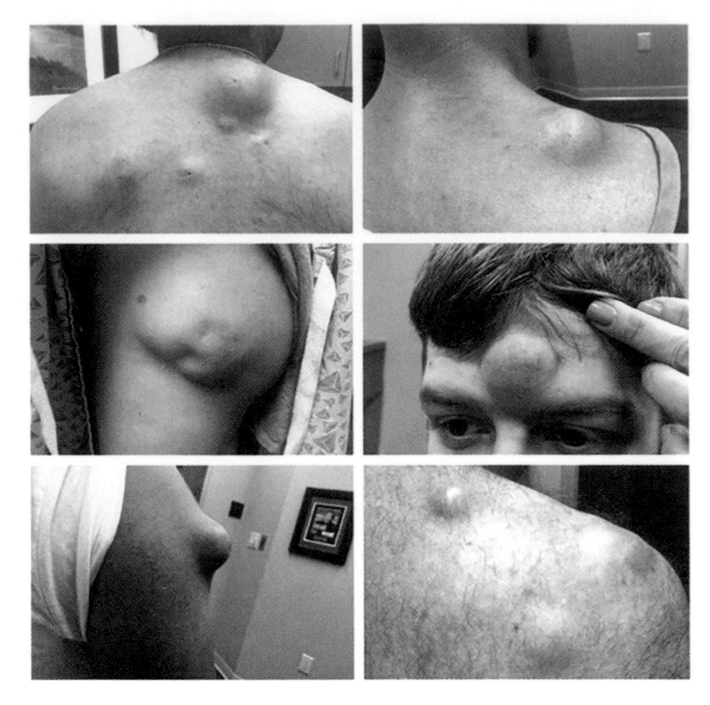

Various epidermoid cysts.

or disturbed, which is the primary reason people seek removal. Two of the most common types of cyst that occur under the skin's surface are epidermoid and pilar cysts.

Epidermoid cysts are probably the most common tumor of the skin. (Bear in mind that when I use the word *tumor,* it does not automatically mean something malignant; it's just a term we derms use to describe a growth under the skin, no matter the size.) You usually recognize it as a bump on the surface of the skin, with no major changes to the surface of the overlying skin, and as you will hear me mention in my videos, it is "mobile under the skin." This is an important point. In general, a growth that you can shift from side to side even though it is under the surface of the skin is most likely benign and not life threatening. Most commonly, it is either a cyst or a lipoma (which I will discuss later). A growth on your skin that is bound down, meaning it's stuck to your body and doesn't shift back and forth easily when you push it around, is more suspicious and potentially a source of concern and should certainly be shown to your physician for further evaluation.

If you look really closely at an epidermoid cyst, you may see a small pinpoint opening, often near the center of the dome. This looks like a little blackhead and is what we call the punctum. You may recognize this if you have a cyst and try to squeeze it. The punctum may extrude yellow, pasty contents the consistency of cheese, with a sharp, pungent smell. This is macerated keratin, otherwise known as wet, dead skin cells. Imagine what an accumulation of damp, dead skin cells collecting in an area for many years may smell like, and you can imagine what a cyst can smell like.

So why do cysts happen, anyway? Well, they can happen anywhere but are often found on the face, neck, and the upper body above the waist. They can occur because of acne, when a follicle gets plugged with enough debris. They can even occur due to trauma, where part of your superficial skin accidently gets pushed down under the surface. It could even be just from bumping into a pointed corner or from someone poking you with a sharp pencil. The skin that is trapped underneath forms a tiny sac or balloon. In the same way that our skin constantly sheds dead skin cells, so does this little sac of skin. But instead of the dead cells flaking off onto the floor, they fill the submerged cyst, causing it to enlarge. And that's why cysts can continue to grow.

Interestingly, after removing literally hundreds of cysts over the last few years, I've noticed that cyst contents can range from the whitest of white to the blackest of black and many colors in between. I believe that people with a little more pigment in their skin shed dead skin cells that are darker in color, and therefore the cyst contents can be shades of gray. But they can also have cysts full of bright-white contents. I don't recall ever removing a cyst with dark debris from a patient whose complexion is extremely light.

If you have watched my videos, you know already that the only way you can remove a cyst definitively and ensure it doesn't grow back is to excavate the entire cyst and its sac. Because if any part of the sac is left intact under the skin, there's a good chance it will regenerate. Also, if an epidermoid cyst is not removed entirely the first time, a second attempt at removal becomes a little more challenging. This is because the cyst can grow back surrounded by scar tissue. Imagine a little balloon under the skin that gets partially removed but still grows back. However, it grows back a little misshapen, maybe bumpier, like one cyst bubble that has grown other bubbles around it. A multiloculated cyst, as this is called, is not only more difficult to excise but also more likely to recur.

I've seen some pretty darn big cysts in some unusual locations. But I think that, overall, lipomas have the opportunity to get bigger. Because the size a cyst gets is dependent on what it's encasing can handle, and there is an eventual limit to their size. Just like blowing up a birthday balloon, the cyst can become overfilled to the point where its wall ruptures. This brings about inflammation, swelling, and pain.

When a cyst becomes inflamed and gets colonized by bacteria, then it is called an abscess. There is an important difference between an inflamed cyst and an abscess that arises from an infected cyst.

Don't Squeeze the Cyst!

It's tempting to squeeze your cyst, but it's not a pimple and should not be squeezed. Let me tell you why: Every time you traumatize your cyst by squeezing it, there is an opportunity for it to become irritated and inflamed. If the cyst wall tears or sheers under the skin, whether due to your accidently injuring it or purposely squeezing it, the internal contents of the cyst escape through the breached cyst wall and come in contact with the tissues surrounding it.

Trust me: your skin won't like this. It will mount an immune response to fight off these foreign cells, called a foreign-body reaction. Inflammatory cells cause swelling, redness, heat, and pain in the area, and this is really just your body recognizing that something is under your skin that shouldn't be there and wanting to eliminate it. This causes increased pressure under the skin, which manifests as pain. It can really hurt and look ugly.

Interestingly, most people and even many physicians automatically believe that this is a sign of infection. However, in most cases, if we actually take a bacterial culture of the area, it will be sterile and show no evidence of any bacteria inhabiting the area. What's happening is purely an immune response: your body scrambling to protect itself from these wet, dead skin cells it perceives as foreign invaders that have escaped from the cyst sac. So it's technically incorrect to call a red and angry and painful cyst infected, and, in many instances, antibiotics are not needed. We just need to get these inflammations out from under the skin's surface. We need to do what's called an I&D, or incision and drainage. Once we relieve the pressure the inflamed cyst is causing under the skin, patients feel better almost instantly.

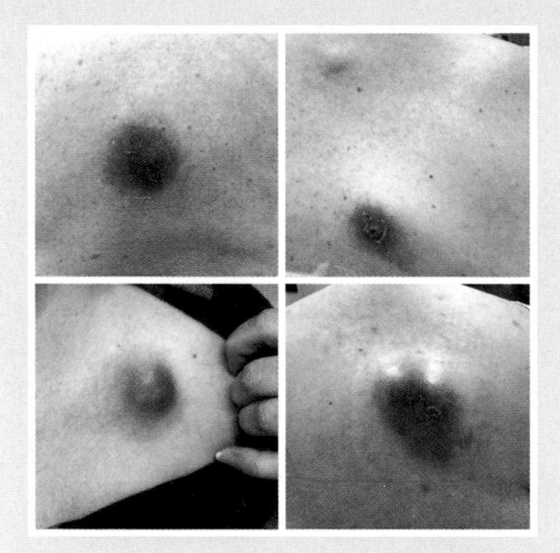

Inflamed epidermoid cysts.

How to Prevent Them (If Possible)

We can't prevent them, but certain factors increase the likelihood of their appearance. A history of acne, injury to the skin, being past puberty, and certain genetic disorders can increase your risk of developing such unpleasant bumps under the skin. I guess my best advice is to learn how to recognize one and leave them alone or get them removed surgically.

Treatment Options

Most cysts, harmless as they are, don't require treatment because they are in no way life threatening. Removal of the sac ensures that it doesn't grow back, as it is extremely unlikely they will go away on their own. There are really two main reasons to get cysts removed:

1. Your cyst is on a part of your body where it is easily irritated, such as on your back, and you lean against it often; or along your waist, so that the waistband of your pants constantly rubs on the area. You don't want to risk the chance of its becoming irritated and inflamed. Not only is an inflamed cyst very painful, but it can eventually heal with a pretty ugly and permanent scar.
2. It forms on an area of your body that is visible to others, and it's a source of embarrassment. If you have a large cyst or even a small one on your face, you wonder if people are looking at you in the eyes when they speak to you, or are they staring at and speaking to your cyst?

What You Can Do at Home, Where Applicable

Sometimes you know the instant that your cyst will turn red and irritated: perhaps you accidently banged it against something because you were in a hurry getting ready for work. Or perhaps you or your significant other couldn't keep your hands off of it and decided to give it a big squeeze. Whatever the cause, if your cyst appears red and inflamed, doctors usually advise applying warm compresses to the area, to help encourage the inflamed cyst to come to a head and drain—kind of like a giant pimple does. If it becomes red, hot, and painful, please seek the advice of your doctor. You may need to have it drained to relieve the pressure and pain.

What You Should Not Do at Home

Don't squeeze it! Keep. Your. Hands. Off. If the cyst ruptures under the skin, pain and swelling will follow shortly.

When to See a Doctor

See a health professional right away if any complications or changes occur in the size of the cyst, or if it gets inflamed, changes color, or appears to be infected. A doctor can treat it with corticosteroid injections to minimize redness and irritation, might prescribe antibiotics if an infection is suspected, and may do an I&D to relieve discomfort. If you want to have the cyst removed for cosmetic reasons, and it is not irritated or inflamed, the process is very simple. (See below.) If you don't know what it can be like, watch one of my hundreds of videos on YouTube of me removing epidermoid cysts!

Healing Time/Results, or "What to Expect"

To remove the cyst, the doctor's first step will be to numb your skin with local anesthesia. Then she or he makes a small incision through the skin over the surface of the cyst. With luck, the cyst wall is strong and the cyst can be dissected away from the surrounding tissue intact as one perfect ball. Often this is not possible, however, and the cyst wall is friable and easily punctured, so the contents are squeezed out and effort is made to remove any remaining cyst wall. In the worst case scenario, for a cyst that has ruptured previously and scar tissue is present, a larger amount of tissue is excised in the shape of an ellipse to remove all cyst contents, lining, and scar tissue. This will result in a larger surgical scar.

PILAR CYSTS

Upon examination, a pilar cyst (also known as a trichilemmal cyst, an isthmus-catagen cyst, or a wen) looks identical to the more common epidermoid cyst. The difference is that 90 percent of pilar cysts occur on the scalp.[6] The pilar cyst wall is thicker than the epidermoid cyst's, so it's more likely to pop out whole. I often compare the thickness of the pilar cyst wall with that of an olive, and the thinner wall of an epidermoid cyst with a grape skin. The internal contents tend to be smoother, but it is also a benign growth. It is fairly common to have more than one pilar cyst on the scalp, and treatment is generally done because people don't like the way they look.

Fun fact: many physicians other than dermatologists call both epidermoid and pilar cysts "sebaceous cysts" because they contain what looks like a sebaceous substance, a waxy or oily fluid or paste, but this is actually an incorrect term. Instead, these cysts are made up of keratin, the stuff that hairs and the top level of the skin are made from. The lining of a pilar cyst consists of cells similar to those found in the bottom of hair follicles. They occur because, for some reason we don't quite understand, cells that are normally near the surface of the skin get into deeper parts of the skin where they multiply, form a sac, and make keratin.

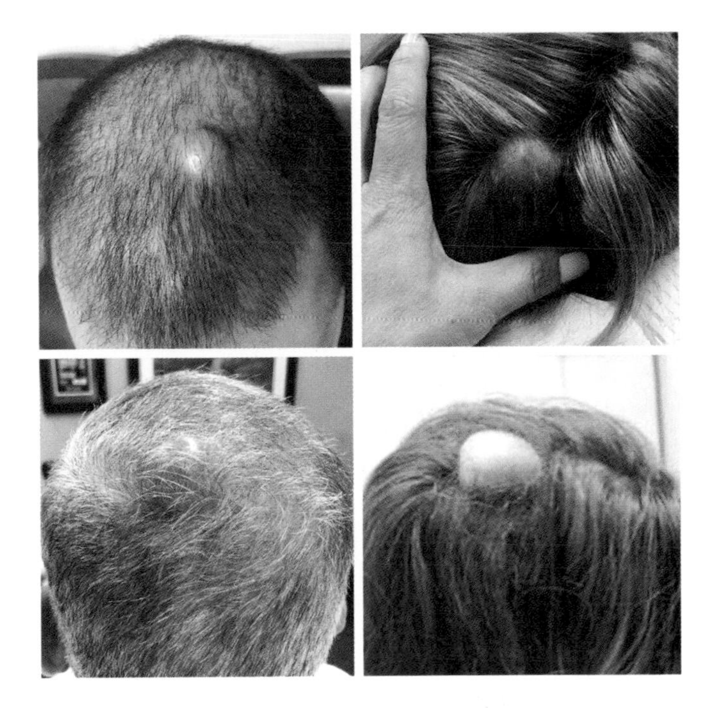

Pilar cysts.

How to Prevent Them (If Possible)

It is not possible to prevent pilar cysts. I joke to my patients that I think it is a sign of genius when you get pilar cysts. I think they know as well as I do that I'm just reassuring them in a joking way that they are normal!

Treatment Options

If you want your pilar cyst removed, you would need to schedule an appointment with a physician who can excise it under local anesthesia. I have actually had some patients admit to having removed their pilar cyst themselves, but I personally can't imagine the pain that would involve. And the risk for infection! Don't do it yourself, please!

What You Can Do at Home, Where Applicable

Try to leave your pilar cyst alone. As long as it doesn't bother you and is not noticeable, it can happily coexist with you, going on that wild ride we call life!

What You Should Not Do at Home

No popping! No squeezing!

When to See a Doctor

Pilar cysts are harmless, and they rarely become sore and painful. But if you feel uncomfortable with a pilar cyst because it's annoying or embarrassing, it's time to talk to a pro about your removal options. If they get aggravated by your hairbrush, or they are on pressure areas of your scalp, meaning they grow right where you may lean your head on your pillow at night or where a helmet would easily rub and irritate, these are perfectly good reasons to get them removed. Interestingly, I tend to see the biggest pilar cysts on the top of people's heads because these are not areas that are disturbed when you sleep, plus many people can hide them with a big hair comb-over. Pilar cyst denial is truly a thing.

Healing Time/Results, or "What to Expect"

If your pilar cyst is excised, usually the sutures are removed in seven to fourteen days. The area may feel a little sore and bruised for a few days, but nothing that requires prescription pain medications.

ABSCESSES, FURUNCLES, AND CARBUNCLES, OH MY!

I feel like those of you who are major popaholics get a little giddy when I say any of the above words, but for someone who actually has one, it is no joke; abscesses, furuncles, and carbuncles can be *painful*. There is some misunderstanding and disagreement about the definition of these terms, even among medical professionals, so let me tell you what I think, coming from someone who has seen more abscesses and the like in the last few years than an obsessed popaholic can even dream of.

Remember that by definition, an abscess is a collection of pus trapped under the skin. The word *boil* is used by many to describe abscesses, furuncles, and carbuncles, probably because it's one of those words that perfectly describe what you imagine them to look like in real life. Abscesses and furuncles, which resemble each other, are both collections of pus that are "walled off" and trapped under the skin. An abscess can appear anywhere on the body, whereas, by definition, a furuncle involves a hair follicle, so they occur only on hair-bearing areas of the skin. Last but not least, a carbuncle is a collection of multiple furuncles; these furuncles can even connect under the skin, forming tunnels of pus with multiple openings that drain the fluid onto the surface of the skin.

When you see me treat abscesses on my YouTube channel and other social media, you are likely seeing what was originally a cyst that has become inflamed so it is swollen, red, and painful, and filled with pus and broken-down, partially liquefied cyst contents. But abscesses develop from other situations, too. For example, if a foreign body gets trapped under the skin—say, a big thorn or a shard of metal—there's the potential for an abscess to materialize in these areas as well.

Furuncles and carbuncles are red, swollen, painful, and inflamed because there is an active bacterial infection going on in the skin, usually due to the bacterium *Staphylococcus aureus*. However, the distinction is that an abscess is a more general term, and there can be "sterile" abscesses, with a cavity of pus trapped under the skin but no bacterial infection present. Remember that pus is composed of white blood cells that the immune system has sent to a particular area of the body to fight off something, be it a ruptured cyst, a foreign object, or a bacterial invasion. The presence of pus does not mean that there is infection.

It's Alive!

S. aureus lives on *all* of us. Many people are frightened of this bacterium, but it is normal flora, meaning bacteria that normally inhabit our skin. It also lives in our nostrils and mouth. So when people tell me how supervigilant they are about keeping their skin clean to fend off a staph infection, I bite my tongue and keep quiet, because I know it will likely upset them to learn that staph lives among us and on us!

How to Prevent Them (If Possible)

Good hygiene is important in preventing these and many other skin conditions. But I have seen these bumps in people with impeccable hygiene, so don't believe the myth that these occur only on dirty, poor, homeless people. Most furuncles and carbuncles are caused by the bacterium *S. aureus*, which typically enters the skin through a hair follicle, small scrape, or puncture (although sometimes there is no obvious point of entry). Accordingly, keeping clean and washing your hands after any kind of activity, especially public activities (riding the subway, shopping, and so on), is important. Your mother was right: wash your hands as soon as you come home!

Treatment Options

Doctors will often prescribe antistaphylococcal antibiotics. As mentioned above, these growths can also be drained with an I&D. Draining a painful abscess, furuncle, or carbuncle can often relieve pain and discomfort immediately.

What You Can Do at Home, Where Applicable

If you feel an abscess or furuncle growing, apply warm compresses, because this will speed up its eventual resolution. Warmth will encourage it to "come to a head" or become more superficial in the skin. Your body is trying to push the contents of the abscess out from under your skin, and this is essentially what has to happen for this to resolve completely. Try taking a hot shower as well, which can also encourage its progression. (And if the abscess drains, this may lead to a less messy cleanup.) Please! If you are concerned, in significant pain, or have developed a fever, call your doc ASAP!

What You Should Not Do at Home

Don't try to puncture one of these bumps yourself, as the risk of infection increases the more an area is manipulated, especially if not done under sterile conditions.

When to See a Doctor

If you have an abscess, furuncle, or carbuncle, you should probably see a doctor who can relieve your pain and suffering, but the abscess also has to be ready to be incised and drained. It's kind of like being pregnant: if the baby is not ready to come yet, the doctor is gonna send you home. Similarly, if the abscess is still forming and not ready to be drained, we will probably prescribe antibiotics and send you home for a couple of days to wait for it to be "ready."

Healing Time/Results, or "What to Expect"

Healing time depends on the size of the abscess and the success of the I&D. If the abscess was drained properly, then you should feel better pretty quickly. If there is infection present, often we have to leave the drained abscess open to allow it to heal from the inside out, and this can take a while. This can be a hassle but shouldn't be really painful.

ERUPTIVE VELLUS HAIR CYSTS AND STEATOCYSTOMAS

I knew very little about these two conditions until this whole Dr. Pimple Popper phenomenon really started. Of course, I had heard of and seen them before, but never really treated them, and certainly I see many more of them now than I ever thought I would in my life. This is one of the things that makes this whole Dr. Pimple Popper thing so fantastic. It's like all the planets have aligned, and everyone wins!

Those of you who watch my social media have discovered and appreciate how amazing and surprisingly unexpected these types of pops can be. My wonderful patients with these growths benefit because they know they can see me and won't be judged by me and the viewers, and will be able to have these growths removed if they want for free or greatly discounted when every other doc has told them no. And I have benefited because these patients come from near and far knowing that I'll likely remove the bumps that many of them absolutely detest and that the removal will make them feel good about themselves. I get to help increase their self-confidence and happiness. That's the best gift I can possibly receive as a dermatologist and human.

Okay, let's get real about these pops! Eruptive vellus hair cysts (EVHC) are firm, flesh-colored or blue-gray bumps that appear most commonly on the chest, back, and upper arms. These growths are small—usually 1 to 4 millimeters—but what they lack in size they make up for in numbers, and a person can have hundreds of them. EVHCs usually pop up on the skin between ages seventeen and twenty-four, sometimes have a familial link, and affect everyone equally. The small cysts contain coiled-up vellus hair, the very soft hard-to-see hair found on the heads of newborn

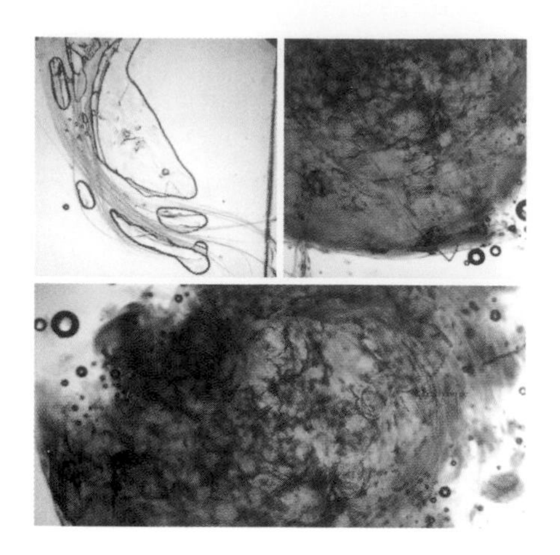

Microscopic view of coiled vellus hair within an eruptive vellus hair cyst.

babies and on the cheeks and temples of adults. The cysts are pretty cool to look at under the microscope: all those tiny, fine hairs coiled tightly within a skin protrusion that resembles a pellet of birdseed. EVHCs can have a central area of umbilication, almost like a punctum. Steatocystomas may at times have vellus hairs, and EVHCs may have sebaceous glands (oil glands) in their lining, which leads some dermatologists to believe these two conditions may lie along a continuum and be related. Treatment is gentle extraction.

Steatocystoma multiplex is found in multiples, and are uniform yellow cystic papules usually 2 to 6 millimeters in diameter, located primarily on the chest, upper arms, armpits, and thighs. The majority of cases show dermal lesions, but multiple subcutaneous masses resembling multiple lipomas can also be present. Bumps usually appear in adolescence or early adulthood, probably because sebaceous activity is at its peak then. Sometimes larger steatocystomas are prone to rupturing and discharging pus (suppuration) and can cause scarring and pain.

Steatocystomas typically contain a syrupy yellowish, odorless, oily material. If they are inflamed or infected by bacteria, they can develop a foul odor.

This is probably the closest thing to a true sebaceous cyst—the term that many people mistakenly use to describe the more common epidermoid cysts. Treatment is removal with small incisions and extraction, with particular care for treatment on the trunk because of the increased chance of poor cosmetic results and/or scarring.

How to Prevent Them (If Possible)

How to prevent these little cysts is a mystery. I don't think there *is* a way to prevent them; some people are just destined to get them. Luckily, remember, they don't harm you in any way.

Treatment Options

While treatment of these cysts is not a medical necessity, the bumps don't disappear or reduce in size or scope on their own (except in 25 percent of children who have

EVHCs). If we extract the cysts, there is a chance you won't get new ones—meaning we can get rid of them for good. Beneficial conservative measures include daily use of topical retinoids (tretinoin 0.05 percent cream daily or tazarotene 0.1 percent cream daily) or keratolytics (12 percent lactic acid lotion or 10 percent to 20 percent urea cream).[7] These topical products can possibly exfoliate the surface overlying the cysts, and if they are superficial enough, maybe then they can be squeezed out. However, in my experience, I have never heard of this being successful, nor do I think it's possible.

I'll always remember my second patient who came in with steatocystomas and EVHCs, all the way from the state of Georgia! She is a fellow physician, and one of the sweetest people I've ever met. It was humbling that she trusted me to remove her steatocystomas and EVHCs, but few dermatologists where she lived had much experience in the thirty- to sixty-minute procedure. And she understands, like I do, that health insurance doesn't pay for the removal of these bumps. She knew that if she saw a dermatologist in her area, they would certainly be capable of removing these, but wouldn't have much experience or desire to do it because it's just. Not. Done.

EVHCs and steatocystomas have been something that people just have had to deal with, and many who have reached out to their physician for help have found that they will refuse to do it or proceed only halfheartedly. And I say this because I was the same way before all this popping business began. Why would I spend thirty to sixty minutes trying to wrestle out these tiny slippery cysts and hard bumps like greased-up birdseed from under the skin when this still leaves the patient with a scar, and I can't even bill insurance for the procedure? How much would this cost for my time?

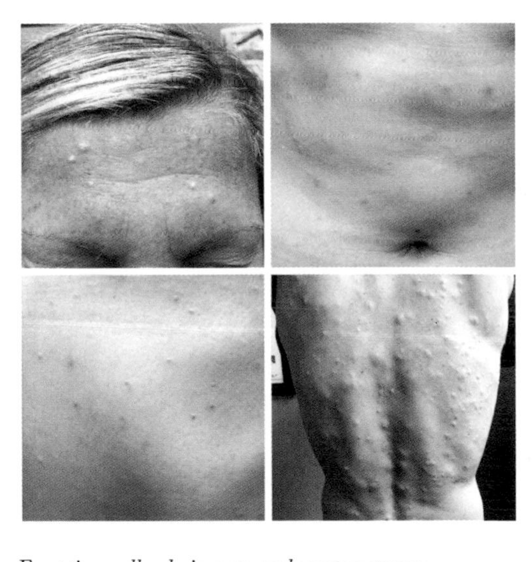

Eruptive vellus hair cysts and steatocystomas.

It could cost $500 or it could cost $5,000, depending on the time involved! Well, perhaps less now partly because I have so much experience and can do it more quickly. I'm sure if you looked back at my first EVHC videos you could see how my skill has progressed. I have learned so much about this skin condition that in the past I've largely ignored because it poses no medical danger. I've realized that removing them means so much more to those who live with them. The scar that is left and is unavoidable is really nothing to them. I see their personality brighten, and their feelings of new contentment and, really, happiness. It's an amazing thing! I'm lucky indeed.

What You Can Do at Home, Where Applicable

Don't pick at these areas, let them be.

What You Should Not Do at Home

No matter how strong the desire, please don't scratch, squeeze, stab, or otherwise engage our friendly EVHCs in an at-home dermatological weapons fight. You will always lose this battle—and probably end up with an unsightly scar!

When to See a Doctor

If one gets inflamed or even infected, let your doctor know. You may need an intralesional corticosteroid injection to calm it down, much like we dermatologists do to soothe an angry pimple, or your physician may prescribe an antibiotic if he or she suspects infection. When you've run out of conservative options and still want the EVHCs removed, your doctor can remove the cysts surgically by excision, curettage, cryotherapy, or laser. Fair warning: it may be difficult to convince your doctor to remove these, since it's not medically necessary, and we take an oath to "do no harm." Some may argue that leaving a scar and increasing the risk of infection and other complications by removing these is not necessary and is grounds for refusal.

Healing Time/Results, or "What to Expect"

If sutures are placed, they will be removed in five to fourteen days, depending on the area and the type of suture used. My general suture removal guideline is that if interrupted sutures are placed on the face, I take them out in five to seven days; on the body, seven to ten days. If buried subcuticular sutures are placed, these are removed in fourteen days.

Steatocystoma Superstar: Momma Squishy

I remember Momma Squishy's first appointment. We didn't record that visit, but now I wish that we had, because you can really see how we quickly and comfortably we went from being mere acquaintances to very dear friends. Don't worry, her first office visit didn't include any extractions, so you didn't miss any good pops from her. She had initially come in for a consult, so we didn't have the proper time allotted to do any extractions. At first, I wasn't even positive if steatocystoma was the correct diagnosis.

Momma Squishy is really the first person I have ever seen with quite an extensive number of large steatocystomas scattered over most of her body. She absolutely detested these bumps and wanted as many of them removed as possible. To do so, though, would require quite a number of very time-intensive visits, and I was concerned how much this would cost her—probably tens of thousands of dollars. I'm sure this was a deterrent for her as well. She had seen other physicians who reassured her that these bumps are benign, but no one had offered to remove them for her.

She found me, and, luckily, my office is only about an hour away from her home. I was a little concerned about filming some of her extractions for my YouTube channel, since many of them were on her buttocks and I wanted to make sure *she* would be comfortable knowing that her tush could be on display to the world. Also, I wanted to make sure that she knew and accepted what the resulting scars would look like after we removed these bumps. Would the scars be just as unacceptable, or, worse yet, would she be even more unhappy with the scars than her steatocystomas?

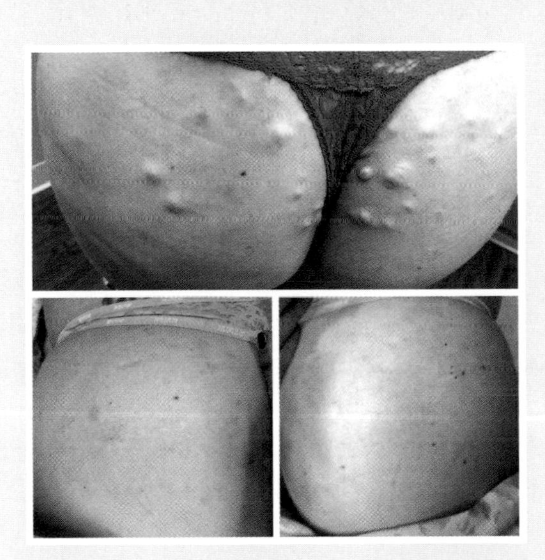

Mommy Squishy's buttocks before and after treatment.

It's people just like Momma Squishy who have taught me that it can be a real and significant improvement to rid your body of the crazy lumps and bumps under the skin that emit greasy, buttery, yellowish ooze, regardless of any scarring that may result. I've learned that the physical toll from the unsightly but harmless bumps isn't nearly as great as the emotional anguish they can impose. Some patients, frustrated that they can't find a doctor to extract them, take matters into their own hands, greatly increasing the risk of infection and scarring. Never try to remove these cystic lesions yourself. They are *way* too deep to remove without anesthesia and sterile instruments!

I think Momma Squishy might be *the* most adored person on my channel. She has an absolutely lovely personality and outlook on life. She is a fantastic mother, wife, and friend. Fans love to watch our relationship with each other deepen, and I think many people watching feel like they are actually in the room with us, like a bunch of close girlfriends just catching up on life. And the cherry on top for all of us is what a *huge* popaholic Momma Squishy is herself! She gasps and makes exclamations of love as she watches her own steatocystomas being removed. She professes out loud the love that many popaholics who watch my videos feel but may be afraid to say. All of us are *so* lucky to have Momma Squishy in our lives!

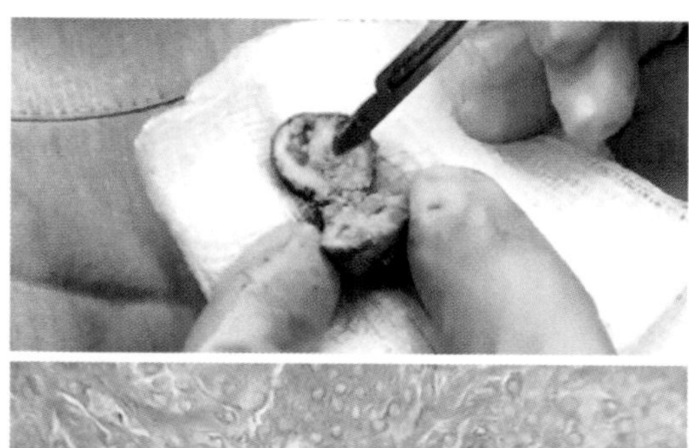

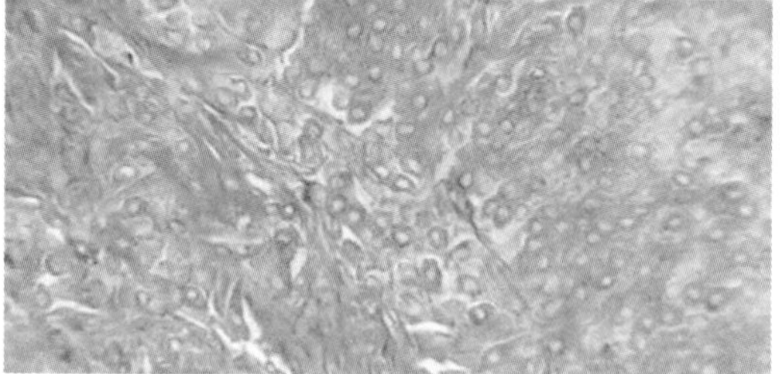

Top: Pilomatricoma cut open to see chalky contents.
Bottom: Shadow cells seen under the microscope.

PILOMATRICOMAS

If you wanna be fancy, call it by its other name: calcifying epithelioma of Malherbe. Pilomatricoma is an uncommon but harmless hair follicle tumor derived from hair matrix cells. We often diagnose it in young children, but we've also seen it in adults young and old. It is slightly more common in women than in men. The cause of pilomatricoma is a localized mutation in the hair matrix cell. They're usually found on the neck and on top of the head but can be found anywhere on the body. They are hard nodules under the skin that don't usually give rise to many symptoms, but they can be tender and sore. It's pretty unusual to get more than one of these. Pilomatricomas can remain the same size for many years and then grow larger. Complications are rare, although a small number of cases have led to cancer of the area. Dermatologists can sometimes feel the difference between pilomatricomas and malignant tumors under the skin: pilomatricomas are a little harder. This is not surprising because when removed, they can look like chalky little rocks that were trapped under the skin.

Sometimes I suspect a growth could be a pilomatricoma before I remove it, but usually I start to suspect it's a pilomatricoma only when I begin trying to excise it, and it comes out much differently than a cyst. Really firm, but it breaks apart easily and is clumpy—similar in consistency to sticky, crumbly dried-up toothpaste that cakes around the cap of the tube.

How to Prevent Them (If Possible)

There is no known way to prevent them.

Treatment Options

Pilomatricomas don't have to be removed, but if this is desired, they must be removed surgically, and if they are not removed completely, they can recur. They are really interesting to see under the microscope, and the presence of "shadow cells," or light pink cells that are often missing a nucleus, seen here will confirm the diagnosis. This is because there is calcification and ossification within pilomatricomas, so parts of it remind us of cartilage and bone.

What You Can Do at Home, Where Applicable

There is no home remedy for pilomatricomas.

What You Should Not Do at Home

Please don't pick at or pop these bumps, as doing so can lead to infection and redness.

When to See a Doctor

When the appearance of these bumps becomes unsightly to you, or if they are tender and sore, it's time to see a doctor. If any growth on your skin doesn't move around easily but is bound down, if it is growing steadily and quickly, or if it breaks down and bleeds easily, please see your doctor to have it evaluated.

Healing Time/Results, or "What to Expect"

Sutures are removed in seven to fourteen days, depending on how large the growth is and where it's located.

LIPOMAS

This benign growth is made up of fat cells in a thin, fibrous capsule, and is usually found just under the skin in the subcutaneous space that houses our fat cells. I describe them to my patients as a fat cell (adipose cell) that decides to have a party and clone itself over and over. It's a clonal collection of identical fat cells encased in a pseudocapsule, so slightly separated from the rest of the fat on our body.

Lipomas can be found anywhere on the body, including your torso, upper thighs and arms, and armpits. You can develop one or more lipomas simultaneously; some people have literally hundreds. We don't entirely understand what causes lipomas, but they do have a genetic connection in that they seem to run in families. Minor injuries can also trigger their growth. They are usually pretty small (1 to 3 centimeters) and can be felt just under the skin—but I have seen and treated very large examples. These are movable, with a soft, rubbery consistency, but they usually aren't painful, and they can remain the same size for many years or grow slowly. Lipomas often appear during middle age and are just slightly more common among men.

Lipoma . . . or Not?

If you have what everyone says is a lipoma but it's painful, you may have a rarer variant called an angiolipoma. This growth is also benign, but under the microscope there are more blood vessels traversing the lipoma, therefore giving it this name.

From my perspective, lipomas are actually pretty challenging but fun and rewarding to remove. Some who watch my videos are initially fearful or grossed out by watching a lipoma-removal video, but then grow to love them like I do. They are particularly satisfying to watch pop out whole and the procedure can be pretty simple and quick when this happens. Some people are just initially leery of watching them because they are often situated more deeply under the skin, so the removal looks more invasive and traumatizing and pain inducing, but I promise you it's very safe and without any major postoperative pain or discomfort.

How to Prevent Them (If Possible)

Researchers and doctors have yet to find a way to prevent lipomas.

Treatment Options

First of all, to make sure your doc's visual diagnosis is correct, you may have to undergo an imaging test (ultrasound). Like many of the conditions I discuss here, removal is considered a cosmetic procedure and may not be covered under insurance. Insurers sometimes make an exception if the lipoma is infected and/or painful or the diagnosis is uncertain. Most lipomas can be removed with a local anesthetic in the doctor's office. The surgeon makes an incision in the skin, removes the growth, and stitches the incision closed. However, if the lipoma can't be accessed through a simple incision in the skin, it may need to be removed in a hospital operating room under general anesthesia.

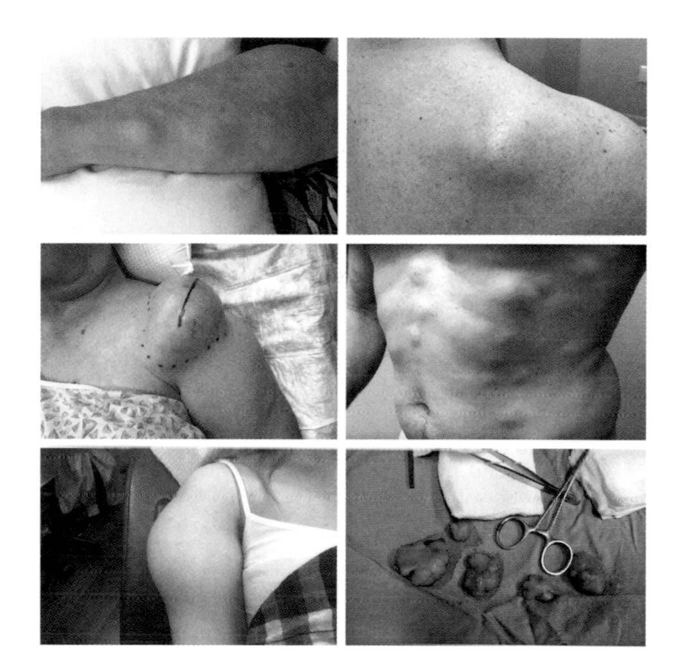

Lipomas come in all shapes and sizes.

The Difference Between a Lipoma and a Keloid

You may think lipomas and keloids look identical, but to a dermatologist, they appear and feel very different. A lipoma, a mobile growth under the skin, often causes no change to the surface of the overlying skin, whereas a keloid is rubbery and firm, and projects from the surface.

What You Can Do at Home, Where Applicable

There is nothing you can do to prevent lipomas. They just happen. Probably to keep me in business . . . only kidding!

What You Should Not Do at Home

You certainly should not attempt to remove a lipoma on your own!

When to See a Doctor

If the growth bothers you or gives you any pain or discomfort, see a physician. He or she should look at any lump or bump on the skin to eliminate concerns about something more dangerous.

Healing Time/Results, or "What to Expect"

If your lipoma is surgically removed, you may be bruised and be sore in the area for a couple of days. Sometimes a lipoma is situated below muscle, and if this is the case, there can be a longer healing time. Healing time is also dependent on the area that the lipoma is removed from. If sutures are placed, they are usually removed within seven to fourteen days.

The Final Farewell

Do you think it would be strange if you wanted to see and maybe even hold your cyst or lipoma right after it was removed from your body? Well, if you're a popaholic, you probably don't think so and actually would be disappointed if you didn't get the opportunity. I usually ask my patients if they want to see the cyst, lipoma, or big blackhead that came out of their bodies, and most of the time they say yes. Their response is usually something like "Wow!" or "That's crazy!" or "Oh, disgusting!" We all laugh and say goodbye to their little friend. Some people actually want to hold it. And I think that's cathartic for the patients; it gives them a chance to take control and get the upper hand over this bump that has caused them embarrassment or even pain. It's like: "Look! I overcame you! You didn't get the best of *me*, Mr. Lipoma!"

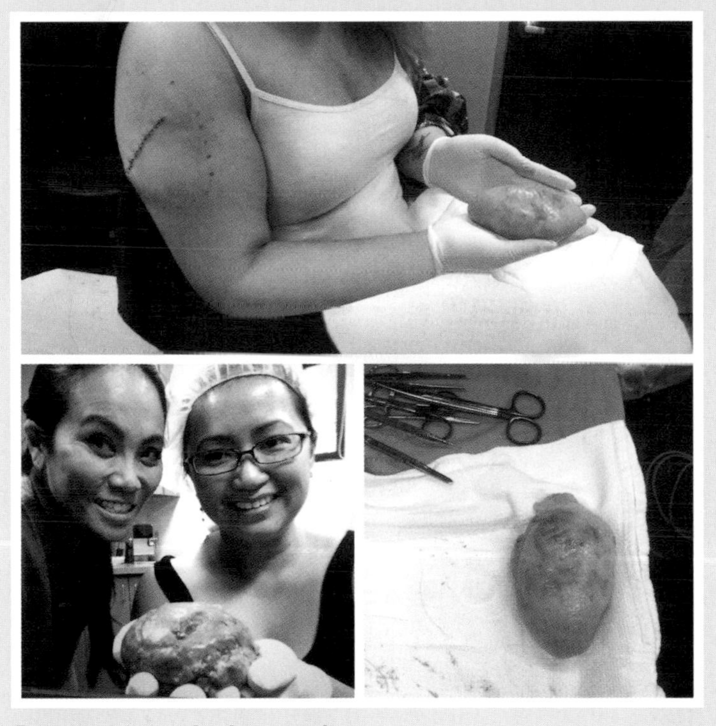

Patients posing with what popped.

COMMON SKIN CONCERNS ON THE BODY

SKIN TAGS

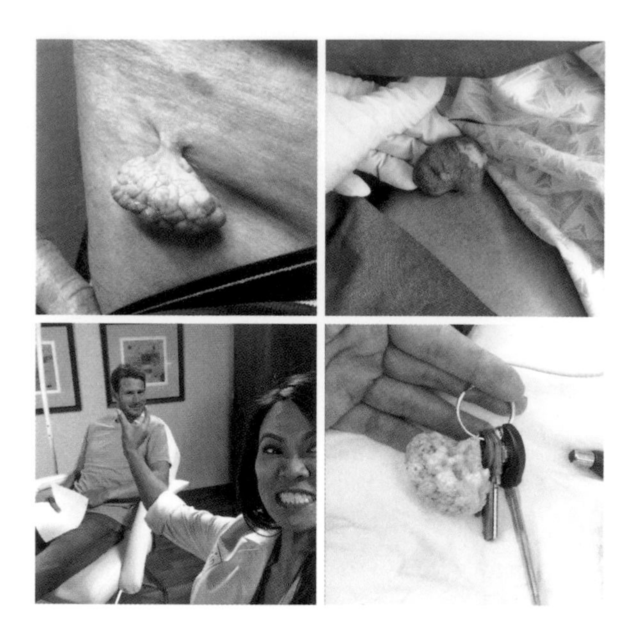

Giant skin tags and my appearance on Tosh.0, *where I was given a skin tag key chain.*

These benign, fleshy, wobbly skin growths are so common that almost half of all adults have one. Skin tags come in shades of pink, a range of flesh tones, and brown. We describe them as being pedunculated (attached to the body by a thin stalk of skin) or sessile (attached by a wider base of skin). Their small size measures usually between 2 and 5 millimeters but of course there are exceptions to these general rules. They are usually found on the neck, chest, and back. People often ask why they get skin tags, and I say that it's sort of like when a sweater pills because of areas that may rub on others. Skin tags tend to occur in skin folds, where it's likely that skin rubs against skin, on the neck, eyelids, armpits, groin, and under the breasts.

How to Prevent Them (If Possible)

There really isn't any way to prevent skin tags other than reduce the areas of skin rubbing against skin. If you are overweight, it is more likely that you have more skin that rubs on skin, so losing weight may help minimize this. Of course, this is harder to do than it is to write about!

Treatment Options

These painless, harmless skin tags usually don't require treatment, but many people request removal. I've certainly heard of people taking their tags into their own hands, attacking them (after deep breaths and mental preparedness) with their own nail clippers or manicure scissors. But they often bleed like crazy! Dermatologists have more humane ways of removing tags. The main problem is that this is not usually covered by health insurance. (I know: How many times do I say that in this book? But it's not my fault!) Most tags can be removed by scissor excision, cryosurgery (freezing), or electrocautery (burning). Your doctor might apply an anesthetic cream or administer local lidocaine injections to ease the pain if your tags are large or if you are getting multiple skin tags removed at once.

My preferred method is to use custom scissors that are serrated so they grip these wily, rubbery tags at the base. Then I use aluminum chloride, which stops bleeding as it is a hemostatic agent, and an electrocautery tool to help to minimize the bleeding. If you look at them under the microscope, you can see there is a healthy blood supply to your skin tags. Viewers of my YouTube channel know that some people grow pretty huge skin tags. I mean as big as a bite-sized cauliflower floret or even a golf ball!

I was once featured as a "CeWEBrity Profile" on Comedy Central's *Tosh.0,* and they showed a video of one of the biggest skin tags I've ever seen. They joked that I made that skin tag into a key chain and gave me a prop key chain. Well, the joke was on me, because I took that key chain home and kept it as a memento, until a couple days later, when one of my children came into my room, sniffed the air, and announced that something must have died there. That prop of a skin tag was a piece of cauliflower they had painted with flesh-colored paint! I had tucked it away in my bedside drawer!

What You Can Do at Home, Where Applicable

Take extra precaution and be gentle in areas where the tags exist. Skin tags can get irritated by clothing or jewelry or by anything that rubs against them. Obesity is a factor here, so it's important to know that weight loss may slow the incidence of new tags. Some people tie dental floss around their skin tags to strangulate them; this can be successful with smaller ones, but it becomes more difficult (and more painful) with larger tags. Tying them off will cut off the blood supply (if this method is successful), and the skin tag should turn black and eventually fall off. Works if you can walk around for a few days with dental floss hanging off of you.

What You Should Not Do at Home

Don't pick! Remember they bleed easily if snipped or picked off.

When to See a Doctor

See a dermatologist to exclude other, potentially harmful diagnoses and to have the skin tag removed if it becomes painful or appears to be changing. In rare instances, a skin tag can pivot at the base and cut off its blood supply on its own, turning the tag red, dark brown, or black. In these cases, they may fall off and resolve on their own.

Healing Time/Results, or "What to Expect"

Skin tags treated with cryotherapy (freezing with liquid nitrogen) or electrosurgery will fall off after a few days. Liquid nitrogen is –195.79 degrees Celsius or –320 degrees Fahrenheit—and that's pretty darn *cold*. Essentially, we use it to apply frostbite to a superficial area of skin. The longer liquid nitrogen is applied to an area, the deeper it penetrates, so your dermatologist's goal is to treat *just* the lesion and nothing else. If you treat an area too aggressively, you can actually destroy normal cells, including melanocytes (pigment cells), and this can leave you with a permanent white spot!

This is why, when we treat something on the face with liquid nitrogen, I always caution my patients that it's better to undertreat slightly. I'm happy to do a little more later if needed, as opposed to treating this bump too aggressively and leaving them with a permanent white spot! Even after removal, the growths might return, and new ones might appear in other areas. Treatments can be expensive because skin tag removal isn't medically necessary, and many insurance companies don't cover the cost.

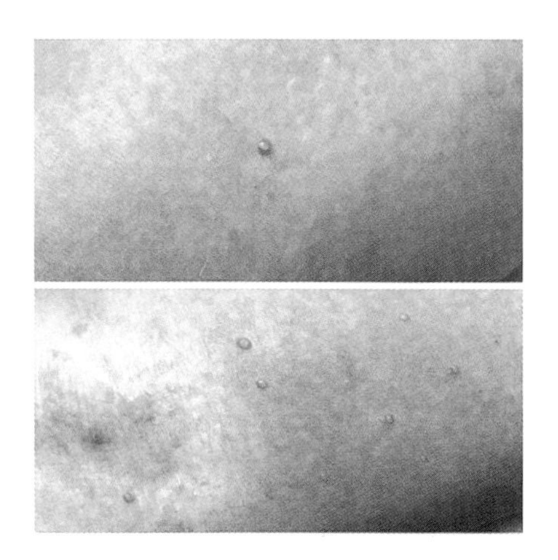

Molluscum contagiosum on the forearm.

MOLLUSCUM CONTAGIOSUM

This skin condition appears as small pearly-white, clear, or beige-colored bumps/papules. The center of the bump is often indented. These growths can be single or appear in groups or clusters. The culprit behind the infection is a virus, molluscum contagiosum, that is easily spread by contact but is not life threatening. Technically, it's considered an STD (sexually transmitted disease), but it's not the same thing as genital warts or herpes. That's because the virus commonly spreads through skin-to-skin contact, including sexual contact or touching the bumps and then touching the skin. Touching an object that has the virus on it, such as a towel, can also spread the infection. We often see molluscum contagiosum on the trunk, face, eyelids, or genital area. The lesions are also common in young children attending day care because the virus is spread through touch, and we all know that toddlers touch everything! The bumps can become inflamed when scratched (and toddlers will often scratch them) and turn red and sometimes get secondarily infected.

It may be hard to pinpoint the cause of the bumps because the time between exposure and bumps appearing is usually two to seven weeks but can take up to six months. If you're healthy, your body will eventually figure out that these are present, and once your immune system is alert, it will destroy them even if you leave them untreated. The problem, though, is that you never know if that will be in a week, a couple of months, or even a year or so! It's hard to tell a parent that their child can just live with these bumps on their arms or, worse, on their face, since this is especially distressing to the parents as well as the kids. However, people whose immune system is compromised, due to disease or certain medical treatments, may have larger and more numerous bumps, and these do need special intervention.

How to Prevent Them (If Possible)

Since molluscum contagiosum can be spread through touching infected objects or by skin-to-skin contact, good hygiene is essential to avoiding these bumps. It goes without saying that day care center staff need to be vigilant about cleanliness. Sometimes day care centers won't allow a child with known and active molluscum to come to school for fear of passing the virus on to others.

Treatment Options

Your doctor can freeze off the bumps with liquid nitrogen, which is called cryotherapy or cryosurgery. She can also scrape them off, which is called curettage. Certain topical chemicals can also remove the bumps, and include cantharidin and imiquimod. Topical creams and liquids for treating warts may also be used. But many people (including children) may not even need treatment because molluscum contagiosum usually goes away on its own.

Beetle Juice!

Cantharidin is synthetic blister beetle juice. There's an actual beetle that can elicit blisters on the bottom of the feet when it's stepped on and squashed, and a synthetic form of its blister-causing chemical called cantharidin is used to artificially create a blister purposefully. It's placed on a molluscum bump and induces the formation of a blister on the skin it comes into contact with over the next few hours.

What You Can Do at Home, Where Applicable

Keep the area clean, bandage over the bumps, and cover them with clothing to keep yourself from scratching them and to prevent others from touching them. They can actually spread across your skin and increase in number when you scratch them, a phenomenon called Koebnerization.

What You Should Not Do at Home

Try not to scratch them. Do not share towels or washcloths. If the bumps are on your face, avoid shaving if at all possible. If the bumps are in your genital area, avoid sexual contact until after you've been treated, or else you run the risk of transmitting them to another person.

When to See a Doctor

If the bumps are bothering you, if you're scratching them and breaking the skin, if they keep increasing in number, or if they are on areas of your body of concern to you, please see your doc.

Healing Time/Results, or "What to Expect"

If treated, healing time is generally two to four weeks. Keep the treated areas out of the sun for the first couple of weeks after treatment so that the area will improve more quickly.

WARTS (FLAT WARTS, REGULAR WARTS, PLANTAR WARTS, GENITAL WARTS)

Ah, yes, the wonderful world of warts! A wart is a skin growth caused by some types of the virus called the human papillomavirus (HPV), and can be easily spread. HPV infects the top layer of skin, usually entering the body via a break in the skin. The virus then causes the top layer of skin to grow quickly to form a wart. One problem with warts is that you can reinfect yourself just by touching the wart and then touching some other part of your skin. Not only that, but you can give other people warts by sharing things like towels, razors, and other personal items that come in contact with your skin. It can take a long time, sometimes months, before you notice a new wart.

Most warts go away on their own within months or years. Warts can grow anywhere on the body, and there are different kinds. Common warts grow on the hands and plantar warts grow on the soles of the feet. This is my spiel when I see someone with warts. I always heave an internal sigh when I say this because I've done it so many times. Here goes:

Warts are caused by a virus that is all around us. For some reason, sometimes our body does not recognize that there is a virus living on us; it is flying under our immune system's radar. The wart grows. Really, it's up to our immune system to figure out that there is a virus living on our skin, and when it does, the wart disappears. However, we don't know when this day will come. It *will* happen, though, if you are a healthy person with a healthy immune system. In other words, I've never had a ninety-year-old tell me they've had this one stubborn wart since they were nine years old. And this is the problem: If you google "How to treat warts," you will find hundreds of treatment suggestions. But if there was one great way to treat a wart, there would be only that *one* way. The fact that there are hundreds of possible options should tell you there is no single great way to treat warts.

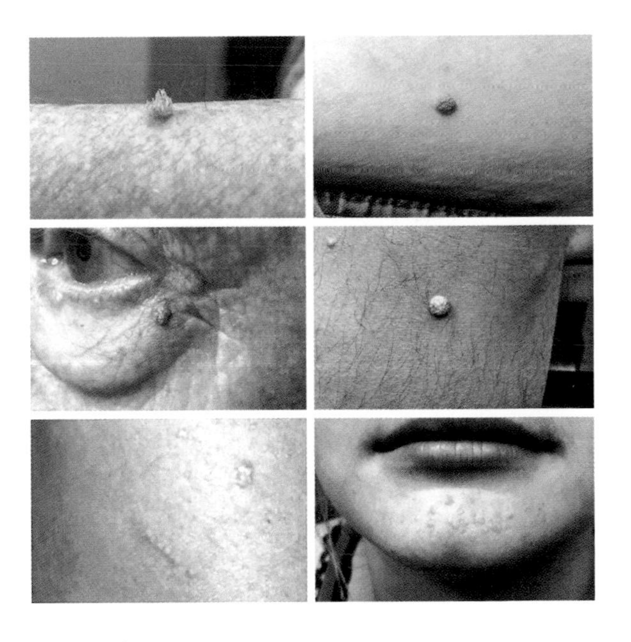

Common verruca. Bottom left: A phenomenon called Koebnerization. Bottom right: Flat warts, aka verruca plana, on the chin.

How to Prevent Them (If Possible)

Wart viruses are out there in our environment. When you're at the gym or staying in hotel rooms, wear your slippers or flip-flops. Exposing your feet increases your chances of picking up the virus from the floor. Wash your hands, keep clean, but please don't let it make you crazy. I had a wart recently. *Me!* I treated it, and it went away eventually, but it took three to four months. And I consider myself lucky that it lasted only that long!

Treatment Options

Warts are ugly (I have yet to meet a beautiful wart), and if they are itchy or spreading, you can treat them with topical therapies, both prescription and over the counter, or with an injection of medicine administered by a doctor. Freezing the wart (cryotherapy) or removing the wart with shave removal (curettage) are other possible treatments. Unfortunately, these wart treatments don't always work because the strategies used don't treat the underlying cause of the wart: the virus. Other treatments, such as topical imiquimod and direct injections of Candida antigen into the wart, are methods used to try to grab the attention of your own immune system. Conceivably, if your body suddenly realizes that there is a wart coexisting on the body, the immune system will get to work and get rid of it. So if this works, one day you may wake up and notice the wart has vanished.

Your Doctor Should *Never* Laser Off a Wart!

Using a laser pulverizes the virus particles but then releases them into the air. In the past, laser treatments led other people in the treatment area (patients and staff) to develop warts on their nostrils because they breathed in the wart viruses released into the air!

What You Can Do at Home, Where Applicable

My best advice (and what I did when I had a wart recently) is to use an OTC salicylic acid treatment or even cover the wart with duct tape. You can get both of these products over the counter. A topical salicylic acid bandage can soften the wart to help peel it off, and we actually don't know why duct tape works, which goes to show you how difficult and frustrating it can be to remove warts.

What You Should Not Do at Home

Please do not try to cut off the wart on your own. The black dots you see if you look closely at your wart are actually little blood vessels. If you cut them, they will bleed, and you risk scarring and infection.

When to See a Doctor

See your doctor when the warts are growing and spreading, are painful, or are unsightly.

Healing Time/Results, or "What to Expect"

It can take several weeks or months or even years for warts to disappear with topical treatments. If the wart is burned off, it can take several weeks to heal, and you may have a small scar. Remember to expect that you may need multiple treatments, and even then, the wart can still be stubborn and remain!

KERATOSIS PILARIS

Keratosis pilaris (KP) is common and harmless, but it does cause annoying small, hard, ruddy bumps or papules that make your skin feel a bit like sandpaper. These bumps usually occur on the upper arms, thighs, and buttocks, sometimes with redness or swelling, and occasionally on the cheeks of your face. KP can cause itching, but other than that, there is not a lot of discomfort or pain associated with the condition. It starts to show up in childhood or during the teen years, but usually becomes less severe with age—although some people deal with it to some degree well into their fifties.

A buildup of keratin, or skin cells, is the cause of KP. The buildup blocks the

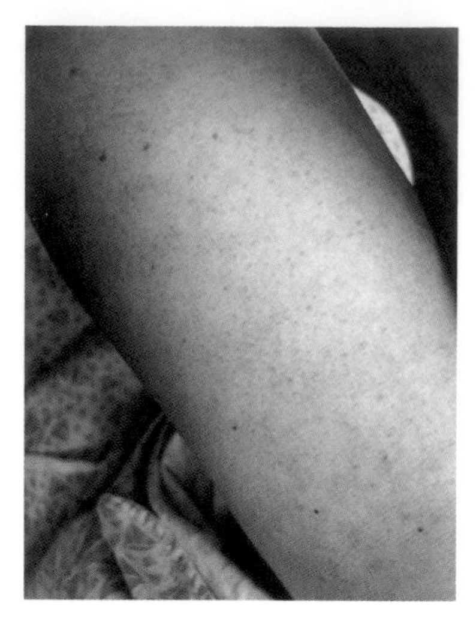

Keratosis pilaris on the upper arm.

opening of a hair follicle, and a bump occurs. It's actually a form of dry skin, so it's more common in people who have dry skin, and it's often worse and more noticeable during the drier winter months. Two things bother people the most when they have KP: the bumpiness (when they run their hands over the upper arms, the skin is not smooth) and the redness (they see fine, almost pinpoint red or brown bumps on the skin, which makes their skin look splotchy and uneven in pigmentation). This is something that many women planning to get married agonize over because they want to wear their fairy-tale strapless wedding gown and hate the red, blotchy, and bumpy appearance of their arms. I'm willing to bet this is one of the main reasons some brides opt for a shawl or long sleeves to cover their upper arms.

How to Prevent Them (If Possible)

You can't prevent keratosis pilaris. It really depends on your skin type and what your parents passed down to you. Don't blame yourself!

Treatment Options

Unfortunately, this is not one of those skin conditions that you can treat and "cure." Instead, you should be proud you have identified it for yourself, understand why you have it, and learn ways to keep it from getting worse, or little tips and tricks to try to make it look better—albeit sometimes temporarily, as it will likely return.

What You Can Do at Home, Where Applicable

Two approaches can be taken to improve the appearance of KP: minimizing the bumpiness and minimizing the redness.

First, use a humidifier to add moisture to your air at home, since dry skin definitely makes KP worse. Topical exfoliant creams and lotions help slough off dead skin cells from the surface of your skin efficiently and, if used regularly and consistently, can help minimize the bumpiness felt in KP. These include products that contain alpha hydroxy acid, lactic acid (such as AmLactin, available over the counter), salicylic acid, or uric acid. There are prescription varieties with the aforementioned ingredients that your dermatologist can prescribe for you. You can also find salicylic acid products in the acne treatment section of the drugstore, and these can be helpful in the same way. Pairing an exfoliating cleanser with a mechanical brush such as the Clarisonic can be helpful too, to try to buff the bumpiness down. My SLMD Skincare line includes salicylic acid body spray and body wash that are excellent treatment options for KP.

Topical retinoids and chemical peels can also help prevent hair follicles from plugging up. Retinoids include products with the ingredients retinol, tretinoin (Avita, Renova, and Retin-A), and tazarotene (Avage and Taxorac). Topical retinoids, however, can irritate your skin or cause redness or peeling, so decrease frequency of use if this happens. If you're pregnant or nursing, or are considering becoming pregnant, avoid topical retinoids. Chemical peel acids may also cause redness or a slight burning, so they aren't recommended for young children. You should likewise decrease the frequency of use or even stop such products at any age if they irritate your skin.

The redness from keratosis pilaris can be minimized by applying over-the-counter hydrocortisone creams, but these cannot be used over the long term. I recommend using a hydrocortisone cream for the week or two before a special event. In other words, don't just try slathering different products on your arms to clear up your KP days before a big event, because you may run the risk of irritating your skin even more and making things look worse. Try the different treatment options listed above beforehand and gauge your skin's reaction. See if there is noticeable improvement well ahead of showing off your smoother, less blotchy arms.

What You Should Not Do at Home

Avoid picking at or scratching KP. Don't take long, super-hot baths or showers, as they are drying to the skin (and dry skin makes KP worse).

When to See a Doctor

If the bumps become unsightly, itchy, or open and red, see a doctor.

Healing Time/Results, or "What to Expect"

It takes several weeks to see results with topical treatment.

ACANTHOSIS NIGRICANS

While not technically a bump, acanthosis nigricans is distinguished by areas of dark, velvety sections of discoloration in body folds and creases such as the back of the neck, armpits, and groin area. These *can* thicken the skin and certainly make people who have it very self-conscious. Skin tags are often found in the same area as well. This condition normally happens most commonly in people who are overweight or suffer from diabetes, both type 1 and type 2. Overweight children who develop acanthosis nigricans are at higher risk of developing type 2 diabetes than those who do not develop the skin condition. In rare instances, the appearance of acanthosis nigricans can be a warning sign of a cancerous tumor in an internal organ, such as the stomach or liver. In most cases, though, this is just a condition that is aggravating and embarrassing to the person that has to live with it. People tell them that their neck looks "dirty," and they are self-conscious about raising their arms because their armpits are "much darker than they should be."

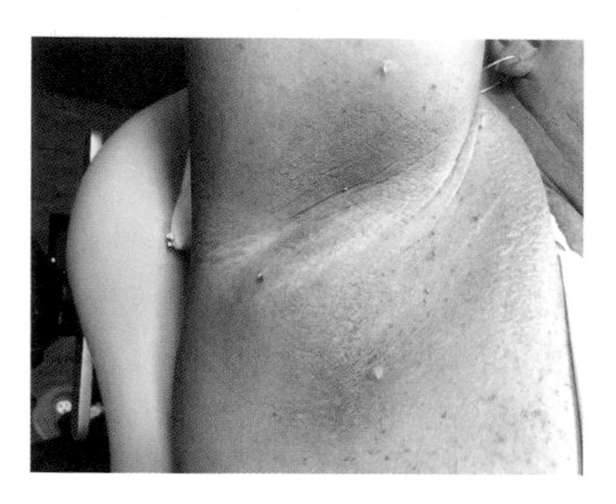

Acanthosis nigricans in the armpits.

Many people who have acanthosis nigricans are insulin resistant. Hormonal imbalances and other disorders can also cause the condition to appear. Women with ovarian cysts caused by hormonal problems can develop the condition. An underactive thyroid gland or issues with the adrenal gland can also cause it to develop. Medications including high-dose niacin, birth control pills, and prednisone and other corticosteroids can also be a cause of acanthosis nigricans. It can also sometimes accompany lymphoma or when a cancerous tumor begins growing in an internal organ. If you suspect acanthosis nigricans, see your doctor, as it could be a sign of one of these serious underlying problems.

How to Treat Acanthosis Nigricans

Unfortunately, there is no specific treatment for the condition itself. However, you may be able to treat the underlying causes of acanthosis nigricans. For instance, if you are overweight, normal color and texture of the affected areas could be restored by losing weight. If the condition seems to be related to a medication or supplement you take, talk to your doctor about switching meds or eliminating the supplement. If a cancerous tumor is the cause, surgically removing it can often clear up any skin discoloration. Topical solutions can also help. Prescription creams can lighten or soften the affected areas. Topical antibiotic and oral acne medications can, in some cases, improve the appearance of acanthosis nigricans. Laser therapy may reduce the thickness of skin that is related to the condition.

HIDRADENITIS SUPPURATIVA

I get questions *all* the time about hidradenitis suppurativa (HS), a very complicated inflammatory skin disease that certainly is a source of frustration, pain, and embarrassment. I'll bet that people who develop hidradenitis suppurativa really wish their apocrine glands would just disappear, since they can cause HS sufferers many problems. HS is characterized by blackheads, whiteheads, pustules, and recurrent boil-like nodules and abscesses that are extremely painful and embarrassing, since they often unpredictably ooze a pus-like discharge. They can even burrow under the skin, creating sinus tracts, almost like a gopher who pops up in various areas, digging different tunnels in different directions under the skin. These difficult-to-heal open wounds, or sinuses, lead invariably to scarring.

Apocrine glands on the human body are concentrated in the armpits, the groin, and the external auditory canal of the ear, as well as on the areolas. They don't become active until puberty. Interestingly, secretions from these glands in humans serve no known function, whereas in other species, they have a protective or sexual function, or regulate body temperature. Pretty fascinating, huh?

Hidradenitis suppurativa is also known as acne inversa. The condition often starts at puberty and is most active between the ages of twenty and forty; in women, it can resolve at menopause. Hidradenitis can affect a single area or multiple areas in the armpits, neck, inner thighs, groin, and under the breasts. Anogenital involvement most commonly affects the groin, perineum, mons pubis, buttocks, and perianal folds, in addition to the vulva in females and the sides of the scrotum in males.

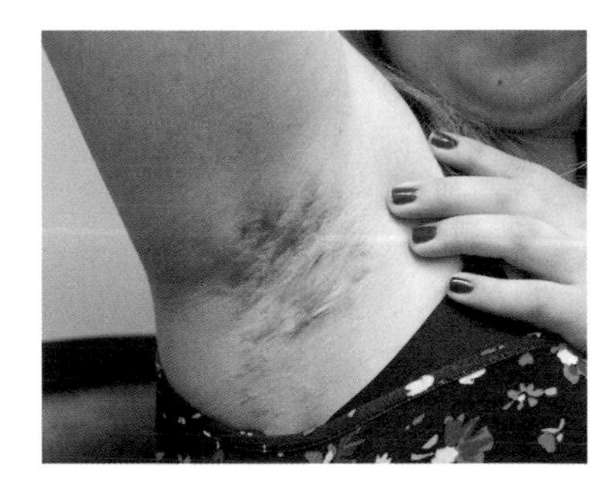

Mild inactive hidradenitis suppurativa.

Signs and symptoms of HS include:

- Open and closed comedones
- Painful, firm papules and larger nodules
- Pustules, fluctuant pseudocysts, and abscesses

- Draining sinuses linking inflammatory lesions
- Hypertrophic and atrophic scars that can often distort the appearance of the area involved quite dramatically

Many patients with hidradenitis suppurativa also experience acne, excess hair growth on the body (hirsutism), and psoriasis.

We don't actually know what causes hidradenitis suppurativa, but it is categorized as an autoinflammatory condition. For some reason our body is attacking itself and its own apocrine glands.

What does this all really mean to you if you suffer from this condition? Unfortunately, not that much. In fact, it may make you lose hope that you can be cured. Well, there are a few things you can do, and as I always say, a key to understanding a skin condition that you have is education, really learning about it. Knowledge gives you a sense of control and is the best way to start figuring out what can be done to make things better.

This skin condition can be quite devastating, both physically and emotionally. It is chronic, often feels as if it's unrelenting, is painful, can be smelly and messy, and can lead to depression and potentially severe debilitation. You may wonder why I include this subject in my book since it's not a really common condition. It's because *so* many of you are quietly, secretly living with this condition and feel a sense of hopelessness. I understand this and will try to give you as much information as I can to help.

Treatment Options

Please see a dermatologist if you suffer from HS, for there are certainly medications that we can prescribe to make you more comfortable. You mainly want to prevent or control and calm down the flares and breakouts you get with this condition because these are really painful, uncomfortable, and messy and lead to further scarring. Medicines like acetaminophen can help with pain management. Prescription antibiotics can help with pain and swelling, and help fight the bacteria on the skin that can make things worse.

Local injection of corticosteroids to areas of inflammation can calm down things quickly but temporarily. Surgical excision of areas can be successful, but this can't always be done, depending on the area affected. Nevertheless, this is the best chance for a permanent cure in an area. Interestingly, we have been seeing very promising results from a new class of medicines called biologics, which are most commonly given intravenously or via injection. These medications definitely have to be prescribed and monitored, often have to be administered by your physician, and can be quite expensive, but there is *hope* and I'm sure more progress and developments will be made to figure out how to cure this condition!

THE BENIGN TO THE MALIGNANT

MOLES, FLAT VERSUS RAISED

We all have moles. Moles (nevi, singular nevus) are benign growths that can range in color from pink or flesh colored to the blackest black. They can be smooth, dome-shaped, flat-topped, slightly raised, downright dangly, sometimes jiggly, and even look like a miniature brain. "Common" moles are the typical, boring ones—but in this case, it's good to be boring! These are usually pink, tan, or brown and circular or oval, with clear boundaries and a smooth dome shape. Common moles are often smaller than one quarter inch wide, or the size of a pencil eraser. Some have hair growing out of them, which is normal and even prized in some cultures. If you have hair growing from your mole, this may indicate that the mole is congenital, meaning you were born with it.

A giant congenital nevus, meaning one that is greater than 20 centimeters in diameter, has a 2 to 15 percent increased risk of developing into a melanoma. You would know if you had one of these giant moles, trust me, so if you don't, don't worry about it. Many more people have atypical nevi, aka dysplastic nevi, and people who have unusual-looking nevi like this often have family members who also have different-looking moles. People with many dysplastic nevi, who have family members who

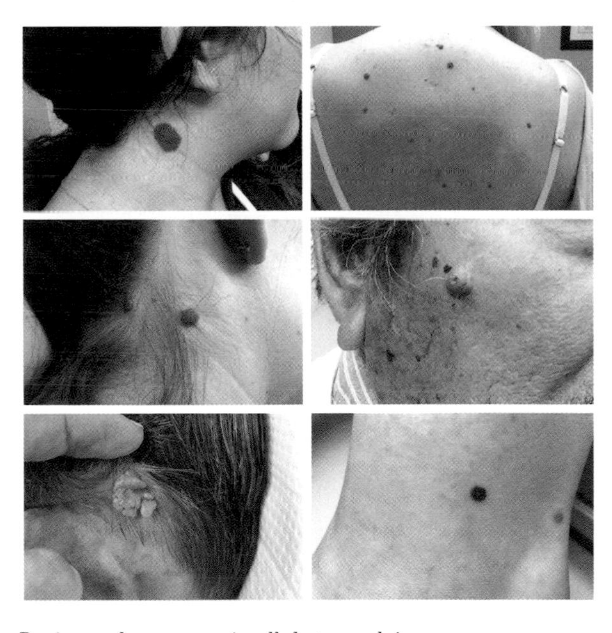

Benign moles can occur in all shapes and sizes.

also have funny-looking moles, are said to have dysplastic nevus syndrome (DNS).

So now many of you may be asking me: Wait, what is a dysplastic mole anyway? How do I know if I have one? I appreciate the moments when patients come to see me scared to death about showing me this spot on their arm that came up quickly and looks dark, crusty, and ugly, and they are frightened about how I will react to it. And I tell them after two seconds of looking at it not to worry—"It's completely benign; you can keep it if you like!"—because it has virtually no chance of being or becoming a melanoma. They look at me with relief, followed quickly by a question: "How can you *tell* so quickly? Tell me how I can tell, please?"

Sometimes I feel like my patients think I'm holding back secrets from them; that I'm not telling them about an easy visual clue I'm looking for—for instance, if a certain pattern in the skin told me the secret of what we have inside our skin. If I *could* tell my patients a secret that would instantly let them know whether a mole was benign rather than life threatening, I surely would! But it has so much to do with education and experience, the story you tell us, and instinct. At home, you can start by referring to the ABCDEs of melanoma (see page 43), but the answer is really not that easy.

Here's what I *can* tell you, and it explains why the role of a dermatologist is so important. We look at moles on a daily basis at work and have seen all types. Hopefully we have both the knowledge *and,* just as important, the experience to know when something is suspicious. Especially with people who have DNS. I always think of that *Sesame Street* segment, the one where they sing this song: "One of these things is not like the other," and they show you four different pictures. Maybe three of them are different balls, like a baseball, a soccer ball, and a basketball. The third image is also a ball shape, but it's . . . an orange. My job is to identify the orange.

How to Prevent Them (If Possible)

There is no way to prevent a mole. I remember during my training, a knowledgeable dermatologist told me that the average person has a hundred moles, and I've repeated this fact to many patients. But come to really think of it, I don't believe this is the case. We all have at least *one* mole, and many of us have more than a hundred. Some we are born with and some appear when we are kids and up to our mid to late twenties, but beyond our thirties, it's uncommon to develop new moles.

Treatment Options

Benign moles don't require treatment, though they may be removed for cosmetic or convenience purposes (when moles get caught on clothing or are in the way while shaving). When we as dermatologists remove moles, we never just discard them in the trash. I always send them for microscopic evaluation, to confirm (ideally) a benign diagnosis. To identify the nature of a mole, your doctor will perform a simple office procedure called a shave or snip biopsy. However, if the mole is large and flat to the surface of the skin, it may be better to surgically excise the mole, which requires stitches and a longer procedure, usually completed under local anesthesia in an office setting.

What You Can Do at Home, Where Applicable

Check your moles every one to two months using a simple ABCDE method used by doctors: Asymmetry, Border irregularity, Color change, Diameter, and Elevated or raised (see page 43). If you notice any changes, see your health professional immediately because it could be a warning sign of melanoma.[8]

What You Should Not Do at Home

Never try to shave off a mole at home. If the mole is cancerous, some of the harmful cells might stay in the skin or even spread. In addition, you could cause an infection or a scar. Don't pick at your moles. Picking may actually increase the risk of malignant transformation. It certainly can distort the appearance of a mole and make it difficult for us to determine with certainty whether it is benign or malignant. And picking can also create an ugly scar!

When to See a Doctor

You should see a health professional if your mole itches, bleeds, oozes, burns, or is painful. Make an appointment as well if you see a change in size, elevation, or color (especially if it turns black) or if a new mole appears after the age of thirty. You may gasp and say, "Wait, I have plenty of moles that have cropped up after my thirties!" Well, a visit to your dermatologist will hopefully alleviate your fears, because there are (unfortunately for us) many other types of growths that can crop up on our skin after our thirties (most commonly solar lentigos and seborrheic keratoses) that look a lot like moles. Your dermatologist can often reassure you as to their benign nature, but the only way we can do this is by evaluating your skin! Ease your mind and practice self-care with a visit to a doctor.

Healing Time/Results, or "What to Expect"

When a mole is removed via shave biopsy, what's left resembles a scrape on the skin: a flat abrasion the size of or slightly wider than the mole that previously resided there. It's an old wives' tale that "scrapes" like this need to dry up to heal well. In actuality, if the area dries up and forms a hard scab of dead skin and dried blood, this forms a wall that makes it difficult for new skin cells to grow and repopulate the area. It's actually best to keep the area moist with antibiotic ointment and a bandage, and it will heal faster this way as well! The red abrasion will eventually, depending on the size, heal and become a small flat white or red or sometimes brown spot about 75 percent the size of the initial lesion. Be patient, but of course let your doctor know if you think it's not healing correctly! Moles can also be surgically removed and sutures may need to be placed.

PRECANCEROUS GROWTHS

A precancerous growth—actinic keratosis (AK) or solar keratosis—is crusty reddish, pink, or flesh-toned skin damage that is often elevated, rough, and has a wart-like appearance. The condition is often referred to in the plural, *keratoses,* because they commonly form in clusters or groups. AKs are considered precancerous because if left untreated, they could develop into a skin cancer called squamous cell carcinoma (SCC). It is caused by exposure to ultraviolet (UV) radiation and so is often found in people who have overused a tanning bed. It's rare, but it can also be caused by overexposure to X-ray machines. So it's not surprising that they often appear in places that receive the most sun exposure, including the face, neck, ears, and shoulders, bald scalp, hands and forearms, and shins.

When they first appear, AKs are frequently so small that people notice them only because they feel the sandpapery sensation on the skin. There may be even more invisible lesions than those that can be seen on the surface. Most often, actinic keratoses develop slowly and are usually smaller than a pea, but depending on the level of damage to the skin, they can reach a size from an eighth inch to a quarter inch. Or multiples can combine, and you can have a large swath of skin that has skin damage at the level of precancer or actinic keratoses. Early on, they may disappear only to reappear later. Occasionally they itch or produce a pricking or tender sensation. They can also become inflamed and surrounded by redness. In rarer instances, AKs can even bleed.[9]

How to Prevent Them (If Possible)

The problem is that you usually develop these decades after the sun exposure that caused them; those AKs you notice in your fifties and sixties have to do with the sun exposure you had when you were in your twenties. So sun protection in your younger years is important.

Treatment Options

Early detection and treatment can eliminate many actinic keratoses before they become skin cancers. There are a few ways to effectively treat AKs, depending on your age and your overall health.

CRYOSURGERY: This technique involves the application of liquid nitrogen by a doctor to the AK. This freezes the tissue. The lesion and surrounding frozen skin may blister and swell about a week after treatment. It eventually crusts over and falls off.

CURETTAGE AND DESICCATION: This involves scraping off or shaving part or all of the lesion, then applying heat or an electrocautery tool to stop the bleeding and potentially kill any remaining AK cells.

TOPICAL TREATMENT: For widespread actinic keratoses, a prescription topical cream, gel, or solution can treat visible and invisible lesions with a minimal risk of scarring. Topical 5-fluorouracil is an example.

Worse Before Better

I tell my AK patients that their spots will look worse before they look better if they use the creams we prescribe to treat them. *Much worse.* Topical treatment with

5-fluorouracil was discovered in an interesting way. Essentially, this same product is used as a chemotherapy agent, administered intravenously, and when people got this treatment for cancer of organs other than the skin, their docs noticed that any actinic keratosis on their skin would get really red and angry, maybe even bleed and get scabby. Then when the medication was stopped, this redness would resolve and many of them would disappear! They made a topical treatment form of this medication to apply directly to actinic keratosis, and even superficial skin cancers, and lo and behold, it worked! So yes, you apply this topical product to your skin usually for three weeks, or as directed by your doctor. The AKs get pretty angry and inflamed, usually within a week or so after beginning treatment. When you stop the medication, these AKs will "calm down" and many of them will entirely disappear.

IMIQUIMOD (ALDARA, ZYCLARA): A form of topical immunotherapy, it stimulates the immune system to produce interferon, a chemical that attacks cancerous and precancerous cells. Your skin reacts in a similar way to how it reacts to 5-fluorouracil, getting red, angry, inflamed, maybe even bleeding, but treatment can really improve the sun damage and minimize the number of AKs you have.

CHEMICAL PEELS AND LASER RESURFACING: While you may be familiar with these techniques as anti-aging strategies, they can also be used to remove superficial actinic keratoses on the face and body by essentially peeling off the superficial layers of skin where the AKs reside. The physician applies trichloroacetic acid, glycolic acid, and/or similar chemical peel acids to the skin, causing the top skin layers to slough off. Laser resurfacing at a lighter setting can specifically and methodically remove the superficial layer of skin as well, and we usually use erbium or CO_2 lasers to accomplish this.

What You Can Do at Home, Where Applicable

These types of spots, once they appear, can't be treated with home remedies. But you can prevent future ones from developing by protecting your skin from the sun and other sources of UV radiation.

What You Should Not Do at Home

Don't pick at them!

When to See a Doctor

If you suspect a precancerous spot or spots, you should see a doctor. If you tend to get these, you may be someone who sees a dermatologist on a regular basis, maybe yearly or even a few times a year, to keep these in check and under control. Remember, the more you have, the more chance you have of one or more AKs turning into a squamous cell carcinoma.

Healing Time/Results, or "What to Expect"

Healing time varies depending on the type of treatment you receive—topical treatments work over time, while more acute treatments can have an immediate effect with a two- to three-week healing time.

MALIGNANT GROWTHS (BASAL CELL CARCINOMA, SQUAMOUS CELL CARCINOMA, MELANOMA)

Skin cancer is the most common of all types of human cancers, period, with one in five Americans developing one in their lifetime.[10] A malignant growth is a cancerous tumor that occurs when cells multiply abnormally. Cancerous tumors take over the oxygen and nutrients that neighboring tissues need to survive. All cancers are malignant, but not all are metastatic.

Metastasis is when a cancer has the potential to spread to other parts of our body, most commonly via our blood or lymph system. Basal cell carcinomas (BCCs) and squamous cell carcinomas (SCCs) are the most common kinds of skin cancers and have a very low potential to metastasize, which is a good thing. Melanoma is a type of skin cancer that can metastasize, and incidence continues to increase, which is why it is discussed so often, and why we advise people—especially those with a high risk of melanoma—to get regular skin exams by a dermatologist.[11]

Let's talk about BCCs and SCCs first, since they are so common. SCCs are more dangerous than BCCs and have a chance to metastasize, although not usually as agressively as melanomas. It's extremely uncommon for BCCs to metastasize; they are slow growing and locally destructive. The good news about these two common types of skin cancers: it's uncommon for them to threaten our lives unless they get too large, but at a large size, it's impossible to ignore them. Once when I was interviewing for a dermatology residency position, I visited a Chicago free dermatology walk-in clinic for economically disadvantaged people without insurance. One young man who came in looked like he had a raw hamburger patty slapped onto the side of his face, near his eye. I thought to myself, "That has *got* to be a skin cancer." (It was a basal cell carcinoma.) *How* could he actually walk around like that? I wondered. Well, the reason he came in was that he was beginning to go blind in that eye! There is something to be said about people's fear of doctors, and yeah, "denial" is not just a river in Egypt!

At any rate, if you have had one BCC, you have a 50 percent chance of developing another one somewhere on your body within the next five years. This is because, we believe, you have reached a certain threshold of sun exposure in your lifetime, and this cumulative damage to your skin has caused you to cross over the threshold and you now have increased risk of developing similar skin cancers. Don't forget that SCCs *do* have the potential for metastasizing but, in general, are not as aggressive as melanoma. I guess if you were to get one of these, the order of "priority" would be BCC, then SCC, then melanoma. But let's give you information to help you keep from getting any of them!

What do these bumps looks like, exactly? Well, it's not really an exact science, but let me tell you how we dermatologists describe these growths. A BCC is a pearly, slightly rubbery-feeling bump on the skin, studded with linear blood vessels. You may think it's a scratch, a bug bite, or even a pimple, but the difference is that a BCC doesn't go away. It grows slowly but continuously, and it may sometimes bleed easily if you rub it with a washcloth or accidently drag your fingernail over it.

SCCs, in general, look a little uglier. Another name for them is "rodent ulcers"—I think you get the point. They sometimes grow quickly, looking like a little volcano with a scab at its peak. Or an SCC can be a rough, almost flat area on the skin, but again, this type of bump tends to bleed more easily with trauma than regular skin, grows, and doesn't go away. Now, these are the most common forms these bumps take, but they can have many different appearances.

Both BCCs and SCCs most often occur on sun-exposed areas such as the face, neck, scalp, and the backs of hands. I joke with men that I can tell they have never had a hippie period when they had long hair covering their ears since they have a lot of sun damage on the upper rim (helix) of the ears. The more sun we have had in our lives, the more increased risk we have of getting BCCs and SCCs. Ultraviolet (UV) rays from consistent long-term sun exposure are the number one cause of skin cancers. Other contributing risk factors are a history of multiple blistering sunburns and chronic use of tanning beds.

You may ask, Why do these need to be removed? Why are they considered malignant and "cancer" if they don't threaten our lives? Well, because they are locally destructive. These two types are unlikely to spread to other areas of the body, but the larger they are, the more problems they cause. If a BCC on the nose is allowed to grow, it can take over the entire nose. If it takes over your whole nose, you will need a prosthetic nose to cover that hole in your head. The larger a skin cancer to be removed, the larger the scar. BCCs in particular are slow growing. They double in size every year, so of course this means the larger they are, the larger they get!

A significant portion of my private practice includes my work as a Mohs micrographic skin cancer surgeon. And it's one of my favorite things to do. When I say that, I sometimes think I sound like a sick and twisted person, since I'm professing my love of "carving on people's faces," but that's not what it's about. Mohs surgery is a specialized technique of skin cancer removal. It's predominantly used to remove BCCs and SCCs, mainly on the head and neck, and the point is to remove the skin cancer while taking as little normal tissue around it as you can. Then, while the patient waits, a technician slices up this tissue very thinly and stains it and places it on a microscope slide for me to look at.

At this point, I'm able to check all around the edges of the skin cancer tissue and also the deep margin to make sure that there are no "positive" edges (meaning no more skin cancer left). If there *is* still a positive margin, I've actually made a little map/diagram of how I've removed this skin cancer, so I can go specifically to where that positive margin is and take a little more from that area. In this way, we remove as little tissue as possible. And the smaller the amount of tissue removed, the smaller the size of the resulting scar (in general).

Of course, we have only so much skin on our nose, or around our mouth or on our cheeks! This technique has the lowest rate of recurrence, with a success rate of 92 to 98 percent. My favorite part of Mohs surgery is the part that requires the most creativity. After you've confirmed that you have removed the skin cancer and you have a "hole" left—what we call a "secondary defect"—now the Mohs surgeon needs to examine the area and decide the best method of surgically repairing and reconstructing the area so that the scar is the least noticeable. I tell my patients: my ultimate goal is that *you* may always know that something was surgically done here, but I want to make

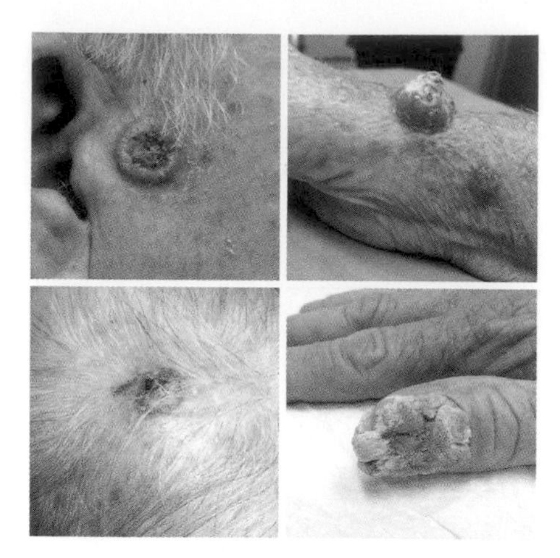

Left: Different presentations of squamous cell carcinoma of the skin.

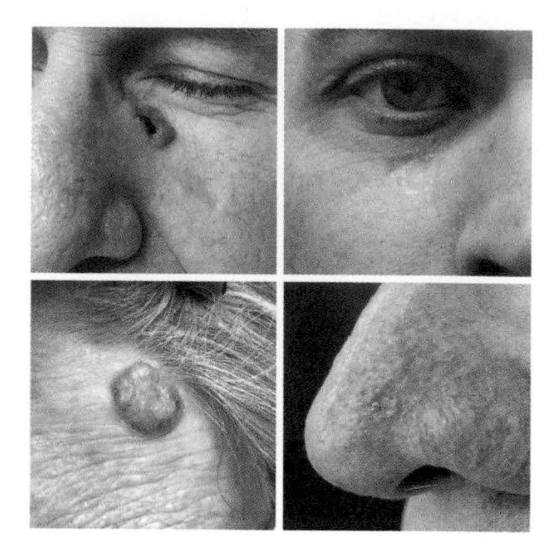

Different presentations of basal cell carcinoma.

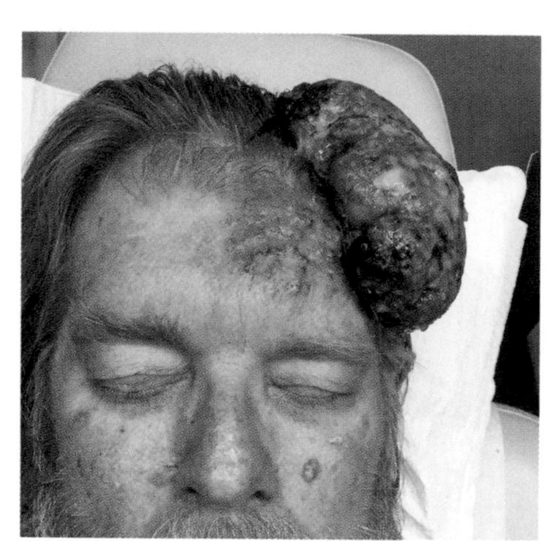

This man has a BCC on his left cheek but came in for the growth on his forehead, which is a melanoma.

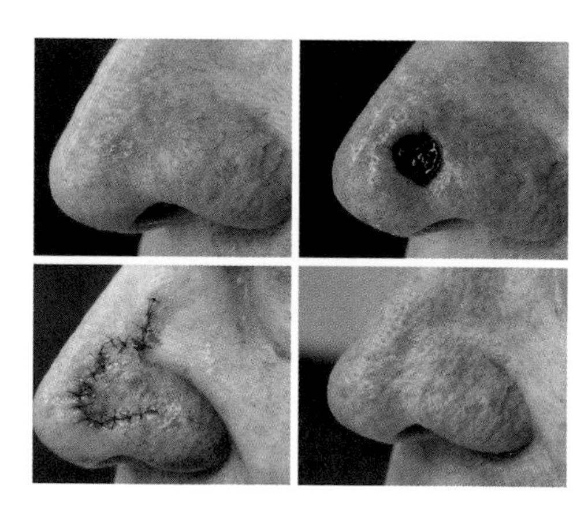

Mohs surgery and repair of a BCC on the nose.

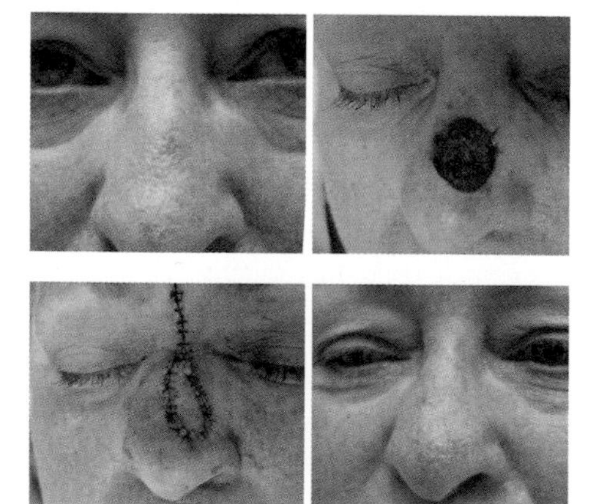

Left: Mohs surgery on a BCC on the nose.

it so that no one else has any idea that you ever had any skin cancer or any surgical repair in the area.

Now, let's talk a little about melanoma, which is the most commonly known and recognized "deadly" skin cancer. Most of us have heard of this kind of cancer, and know that it's a skin cancer that appears on our skin as a weird-looking mole, and that it can be deadly. Any type of life-threatening cancer is devastating, but what is particularly devastating about melanoma is that its peak incidence is during the "prime age of life." One in four persons who develop melanoma are under age forty. The median age of presentation is forty-five to fifty-five years old. While it is the ninth most common human malignancy, it is second only to adult leukemia in terms of loss of potential years of life.[12]

Melanoma, when diagnosed early, is almost always curable. However, a melanoma that is diagnosed late in the game is almost always incurable. This is why dermatologists urge everyone to have at least one body exam in their lifetime. And though sun plays a role in creating it, similar to BCCs and SCCs, melanoma is more likely than the other types of skin cancers to occur where the sun doesn't actively shine.

Some Mohs surgeons perform Mohs surgery on melanoma, but tissue sparing is not a priority here; the guidelines are to take wide margins when you are surgically removing a melanoma. It typically appears in light-skinned people and those who have had a great deal of exposure to the sun, but it can occur in all kinds of people, regardless of skin tone or color. It's more often "off the radar" with darker-skinned persons, so unfortunately it is caught late in many of those cases. Bob Marley, the Jamaican singer-songwriter, died from a melanoma that grew in his toenail bed! He thought it was just a bruise for quite some time, since it turned his toenail a dark purple/black color.

Do Your (History) Homework

Dermatologists often have a questionnaire that we give to our patients at their first visit, and one of the questions is "Do you have a history of or does a family member have a history of melanoma?" I think this should be more specific than a yes or no question. If you are told or you learn that one of your family members has skin cancer, it's very helpful if you find out whether it was a melanoma versus another type of very common non-life-threatening skin cancer. If you have a family history of melanoma specifically (as opposed to BCC or SCC), we dermatologists will look at your moles and likely have a lower threshold in deciding whether to biopsy or remove one of them. This is because we know that someone with a family history of melanoma is more likely to develop one him- or herself.

Let's first discuss melanin, or pigment. Melanin is made by a specific cell that is mainly seen in our skin, called a melanocyte. It protects our body against the harmful effect of UV rays and is distributed to the skin cells to act as a shield and protect our skin's DNA from damage. Sun exposure stimulates the melanocyte to produce more pigment; it's essentially our body's response to danger. This is represented as a tan, but if we have light skin that doesn't produce much melanin, then we burn. Melanocytes can often multiply repeatedly and become a collection of cells called a nevus, or what most of us call a mole. This is a normal process and occurs most often up until our mid to late thirties. In our thirties, this process of creating and growing moles stops, the size and shape of all your moles stabilize, and you rarely develop any new moles, nor should any of your existing moles change much.

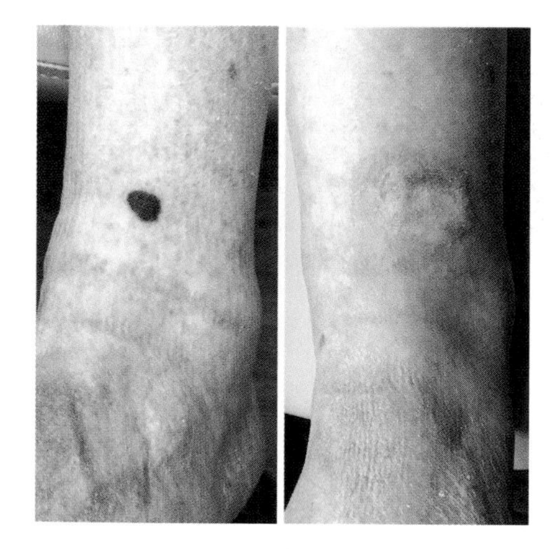

Melanoma before and after removal and replacement with a graft (tissue from his abdomen).

In melanoma, DNA damage (from sun exposure or other factors; even genetics plays a role) causes the multiplying process to progress out of control, leading to continued growth and the potential for the invasion of cancerous cells into blood vessels and lymph vessels. This can lead to the cancerous cells spreading to far areas of the body (metastasis). Melanomas can develop within a previously existing mole but can also occur where there is not a mole present. There are melanocytes not only in our skin but also on our lips, in our mouth, in our genital region, even within our eyes, and anywhere there is a melanocyte there is the potential for a melanoma. They can even be on internal organs, where we can never see them.

The four most common types of skin melanoma are superficial spreading melanoma, nodular melanoma, lentigo maligna melanoma, and acral lentiginous melanoma.[13]

As we saw earlier, benign common moles (nevi) are usually pink, tan, or brown and circular or oval, with clear boundaries and a dome shape, and are generally smaller than one quarter inch wide. Atypical moles (dysplastic nevi) can potentially develop into melanoma. An atypical mole can be larger than a common mole with a different color, surface, and border. It is usually flat with a smooth, scaly, or pebbly surface; an irregular edge; and a mixture of several colors. If a growth or mole on your body appears different from the others, ask a health professional to look at it.

No Place in the Sun

I remember a few years back my husband arranged for a surprise hot air balloon ride in San Diego. It was a beautiful sunny summer day, not too hot and with a steady breeze to chase the clouds from the sky. Our group was to meet in a supermarket parking lot to await a van pickup for transport to the balloon launch site. The van was fifteen minutes late, leaving a group of twenty people, including us, waiting outdoors in the middle of the day with no place to sit. Without saying a word to each other, my husband and I both chose to stand ten yards away from the rest of the group. Not because our intent was to be antisocial, but because we found one young tree that provided a small patch of shade. What shocked me was how automatically my husband and I chose the shade and how everyone else didn't even consider it! I remember that we just looked at each other and shook our heads. I think I muttered under my breath, "Look at all our future patients!"

Recognize if you are a person who may be at increased risk for developing a melanoma:

1. Although all skin colors can be affected, people who have very fair skin and light hair and eye color and who burn easily are at high risk.

2. A family history of melanoma increases the risk of developing one.
3. People with many large, unusually colored, irregularly shaped moles may have a condition we call dysplastic nevus syndrome, and they are at higher risk. This tends to run in families.

How to Prevent Them (If Possible)

The best way to prevent melanoma is to decrease the risk by avoiding the sun, especially when its rays are strongest, between ten in the morning and four in the afternoon. Seek the shade and do not allow yourself to get sunburned. Avoid tanning and UV tanning beds. Wear protective clothing, UV-blocking sunglasses, and a broad-brimmed hat. Use broad-spectrum (UVA/UVB) sunscreen with a minimum sun protection factor (SPF) of 15 every day. For extended outdoor activity, use a water-resistant, broad-spectrum (UVA/UVB) sunscreen with an SPF of 30 or higher. Apply it often, especially before, during, and after water-based activities, when sunscreen can sneak off easily.

The standard advice on sunscreen is to apply one ounce (about two tablespoons) to your entire body thirty minutes before going outside, and then to reapply every two hours or immediately after swimming or excessive sweating. Are you doing yourself or your children a terrible disservice if you don't apply sunscreen thirty minutes before you go in the sun? No! Dermatologists say this not because this makes sunscreen more effective, but because this is how the landmark first study about sunscreens was designed. Don't worry! Apply your sunscreen once you get to your spot (in the shade!) at the beach or pool.

Especially keep newborns out of the sun. It's not recommended that sunscreens be used on babies under the age of six months. Mainly this is because using these products on infants has not been properly studied, and because babies have a higher chance of absorbing products put on their skin. The solution is to cover them up and keep them out of direct sunlight!

If you have a family or a personal history of melanoma, we recommend a full body physical examination by your physician every three to six months. In fact, people with dysplastic nevi who have at least two blood relatives who have both dysplastic nevi and melanoma have the worst prognosis for the development of melanoma. They may actually have a 100 percent chance of developing a melanoma in their lifetime.

Treatment Options

This is in the hands of your dermatologist and/or oncologist. Possible treatments for melanoma include excisional surgery, lymph node biopsy, and chemotherapy and radiation therapy.

What You Can Do at Home, Where Applicable

Early detection is key to overcoming skin cancers. Learn how to check for the early signs of skin cancer to increase your chances of early detection and treatment—and recovery. Investigate the normal moles or marks on your body so that you will know if there has been any change. Using the ABCDEs of melanoma (see page 43), examine your skin head-to-toe every month.

What You Should Not Do at Home

Don't delay a trip to a health professional once you notice any changes in an existing mole, freckle, or other spot. The same holds true if you find a new growth that has any signs of skin cancer. Don't avoid seeing a doctor just because the growth doesn't hurt. It's important that you *pay attention to your instincts*. Too many times I've had a patient come in to show me a mole that they just didn't feel right about, and it turned out to be a malignancy. Trust your instincts, because they are often right.

When to See a Doctor

See a doctor if you notice any new growth or change on your skin. It's important to make an appointment *right away* if you observe any change in the size, shape, or color of an existing mole, or if a new dark area of skin develops.[14]

Healing Time/Results, or "What to Expect"

Healing time and expectations vary for each cancer treatment, depending on how aggressive the treatment was. Open a line of clear communication with your doctor and ask questions regarding how long it will take to heal and what you should expect after your treatment.

Chapter 3

Acne: An Issue for the Ages

MANY FANS OF MY PIMPLE POPPING VIDEOS WERE INITIALLY DRAWN TO them because they were *personally* searching for answers about their own acne. We are all familiar with acne, we have seen friends who have had to deal with it, and the vast majority of us have had at least one pimple in our lifetimes. A few pimples as a teenager, okay, most of us can accept that as normal and brush it off without it affecting our lives much at all. However, to many adolescent and adults alike, acne can be quite emotionally devastating and can have a serious impact on social lives and self-esteem.

I believe a lot of this frustration and sadness surrounding acne stems from the feelings of loss of control. My goal as a dermatologist treating someone's acne is to give my patients a sense of control back, make them feel that they *can* successfully treat their acne and clear their skin up. And I believe that to gain control, people must be educated. If I can teach you how to best identify *what* you have on your skin and *why* it's happening, then you will understand what treatment options work best for you, and your sense of control will be reestablished. This is the best way to find the treatment that will work for you.

Acne is an extremely common skin complaint in the United States—heck, in most of the world. In America, it affects up to fifty million people every year. A staggering 85 percent of young people between twelve and twenty-four experience some degree of acne.[1] Acne breakouts peak in most people during their teenage years, but, alas, men and especially women wrestle with adult acne.

The term *adult acne* should be an oxymoron, but unfortunately, it is not. What dermatologists call "adult-onset acne" can affect people well into their thirties, forties, and fifties. Women tend to get adult acne more often than men do, and I'll explain why. No matter a person's age or sex, the impact of acne extends well beyond the physical and visible manifestations. It can be quite traumatic and lead to lasting lack of confidence and self-esteem and bouts of depression and anxiety. This is why acne should be treated, not just to eliminate its ugly and painful bumps.

Some may say, don't worry about your acne, you'll eventually outgrow it, it's just part of growing up. Or, it's just an annoying skin condition but it's not gonna threaten your life in any way, so why waste your time treating it? Does someone with just a handful of blackheads on their nose need treatment? What about someone with a severe form of acne that causes extremely painful, ugly mounds of dark crust to form on their forehead, cheeks, chest, and back?

Certainly, the more aggressive the acne, the more likely you are to suffer from discomfort and other adverse effects like increased risk of infection and scarring. *Equally* important, however, is the risk of developing emotional scars, which are just as debilitating and painful. Remember, acne tends to hit the hardest during a vulnerable part of our lives—during puberty, our teenage years. This is a time when most of us are in our most "awkward" stage anyway: we easily trip over limbs that seemingly grow inches overnight, our voices switch octaves uncontrollably, we discover we are physically and emotionally attracted to others, and we often feel gawky and uncomfortable in our own skin. Days can be described as just a string of embarrassments about this body that we are trying to get accustomed to.

Adding a terrible acne breakout to this can have a huge impact on the way we relate to others and to the world during a time in our lives when we're taking the first steps toward establishing relationships with people outside of our own protected family nest. An acne breakout can be the difference between going to the school dance with friends or staying home alone feeling ashamed of our skin. Having pimples can make us very self-conscious when we already have a hundred things to feel unsure or confused about, and being embarrassed about our acne can cause many of us to hide away, which can really affect the development of our personalities.

In this section I want you to understand what acne is and be able to identify each

Levels of acne severity, top to bottom: early comedone, later comedone, inflammatory papules and pustules, acne cysts and nodules.

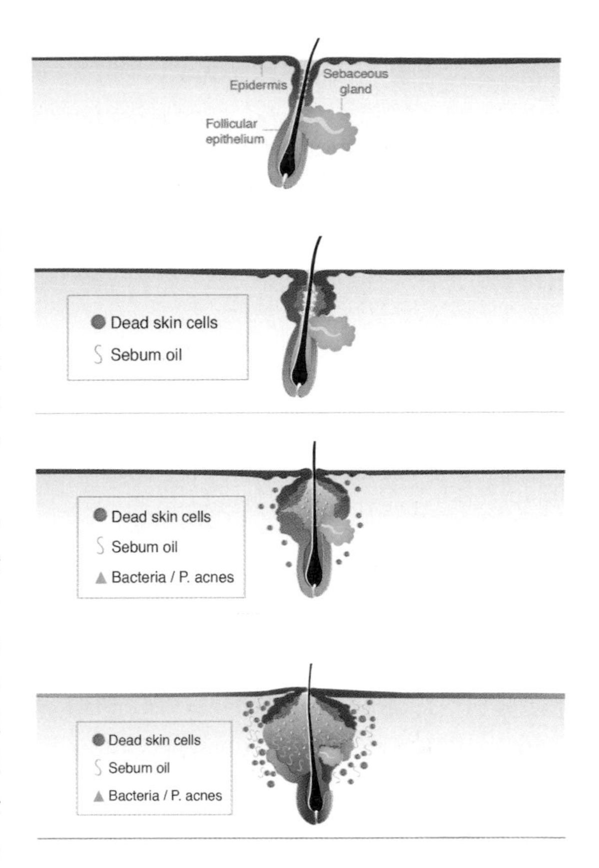

type of acne and its cause(s). This is the key to gaining the upper hand on your acne, to control your acne instead of letting your acne control you. I'll give you the right information to help you whether you get one small solitary Mount Vesuvius pimple once a month or you have acne conglobata, the most severe and potentially physically debilitating form of acne.

What is acne, exactly? Acne (aka acne vulgaris) is an inflammatory skin condition that arises in the pilosebaceous follicle. A hair follicle is composed of a pore/opening on the skin's surface and underneath the skin, the hair bulb with a sebaceous gland (oil gland) connected to it. The oil gland empties into this pore, and even though it's a hair follicle, no visible hair may grow out of it because the hair can be very, very fine. Hormones control the activity of our sebaceous glands and cause them to enlarge and become more active, producing more sebum (aka oil). This sebum mixes with dead skin cells inside a widened hair follicle to clog our pores.

There are three main types of acne. You can have one kind or all three. They are listed in the order of severity below.

1. Comedones (blackheads and whiteheads)
2. Inflammatory papules and pustules
3. Cysts and nodules

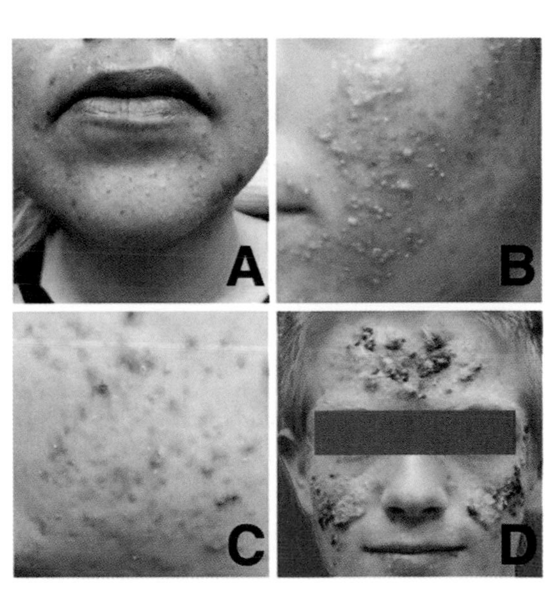

Types of acne: (a) comedonal, (b) papulopustular, (c) papules, nodules, and cysts, (d) severe cystic and nodular.

COMEDONES

Comedones are created when pores are plugged with excess sebum (oil), which combines with keratin (dead skin cells) and dirt or debris from our environment. Comedones are the primary lesions, the building blocks of acne. They consist of two types: blackheads and whiteheads.

A blackhead can also be called an open comedone. It's a clogged pore in the skin that is open and exposed to the air. Blackheads are "black" or dark in color not because they are clogged with black dirt, but because the contents are oxidized (exposed to oxygen), which causes them to darken. They're often found on the face and trunk but can be found anywhere on the body that you have follicles—which is essentially everywhere except for our palms and the soles of our feet. As a dermatologist, I prefer extracting them using a Schamberg-type comedone extractor. Personally, I use an 11 blade (one that comes to a sharp point), but some dermatologists like to use a lancet (a small, short pin).

While a blackhead is an "open" comedone, a whitehead is technically a "closed" comedone. A whitehead hides beneath the skin's surface, and so without exposure to air and oxygen, the bump appears white or flesh colored. Since whiteheads are just under the skin's surface, they often cannot be removed by squeezing or using a comedone extractor alone. Topical tretinoin (in the class of medications called retinoids) can help make these whiteheads easier to remove by softening and thinning the skin overlying the whitehead, but more importantly, retinoids can help prevent new blackheads and whiteheads from forming in the first place. If you can't get a prescription for tretinoin, the next best over-the-counter options are retinol or adapalene, which are also both retinoids. My SLMD acne system includes a retinol serum and can be purchased at SLMDskincare.com. Remember, this is *not* something I advise people to extract at home, because it requires that the surface of the skin be disrupted or broken first in order to expose the whitehead. I know that some of you will still take this too far! Remember that trauma to your skin can lead to infection and scarring.

More Blackhead Superstars: Button Blackhead and Kitchen Sink DPOW

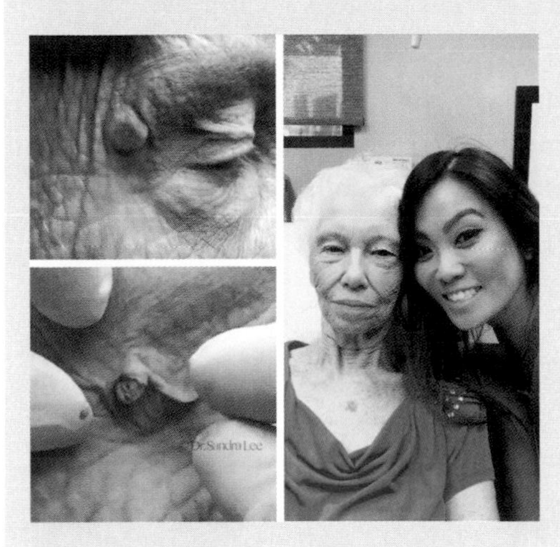

Gerri, who had the button blackhead, and me.

BUTTON BLACKHEAD

Gerri is one of my biggest and spunkiest cheerleaders! I don't know what I've done to deserve all her love! It was really by accident that I found that flat, coin- or button-sized blackhead just lateral to her right eye. And the conversation was just hilarious between Gerri, her daughter, and me as I removed this huge blackhead, which we have argued looks like a smallmouth bass or a squirrel. She makes me laugh every time I see her, and the world is just a better place with her in it.

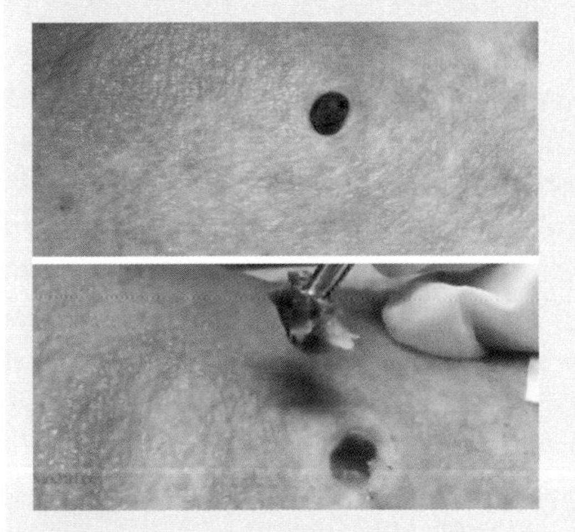

Large kitchen sink DPOW before and after removal.

KITCHEN SINK DPOW

This absolutely adorable mother-daughter duo (the daughter brings Mom in for regular skin checks, since she has a history of non-life-threatening skin cancers) is a study in contrasts. During one visit, I noticed Mom had a very dark, almost black spot on her right upper back, which from afar could look like a suspicious, possibly dangerous growth. On closer inspection, however, it's obviously a huge blackhead, a dilated pore of Winer (DPOW). Now, I understand that many of you wonder how someone could let a blackhead grow to such a large size. Well, in this case I think it becomes evident why when you hear the conversation between the patient and her daughter.

The daughter cannot handle seeing any medical procedures and certainly cannot deal with blood or needles. She did *not* want to look at the blackhead when it was intact, nor when it was removed. And, well, her mother, as she herself professed when I asked her if she has ever seen this huge blackhead on her upper back just behind her right shoulder, responded: "Well, I'm not a contortionist!" Absolutely hilarious. I *love* these two women! The huge DPOW left a noticeable impression in the skin, so later on, we excised this area so that the blackhead wouldn't recur. Sorry, popaholics, we will have to find another blackhead!

This is one of those instances where I am with you guys, that I can't believe she didn't know that this blackhead was there! How could she not feel a bump the size of a raisin? What makes a DPOW particularly satisfying to remove is that much of the time, it looks like it creates so much tension under the skin, and when it finally gives way as this one did, it slips out whole, in its entirety, and leaves cleanliness in its place. This is that one. If you're not quite sure whether you are a popaholic, this one will usually reel you in.

PAPULES AND PUSTULES

Okay, so I told you that comedones are the building blocks of acne. How do these small unassuming bumps that can be fun and downright satisfying for many to squeeze transform into those painful red, embarrassing bumps we all recognize as pimples and zits? Bacteria called *Propionibacterium acnes* (or *P. acnes*) that normally live on our skin invade the plugged pores, which provide the perfect environment for the bacteria to grow and thrive. As the bacteria increase in number, this increases the pressure within the pore, and the mix of oil, bacteria, and skin cells can rupture the comedone. This leads to redness, inflammation, swelling, and pain in the area, and then this becomes that red zit that you hate so much. These are officially no longer comedones but papules and pustules. Acne outbreaks tend to occur in areas where oil glands are plentiful such as the face, neck, back, chest, and shoulders. Outbreaks can also show up on the trunk, arms, legs, and buttocks—really anywhere that we have hair follicles.

Papules and pustules are considered the inflammatory type of acne, and you can see this in mild, moderate, and severe acne. Picking or squeezing these lesions (or any bump or spot on your skin, for that matter) can cause dark spots or even scarring.

Sometimes it's hard to keep your hands away from spots like this, though; they seem so ripe for the picking! But picking causes more problems than it's worth.

Papules are the flesh-colored to pink to red bumps that form when the weakened follicle bursts open. These bumps can be sensitive to the touch. Moderate acne includes the accurately named pustules, which are deeper, reddish pimples filled with white or yellow pus. The surrounding skin can be rooted in inflammation and also tender to the touch. When inflammatory acne papules are really deep, they often don't produce a noticeable bump, but actually form a larger and only slightly raised but really painful lump under the skin. This is what we call a cyst or a nodule.

CYSTIC ACNE

Cystic acne, aka nodulocystic acne, is the most severe form of acne. It is characterized by highly inflamed cysts and nodules. Cysts are deep, painful, pus-filled closed sacs. When ruptured, a cyst can cause further breakouts. Nodules are deep, large, painful swellings that are stiffer and harder to the touch because the inflammation is even deeper under the skin. The inflammation is burrowed so deep in the skin that cysts and nodules can be unresponsive to over-the-counter medications and topical treatments,[2] and even prescription oral and topical options. We are definitely in a no-picking zone here! The increased inflammation associated with both cysts and nodules poses a significant risk of permanent scarring. Scarring is directly related to the depth of damage in your skin. The deeper the inflammation from an acne bump (and cysts and nodules are deeper areas of inflammation), the higher the risk of permanent scarring. That's why dermatologists often recommend more aggressive medications to treat them than standard run-of-the-mill topical and oral acne treatments.

These acne cysts are difficult to prevent. If you have cystic acne, it usually means you've been suffering from acne for a while and have not found effective treatment for it, because it's extremely uncommon to wake up like this after one night. Cystic acne lesions are also most common among teenagers, and especially teenage boys—although teenage girls and adults can suffer from this condition as well. Cystic lesions are hormone related, and the teen years are when hormones are raging. Also, if you have a parent who had cystic acne as a teenager, you're at increased risk for getting it. This type of acne can certainly be extremely frustrating and depressing. Please know that for many people, this type of breakout can't be prevented, *but* you should recognize that if you have other family members who have cystic acne, and you are a teenager with acne-prone skin, you are at risk and should seek advice from a dermatologist as early as you can. This is the best form of prevention. This type of acne cannot be completely cleared up with a change in diet or just washing your face and applying over-the-counter products.

Cystic acne is particularly important to treat because if left untreated, it can lead to permanent acne scarring, which we all know is not life threatening, but is incredibly detrimental to a person's emotional well-being and feelings of confidence. Dermatologists have many treatment options to try—many prescriptions that are effective in treating acne. And we have some "big gun" treatment options, such as isotretinoin (Accutane was the original trade name of this product). Cystic acne is severe enough to even consider isotretinoin as the first line of treatment.

If you have cystic acne, keep your face clean and don't squeeze or pick at these lesions because that can definitely increase the risk of permanent scarring and potential infection. Visit the skincare aisle at your local drugstore, which will have a variety of over-the-counter acne treatment options that may be able to improve your acne, although often over-the-counter options are not usually strong enough to eliminate severe forms of acne. I know, it can be confusing. If you understand why we dermatologists recommend certain products and how they work, this is really key. Please read over the acne treatment section on page 146.

This confusion is also the reason why I developed an acne skincare line, available at SLMDskincare.com, which contains the most effective anti-acne active ingredients available without a prescription. These are products that I myself and other dermatologists would recommend to our own patients. If all this still doesn't work for you, you may need prescription medications, so please make an appointment with a dermatologist—professional help is the best way to prevent long-term, emotionally devastating consequences.

The most important thing to remember is that if you've tried everything and finally made an appointment to see a dermatologist, your acne still won't clear up immediately. Please be patient and try not to get frustrated. Remember, this type of acne did not begin overnight, and cannot be cleared up overnight either. Dermatologist and patient work as a team to figure out the best medications for you.

What Exactly Is the Triangle of Death?

Have you heard about the dreaded area on the face labeled the "triangle of death"? The three points of the triangle are the two corners of your lips and the place right between your eyebrows. Some of you may have been warned that you could die instantly of an infection if you squeezed a blackhead or tweezed a nose hair in this facial region. I was told about this in medical school too, in my gross anatomy class, and I understand why it's called the triangle of death, but I'm here to reassure you that I have never heard of anyone dying from squeezing a zit there!

You see, this triangular area in the center of our face *is* particularly prone to infection because there is a shorter distance for an infection to spread to very important structures, via an area in the center of our head called the cavernous sinus. This space is nestled just under our brain, and important nerves and blood vessels pass through it. Infection in this area can cause cavernous sinus thrombosis (a blood clot) and swelling, which can affect these important nerves and vessels, increasing the chances of meningitis, blindness, stroke, a brain abscess, and even death!

All of this said, we never see breaking news or bold-print headlines announcing, "Another person has died from a pimple on their nose!" In this day and age with our access to doctors, emergency rooms, and antibiotics, a dangerous and life-threatening case arising from pimple popping would be very rare. This doesn't mean you should have at it and start squeezing pimples and blackheads with abandon. If you have a large, sore pimple in this area that is increasing in size and becoming more painful, red, and swollen, the best course of action is to seek out a dermatologist or other physician who may treat you with antibiotics or injections of corticosteroids. As far as at-home treatment, my best advice is to stay on the safe side and try not to pick or squeeze eruptions especially in the triangle of death. A small pimple can be left alone to dry up; a daily swab with rubbing alcohol or over-the-counter acne spot treatment can help.

WHAT CAUSES ACNE?

If you're a teenager, your parents may tell you that acne is just a rite of passage into adulthood. You grow hair in new places, your limbs get long and you may get clumsier, your voice may squeak, and you're unsure about yourself and the world around you. This is probably the most physically awkward time of your life, so yes, acne can just be the terrible cherry on top. If you're no longer a teenager and you're frustrated that you still deal with acne, chances are that you are female and this acne is cyclical (crops up once or twice in a month). Men can get acne as adults, but more often it's the rosacea form of acne. So, why is this *still* happening to you?!

FAMILY HISTORY

Genetics plays a big role in acne. Just as we inherit our mom's blue eyes and our dad's cleft chin, so too can we inherit a parent's skin type. If you have a parent who has oily, acne-prone skin and who had bad acne as a teen, chances are higher you will find yourself in the same position.

HORMONES

Hormonal fluctuations are behind most outbreaks of adult acne in women. Women experience these shifts around their period, when they ovulate (the moment of ovulation when you feel a little twang of pain is called *mittelschmerz*—thank me later for your new ten-dollar word!), during pregnancy and menopause, and when starting or stopping birth control pills. The appearance of acne in the premenstrual phase is related to the drop in levels of the female sex hormone estrogen. I'm sure many of you, like me, don't keep track of when you're going to menstruate—we don't want to be reminded that this takes up a week, a full *quarter* of each month! But I digress. I'm willing to bet that many of you sense you are about to get your period because of the way your skin feels. Along with those food cravings, the mood swings, the breast swelling and bloating, it's common to feel that your skin is just a tad bit oilier, and suddenly you feel a slightly painful bump on your face hovering just under the skin's surface.

Menstruation allows androgens (male hormones such as testosterone that are present in both sexes) the freedom to overstimulate the sebaceous gland, which then overproduces the oil that leads to acne. The movement from female to male hormones can cause more pimples and oiliness of the hair and scalp. Even a newborn can get acne during the movement of birth when a mother passes hormones on just before delivery. Newborns can get acne when the stress of birth causes the baby's body to release its own hormones.

According to the American Academy of Dermatology (AAD), the majority of women with acne have normal hormonal levels, but hormonal testing is recommended for women who have acne in the chin area accompanied by excess facial or body hair, deepening voice, or irregular or infrequent menstrual periods.[3]

LET'S TALK ABOUT STRESS, BABY

Okay, I'm just going to say it, and I think many of you may be surprised: I *don't* believe that stress directly causes acne. However, I do believe when we are stressed, our acne can get worse. Stress can and does suppress our immune system, which can weaken our body's ability to defend against bacteria and inflammation. In response to stress our body will release more of the stress hormone cortisol, which may lead to increased oil production in our skin. So, in my opinion, stress doesn't *cause* acne, but it can *exacerbate* it.

When we're stressed out or anxious, we have a greater tendency to become preoccupied with our acne, absentmindedly picking more at our pimples and oftentimes having less willpower to keep our hands and fingernails off our skin. I guess it's the same kind of anxiety and stress release that people who watch my videos get. There's actually a medical term for this. Acne excoriée is a form of a condition called neurotic excoriations, in which people pick at their skin and can't stop themselves. We believe it's a form of obsessive-compulsive disorder (OCD), and it's a way many of us deal with stress. However, if you have it bad, it can be quite debilitating. Some people pick at their skin to the point where they have gouges all over.

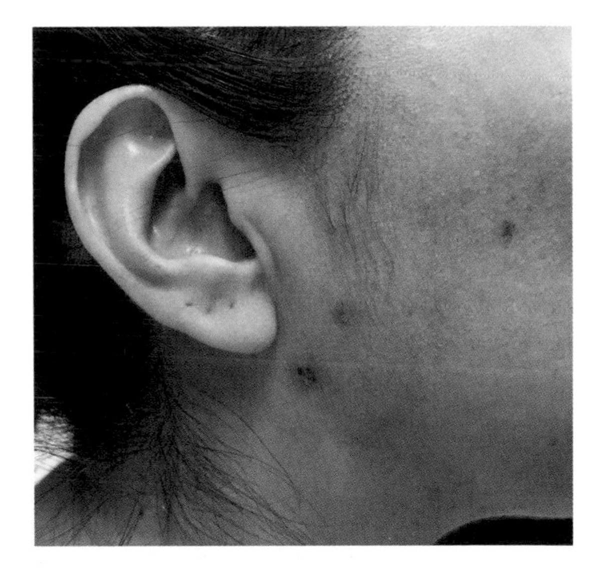

Acne excoriée.

The Strange but True Case of the Chronic Picker

As dermatologists, we learn how to spot someone with acne excoriée, or neurotic excoriations. They have bizarre-shaped scabs (eschars) on their bodies, which tells us they used their fingernails or other objects to pick, scratch, or poke at their skin. Sometimes people will have noticeably more of these lesions on their left forearm if they are right-handed. If they tend to pick at most of the body, upon skin examination we carefully look at their back, because if their skin lesions are due to their own picking and not from a true skin disease, then they will have lesions only where they can reach with their fingernails. Someone with neurotic excoriations may have gouges on their upper and lower back but the skin in the middle of their back, right where they can't reach, will not have a scratch in sight.

SKINCARE PRODUCTS

Many thick anti-aging night creams, certain types of makeup, moisturizers, cleansers, and sunscreens can be making your skin worse. Always look for products labeled noncomedogenic or nonacnegenic—meaning they won't clog pores.

MEDICATION

Acne can be a side effect of some medications, such as those containing iodides or bromides, and oral or injected steroids, including those that athletes sometimes take. Other medications that can cause acne include anticonvulsant medications and lithium. If you suspect that a medication is causing acne or making your acne worse, talk to the prescribing doctor to find out if an appropriate alternative medication is available for your medical condition. However, in my experience, the majority of acne cases are not related to medicine.

DIET

Many people insist that eating certain foods or drinking more water greatly affects your acne. However, this is a controversial subject and there is disagreement even among dermatologists. Some smaller observational studies have determined that milk, especially skim milk, can promote more acne breakouts. Perhaps this is due to the hormones that are added to pasteurized milk. Also, some think there is a link between a high glycemic load (high-sugar diet) and increased pimples. More definitive studies need to be done to confirm or deny these claims. What I tell patients is that if you stayed away from gluten or avoided chocolate and you truly feel that your acne improved dramatically, hey, keep doing it (as long as you get all the necessary nutrition and vitamins in your diet). However, there is no concrete proof that this is the case. If an acne patient's mom asks me to recommend to her child that she stay away from that junk food because it is making her break out, I usually respond, "Pizza causes acne only if you rub it all over your face."

HOW ACNE AFFECTS THE EMOTIONS

Acne is a troublesome skin condition whose effects can manifest psychologically as well as physically.[4] People who have more severe acne tend to experience more extreme moods. People with acne worry that others will have preconceived notions about them, that others will think they don't bathe regularly, are of a lower socioeconomic status, or may even be less intelligent! As a consequence, acne sufferers are at increased risk of depression, anxiety, and suicidal ideation. According to the American Academy of Dermatology,[5] studies show that acne sufferers can experience:

- LOW SELF-ESTEEM: People who have acne tend to internalize negative feelings about themselves. They can even avoid social situations and deny themselves the pleasure of enjoying time with friends and family. This low self-esteem can translate into problems in a professional and social capacity, where a person misses school or work, special events, and even celebrations because of their acne. Teenagers I see in my dermatology office who have bad acne usually come in soft-spoken and shy, often not able to meet you eye to eye. But when you help them clear up their acne, you develop a friendship and relationship with them, and it's so rewarding to watch them lift their eyes confidently, no longer embarrassed by the way they look. It's remarkable when you finally see their personalities shine.

- **DEPRESSION/ANXIETY:** The chronic and inconsistent nature of acne can make some sufferers feel hopeless. Over time, severe or chronic acne can lead to depression. Some even consider suicide. Adult female sufferers of all races fare especially poorly: 71 to 73 percent say they have experienced some degree of anxiety or depression because of the way their skin looks due to acne.[6]
- **SOCIAL ANXIETY DISORDER/SOCIAL PHOBIA:** These medical conditions are characterized by extreme fear and anxiety when faced with interpersonal interactions. Acne sufferers avoid social situations more often than others. One study showed that 45.7 percent of acne sufferers experience social phobia.[7] This chronic avoidance affects one's social, work, and family life.
- **ANGER:** Studies reveal that acne sufferers are more likely to get angry because of their perceived lower quality of life and their frustration surrounding treatment.[8]

Acne patients are encouraged to pay attention to their feelings of anger and other chronic emotional states as well as their quality of life, and to address the severity of their symptoms.

HOW TO TREAT ACNE

Whether acne is found in a teenager or an adult, treatment options are still the same. The main difference is that teenage skin tends to be oiler and more resilient. Adults who have acne usually have skin that more easily gets dried out and irritated by acne medications. If you walk down the drugstore skincare aisle, or watch television or internet infomercials, you know there are plenty of products out there that are supposed to treat acne. In general, the same medications have been available over the counter and by prescription for generations. Some new things have come out, but they are few and far between. We have improved the products, making them more cosmetically elegant, less irritating, and less drying, but the active ingredients remain the same for the most part. But the plethora of products makes it very confusing and frustrating to decide what to do.

Let me try to help you! In general, over-the-counter acne treatments can effec-

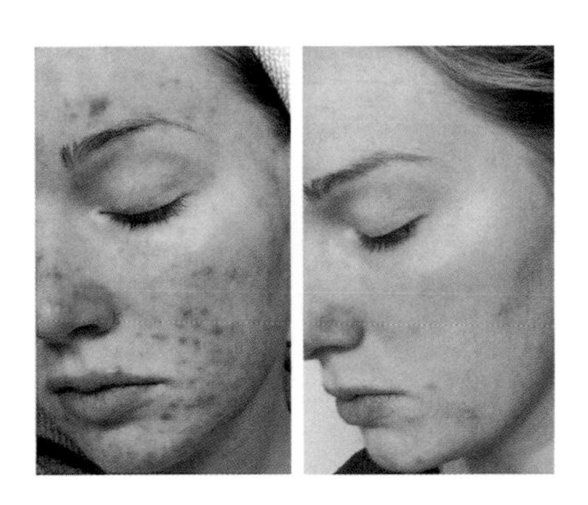

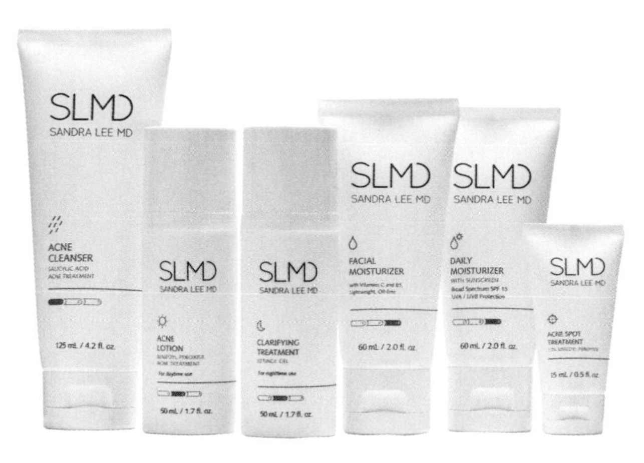

Left: Before and after use of the SLMD Acne System. Right: The SLMD Acne System.

tively treat mild acne and some moderate acne, but if you have moderate to severe acne, and if OTC acne products aren't working for you after four to eight weeks of use, you should seek out the help of a board-certified dermatologist to identify the kind of acne you have. Do you have more blackheads and whiteheads? Your acne may be mild. Do you get brown spots or red spots that persist after your breakouts? This can be a sign of moderate acne. Do you get red pimples or pus-filled bumps, or even purplish, deep-seated, painful nodules under the skin? Your acne is probably severe. Once you identify the kind of acne you have, you can better understand what treatments may work for you and whether you need to seek professional advice.

I understand that many people cannot see a dermatologist for an expert opinion about their acne. Maybe you can't get the time off from work or school to go see a doctor. Or you don't have the income or health insurance to cover the costs of an office visit and prescription meds. Or you don't have a car to get you to a doctor's office. Or you don't have a dermatologist anywhere close to where you live! There are so many reasons people can't see a doctor. That's why I developed an acne skincare line—for people who can't see a dermatologist but who want a treatment that works. SLMD Skincare bridges the gap between seeing a dermatologist and being totally bewildered and confused and frustrated walking down that skincare aisle at the drugstore, wondering what product you should use on your skin to clear up your acne.

Make It Personal

Acne treatment by a dermatologist is personalized. A dermatology visit will include an assessment of most or all of the following when we devise a treatment program for you: your sex; your age; how motivated you are (compliance); your lifestyle, hobbies, or occupation; what treatments you have been on or are currently on and what you think works and, if it doesn't, why; what types of cosmetics or topical products you use; other medication history; menstrual history; family history; whether your skin is oily or dry; and/or your ethnicity (color of your skin). All these factors can come into play when formulating a treatment plan.

OVER-THE-COUNTER MEDICATIONS

Over-the-counter medications can treat blackheads, whiteheads, and mild acne effectively. Some kill bacteria, others work on reducing oil, and some turn over dead skin cells faster. Products with these ingredients are available at most local drugstores and many online stores, including my own: SLMDskincare.com.

Earlier, I discussed the types of acne that we see and included many images. Take a careful look at that information and then at yourself in a mirror to see what kind of acne you have. Then read on to know what type of products will be the most effective for you. If you have more than one type of acne, this is normal! Just know that it may be best to use different medications to target the different types of acne bumps that you have.

Alpha Hydroxy Acids, Such as Glycolic Acid

Alpha hydroxy acids (AHAs) are synthetic versions of acids derived from fruit. They work by gently reducing inflammation and eliminating the top layers of dead skin cells. Their concentration levels determine their efficacy: less than 3 percent of AHAs work as water-binding agents, while greater than 4 percent concentrations (and in a base with an acid pH of 3 to 4) can exfoliate by breaking down the substance that holds dead skin together.[9]

The most effective types of AHAs are glycolic acid (derived from sugarcane) and lactic acid (derived from sour milk). Other alpha hydroxy acids and their origins include citric acid (citrus fruits), malic acid (apples), and tartaric acid (grapes).

In addition to fighting acne, alpha hydroxy acids are also used as topical treatments for extremely dry skin (xerosis), an inherited disease marked by dry, scaly skin (ichthyosis); and melasma, a condition that causes the skin to darken.

AHAs are widely available in several formats, including cleansers, creams, lotions, and cleansing cloths.

Side effects can include dry skin, sensitivity to sun, redness, mild stinging, and irritation. However, it's okay to use glycolic acid during pregnancy.

Beta Hydroxy Acids, Such as Salicylic Acid

These products work by removing the surface layer of dead skin cells that can clog pores. They can also help prevent blackheads and whiteheads from forming. The acids crystallize and settle down within the pore to prevent the accumulation of debris, further guarding against future blackheads and whiteheads.

They are safe for all skin types and shades, and come in washes, creams, scrubs, and even cleansing pads and cloths. Concentrations of the active ingredient are available from 0.5 percent to 5 percent. Just be aware that beta hydroxy acids can cause the skin to dry out, and they can also lead to irritation, especially if they're used in conjunction with benzoyl peroxide. Don't use these products if you're pregnant.

Topical Retinoids: Retinol and Adapalene

Retinoids unclog blocked pores, exfoliate the skin (removing dead cells in the process), and promote the growth of healthy skin. They also have anti-inflammatory properties, which is why you will notice they are listed as a treatment for all kinds and severity of acne. Additionally, they can increase the effectiveness of other topical anti-acne agents because they help clean the area up and allow increased penetration and efficacy of other products like topical antibiotics or topical benzoyl peroxide.

You can buy retinol-based products over the counter in cream, lotion, serum, or oil formats, including products you leave on your face throughout the day or at night. Look for any of these ingredients on a product's label to signal the presence of retinol: retinol, retinaldehyde, or retinoic acid. Retinol is a weaker variant of retinoids, while the stronger variants are tretinoins. Have I confused you yet? Just remember that retinoids for the most part are prescription only—except for retinol and adapalene, the latter of which has recently become available at a lower concentration over the counter—and they are stronger and more effective. If you can't get a prescription, at least get your hands on a retinol.

An added benefit of retinoids is that they have anti-aging properties. They can minimize fine lines and wrinkles, and can even help to prevent precancers, possibly slow down the progression of skin cancers. This all may sound wonderful, but the best benefits are seen with long-term, chronic use, and this ingredient can be irritating to some people, especially if you are prone to dry skin. That's why it's common to start with a low concentration, applying it once every third day (in the evening, as retinoids can be deactivated by the sun). If you tolerate it well, you can increase the concentration as needed and the frequency to daily. If that's too much, though, don't push it. Use only as much as you can to see the benefits without irritating your skin. There is a mild increase in sun sensitivity associated with retinoid use, though sunscreen can minimize this.

Some retinol products target localized areas, such as your lips, hands, and eyes, and the products are marketed this way, telling the consumer that it is specifically designed for a certain area on the body. However, in general, I believe this is only a ploy for cosmetic companies to get you to buy more products. Just be aware of your skin; if, for example, you know that the skin around your eyes is very thin and more sensitive and more prone to irritation, more caution should be used in applying products to this area.

Sulfur

This product removes dead skin cells that block pores. It works well in conjunction with benzoyl peroxide or salicylic acid. It's usually available in spot-treating, leave-on acne products, and it does work best when it is applied to an individual pimple rather than your entire face. It can cause the skin to dry out.

Benzoyl Peroxide

Benzoyl peroxide (BPO) is the most common ingredient in antibacterial cleansers, the first-line OTC treatment for mild acne. This is an ingredient in my SLMD Acne System, and is in many other anti-acne products on the market. This ingredient minimizes acne by killing bacteria and removing excess oil. Use daily to control acne and reduce breakouts.

BPO is available in many types of products such as bar soaps, lotions, gels, washes, creams, foams, pads, and moistened cloths.

Products with benzoyl peroxide vary in strengths from 2 to 10 percent. Start out using products with lower BP concentrations to avoid side effects such as dry, scaling skin or red or burning skin. This is especially true if you have sensitive skin. Additionally, studies show that BPO concentrations of 2.5 percent work just as well as higher concentrations.[10]

Be mindful that BPO is a bleaching agent and can whiten your clothes and/or towels. I like to advise my patients who are using a BPO to stick with white towels and white bedsheets while using this product. If they are applying a BPO to their chest or back, it's best to do so at night so you can wear a white T-shirt to sleep. I would hate for an acne product to ruin your favorite school or work clothes because you applied it to your chest and shoulders and it bleached your clothes.

BPO can also work mildly to improve comedones, which is why results can be even better when BPO is with coupled with certain other prescription acne medications.

> WARNING: Some people can develop irritation from benzoyl peroxide, so if you develop noticeable redness after using this product, you may have this problem, and this product is not for you. Sulfur products are good alternatives.

Azelaic Acid

Azelaic acid is a natural nontoxic acid found in whole grains such as rye, wheat, and barley. It's used to treat both comedones and inflammatory type acne.

It helps peel the outer layers of the skin cells lining the follicle, while also inhibiting the formation of comedones and blemishes. According to the Mayo Clinic, 20 percent azelaic acid cream seems to be effective when used consistently, twice a day for at least four weeks. It can be more effective when used in combination with the antibiotic erythromycin. Prescription azelaic acid (Azelex, Finacea) is an option during pregnancy and while breast-feeding.[11] A lower percentage is available over the counter. One other added benefit is that it may help to lighten postinflammatory hyperpigmentation, the darkening of the skin that happens after trauma, including what happens after an acne bump resolves, especially in people with darker complexions.

Be aware that azelaic acid can irritate sensitive skin or eczema sufferers. Discontinue use and seek medical advice if you experience severe redness, itching, burning, or scaling of the skin.[12]

PRESCRIPTION MEDICATIONS

If over-the-counter treatments are not cutting it for you or if you are suffering from swollen, painful cystic acne, it may be time for a prescription topical or oral treatment. Topical and oral medications may be used together for better results. These treatments also help to prevent acne scarring. Your dermatologist can help you determine the right treatment for your skin.

Topical Retinoids: Tretinoin and Tazarotene

These are stronger variants of the OTC topical retinoids and have the same properties. There are many prescription combination treatments—those that combine a retinoid with another active ingredient, such as benzoyl peroxide or clindamycin or erythromycin. This is meant to increase compliance and make it easier for you to stick to a regimen. You don't want to be trapped in the bathroom all day applying acne treatments, or to clog up your bathroom vanity counter!

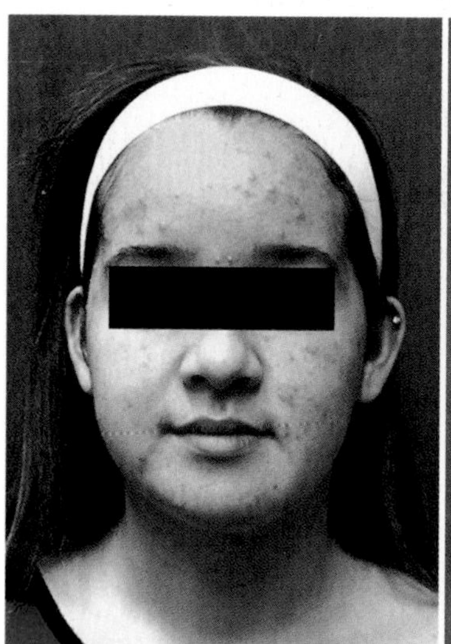

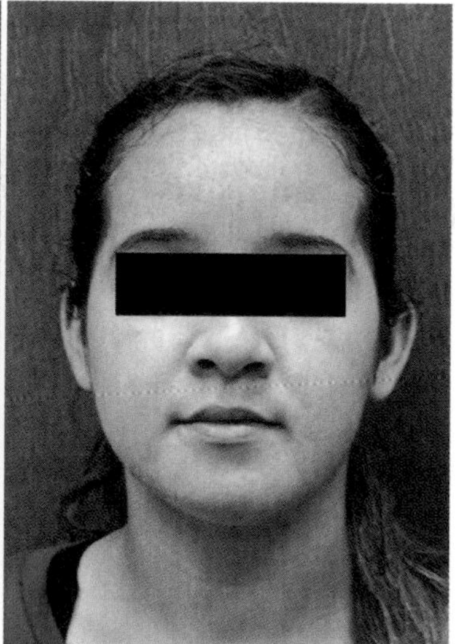

Acne before and after prescription acne medications.

Topical Antibiotics and Antibacterials

Topical antibiotics are commonly used to treat acne because we want to decrease the bacterial count on the skin, since we know that increased bacteria leads to papules and pustules. We commonly prescribe topical clindamycin, topical erythromycin, and sodium sulfacetamide.

Topical dapsone is also a prescription antibacterial. It is well tolerated especially in those with adult acne who tend to be less oily and therefore more sensitive to drying acne medications. One thing to note is that if it is used along with benzoyl peroxide, it can lead to a temporary yellow-orange staining to the skin and hair.

Oral Antibiotics

If you have more moderate acne, dermatologists usually consider starting you on a prescription oral antibiotic. Oral antibiotics treat moderate to severe acne with the one-two punch of reducing inflammation and slowing down the growth of bacteria.[13] The oral antibiotics we prescribe are those that can be effective against *P. acnes*, which is the main bacteria that causes all the problems in acne. Common oral antibiotics include tetracyclines like doxycycline and minocycline. We also will prescribe penicillins, erythromycins, and trimethoprim-sulfamethoxazole (what many of us know as Bactrim).

Side effects differ according to the antibiotic you have been prescribed. These drugs can cause allergic reactions (especially sulfa), gastrointestinal irregularities, dizziness, and increased sensitivity to the sun. A side effect of doxycycline, for example, is esophagitis (irritation of the esophagus that causes trouble when swallowing) and an increased propensity to sunburn. Pregnant women and children should not use tetracycline because it might affect tooth and bone formation in fetuses and young children. Tetracycline and minocycline might weaken the effect of birth control pills. If you don't want to get pregnant, it might be wise to use a second form of contraception when taking these two antibiotics. Some antibiotics can make you more prone to yeast infections. And somtimes none of these medications work because the bacteria on your skin are already resistant to the antibiotic.

Another long-standing issue is that many people don't like the idea of taking an antibiotic for months on end. There are certainly some side effects from long-term use of antibiotics, although the long-term use of tetracycline antibiotics for acne does not weaken the immune system, or induce bacterial resistance, as previously thought. Before you take any medication, seek answers to any questions you may have about your condition or the medication provided. Always be sure to take the medication precisely as directed.

Oral Contraceptives

Using oral contraceptives, aka birth control pills, is an effective way to treat acne in women. The FDA has approved three low-dose-estrogen oral contraceptives that are equally successful: Estrostep Fe, Ortho Tri-Cyclen, and Yaz. They work by balancing the male and female hormones in the body that are responsible for creating acne. The pills contain the female hormones estrogen and progestin (synthetic progesterone), whose presence re-creates harmony in the skin by lowering the amount of sebum-producing male androgens. As we know, the increase in sebum production results in the formation of comedones, the primary lesions of acne, and promotes the growth of bacteria.[14] In other words, the female hormones are a calming force, while the male hormones swoop in and muck it all up. Sound familiar?

Many times, doctors prescribe topical medications or antibiotics along with oral contraceptives for best results in clearing the skin. Be prepared for a couple of surprises. In the beginning of your course of treatment, you might experience some breakouts. In addition, it can take a few months for your acne to clear up. If you are prescribed an oral contraceptive, you should definitely be seeing your gynecologist regularly to monitor you on this medication.

Today's birth control pills have lower medical risks because they contain lower doses of estrogen and progesterone than in the past. That doesn't mean that oral contraceptives are without risks, however. In fact, some are quite substantial: heart attack, stroke, dangerous blood clots in the legs or lungs, liver and gallbladder diseases, migraine headaches, depression, and mood swings.[15] Given the side effects of birth control pills, they should be used to treat acne only if other therapies don't work. These pills are prescribed for acne sufferers who are otherwise healthy and in need of contraception.

Spironolactone

If I see a female patient who complains of acne breakouts that are mainly located along the jawline and on the chin, I immediately pay attention to the timber of her voice. Does this sound a little on the low side? This may sound like a strange thing to do, but what I'm doing is looking for other signs that she may have an increased level of testosterone in her system. I may ask, Do you have irregular periods? Do you notice more hair growth in the beard area (this can happen to us women and is normal, especially in ethnicities with a lot of hair growth, but here I'm asking if they have noticed new hair growth in this area specifically)?

The reason I ask all these questions is because there is a condition called polycystic ovarian syndrome (PCOS), in which women's ovaries grow cysts that secrete testosterone. Now, all of us women have a certain low level of testosterone and this is normal. People who have PCOS, however, can have elevated levels of testosterone and this testosterone triggers acne breakouts in this specific configuration. Spironolactone changes how your skin reacts to male hormones by blocking androgen receptors. This treatment is effective for resistant acne. Side effects include issues surrounding menstruation, breast tenderness, and increased potassium levels in the bloodstream.

Oral Retinoids: Isotretinoin

For very serious acne, your dermatologist might prescribe isotretinoin, an oral medication used primarily to treat severe cystic acne. The original brand name, Accutane, was discontinued; there are now several generic versions and brand names, including Claravis, Amnesteem, Absorica, Myorisan, Zenatane, and Sotret.[16] While this medication is highly controversial for its possible side effects, it is also the only medication that is thought to actually heal acne after five months of treatment. Patients need to be followed closely and the treatment can be complicated, but for acne sufferers who have tried everything else, this pill is everything.

Isotretinoin is a retinoid that comes in pill form. It works by markedly decreasing the production of facial oil (sebum) that leads to severe acne and permanent scarring.[17] By extension, bacteria growth diminishes. A normal course of treatment is four to six months, at a recommended dose of 0.5 milligrams to 2 milligrams per day. An impressive 85 percent of acne patients see long-lasting improvement in that time, along with fewer relapses.

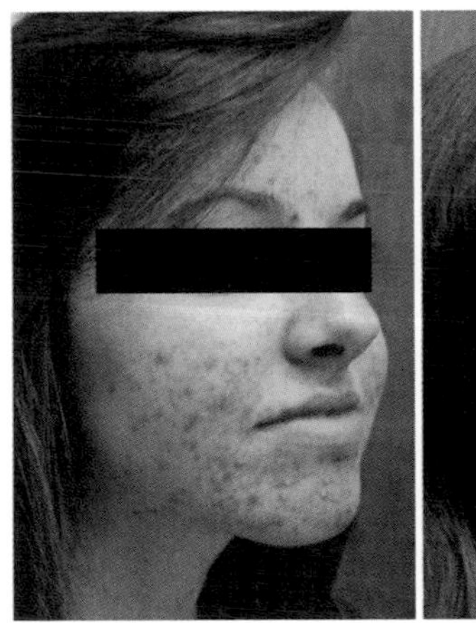
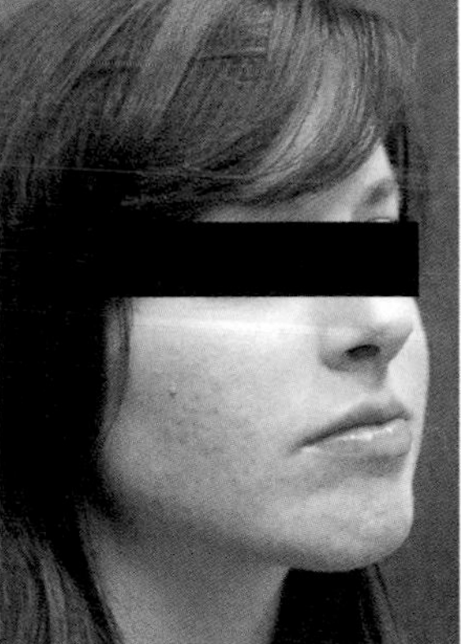

Before and after isotretinoin treatment.

Generally speaking, isotretinoin is considered safe, with a thirty-five-year history of treating millions of sufferers who have experienced fairly mild side effects (facial

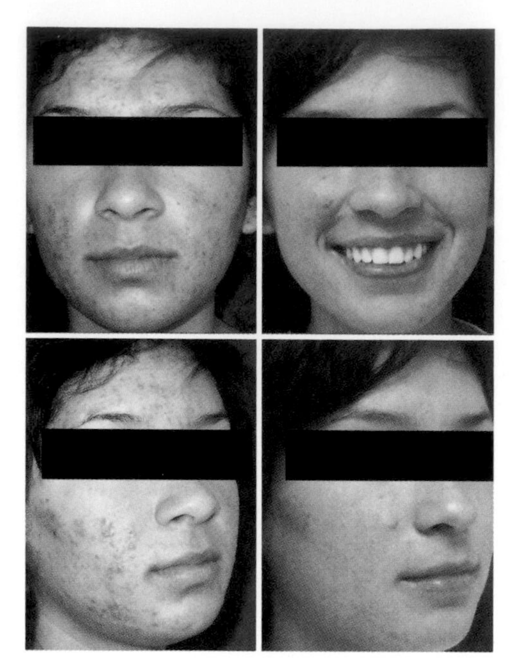

Before (left) and after (right) isotretinoin treatment.

dryness, joint and back pain, itching, rash, and dizziness).[18] Fasting blood tests are monitored monthly to check liver function and triglycerides (substances related to cholesterol), which often rise a bit during treatment but rarely to the point at which treatment has to be modified or stopped.

More worrisome is the high risk isotretinoin has of birth defects if taken by pregnant women. If you're of childbearing age, you need to have two negative pregnancy tests (blood or urine) before starting the drug, monthly tests while on the medication, and another pregnancy test once you're done. Moreover, if you are sexually active, you have to use two forms of contraception, including a birth control pill. This side effect is deemed so serious that experts have created a unique distribution program required to gain a prescription. The patient, prescribing medical professional, dispensing pharmacy, and wholesalers must work together in an online program called iPLEDGE. All parties must meet all requirements to be registered and activated with the iPLEDGE program in order to prescribe isotretinoin.

Other exceedingly rare side effects include inflammatory bowel disease, depression, and suicide. Even though it is unlikely that the medication would lead to these problems, any changes in your bowel function or mood during a course of treatment should be reported to your doctor.

Let me just end this by saying that the decision to use a medication like isotretinoin should definitely be carefully considered if you have severe acne and a real risk for permanent scarring. If I personally needed isotretinoin to clear up my acne, or if one of my sons or my best friend needed isotretinoin, I would have no hesitation prescribing it if there are no contraindications. It does something that no other medication can do. It can potentially completely clear severe acne. It's an amazing medication and it gets a bad rap. Let me put it to you this way: if you took away my ability to prescribe isotretinoin for those who could really benefit from it, I would seriously consider no longer seeing acne patients because there would be no great treatment option for those with severe acne. It would be a terrible loss for acne sufferers.

Cortisone Injections

A cortisone injection/shot, also called a steroid injection/shot or a cyst injection, is a quick and effective way to reduce inflammation and promote healing of active inflamed pimples and severe acne types, including nodules and cysts. This is an ideal treatment if you have a few big pimples, those that you know are starting to come up, are red and pretty painful to the touch, and will likely get a little worse before they resolve. An injection of a very low potency corticosteroid directly into the pimple will likely calm it down, and often the bump will resolve within twenty-four hours. This is certainly what I do to myself when I have a Mount Vesuvius–type pimple that rears its ugly mug on my nose or chin, which happens every now and then. You will need to see a health care provider to get this type of treatment.

PROCEDURES THAT TREAT ACNE

There are acne treatment procedures your dermatologist can offer during an office visit, including:

- LASERS AND LIGHT THERAPIES: These procedures reduce the *P. acnes* bacteria.
- CHEMICAL PEELS: Chemical peels containing glycolic or salicylic acid, Jessner's peel, and others are used to exfoliate the superficial layer of skin, helping to clear out debris from within pores, preventing new blackheads and removing existing ones.

Heat-Based Acne Therapies

You may have seen these devices sold in the cosmetics section of fancy department stores. Sold under brands such as Tria, Tanda Zap, and No! No! Skin, they use the localized application of heat upon an active pimple to make the environment unpleasant and unlivable for the bacteria that cause these pimples. These devices are okay, but certainly won't work for comedones and deep-seated cysts and nodules; maybe it will decrease the duration of an active red pimple by a day or so.

NATURAL INGREDIENTS TO TREAT MILD ACNE

Increasingly, natural products to fight acne are turning up on store shelves. By *natural,* I mean any component derived from a plant, animal, mineral, or microbial source that is found in nature or produced using minimal physical processing. But do these remedies work? Yes and no. Several natural remedies can reduce inflammation and block breakouts, but they aren't as effective as other OTC ingredients produced synthetically or by more complex chemical processes. Below is a discussion of natural acne treatments, for completeness's sake and because I know many people appreciate a "natural" alternative, so here you go!

Tea Tree Oil

Tea tree oil can kill bacteria associated with acne. However, these antibacterial properties take longer to work on acne than benzoyl peroxide does. A study of 124 patients compared 5 percent tea tree oil in a water-based gel with 5 percent benzoyl peroxide.[19] Although the tea tree oil did not act as rapidly as benzoyl peroxide, it did show statistical improvement in the number of acne lesions at the end of three months, and there was a significantly lower incidence of adverse effects such as dryness, irritation, itching, and burning with tea tree oil (44 percent) than with benzoyl peroxide (79 percent). However, tea tree oil can cause contact dermatitis and a worsening of rosacea symptoms.

Zinc

Zinc has both antibacterial and anti-inflammatory properties and it can decrease the production of sebum.[20] Zinc in topical treatments such as creams and lotions may reduce acne breakouts.

Green Tea Extract

Green tea has been used for thousands of years for a variety of skin conditions, including adult acne. It is known widely to decrease inflammation and redness of pimples. According to the Mayo Clinic, a lotion of 2 percent green tea extract helped reduce acne in two studies of adolescents and young adults with mild to moderate acne.[21]

POPULAR MECHANICAL DEVICES TO FIGHT ACNE

Used together with over-the-counter products (and prescription medications too), mechanical acne treatments such as brushes, scrubs, and cleansing cloths can be effective tools for cleaning and exfoliating dead skin cells. Ask your health professional to help you choose the best device for your type of acne. The American Academy of Dermatology explains what these devices are and how they work.

Brushes

Brushes are handheld devices that use an oscillating motion to remove makeup and dead skin cells, deeply cleansing the skin. There really aren't any studies or proof that these motorized brushes can help fight acne. People who swear by these feel they are getting their delicate skin really super clean without damaging it. However, if a motorized brush makes your skin rough and red, it may be doing more harm than good.

Scrubs

Scrubs can contain many types of abrasive particles, such as polyethylene beads (although these have been banned in many countries), aluminum oxide, or ground fruit pits. These may help exfoliate the skin and remove dead skin cells that clog pores. However, using scrubs may cause your skin to become irritated or inflamed. If that happens, try products with smooth synthetic beads (such as polyethylene beads) that are not as rough. Warning: don't overuse scrubs and stop if you develop milia.

Cleansing Cloths

Cleansing cloths provide quick exfoliation in a nonabrasive cleansing form. There are two types of cloths: the first lathers with water and requires rinsing the skin after use, and the second is a premoistened cloth that does not require rinsing after use. These are convenient ways to remove oil and dirt from your face, especially after a workout, so in that way they are useful.

ACNE SCARS

According to the American Society for Dermatologic Surgery (ASDS), acne scars are usually the result of inflamed blemishes caused by skin pores becoming engorged with excess oil, dead skin cells, and bacteria. The pore swells, causing a break in the follicle wall. Shallow lesions are usually minor and heal quickly without forming scars. A deep break in the wall of the pore can allow surrounding tissue to become infected, which leads to deeper lesions. The skin attempts to repair these lesions by forming new collagen fibers, which are not as smooth as the original skin.[22]

Inflammation—particularly the severity and depth of this inflammation—is the key culprit in the development of acne scars. Someone with inflammatory acne, such as nodules and cysts, is more likely to develop acne scars. Also, picking, popping, and squeezing acne increases the inflammation and absolutely raises the risk of scarring.[23]

Acne scars are classified by their appearance. It's useful to be able to recognize and identify them because the type of acne scars you have dictates the treatments that may work for you. This section doesn't include a discussion of hypertrophic scars and keloids, since those scars can occur after any kind of trauma to the skin, not just acne. The types of acne scars are:

- Anetoderma
- Boxcar scars
- Ice-pick scars
- Rolling scars

ANETODERMA (atrophic scars) are really thin. Thinner than your regular skin, so thin that if they are wide enough sometimes you can see the blood vessels underneath the scar. It's common for there to be a loss of pigment in the area, so these types of scars can be lighter than your skin color. The scar appears de-

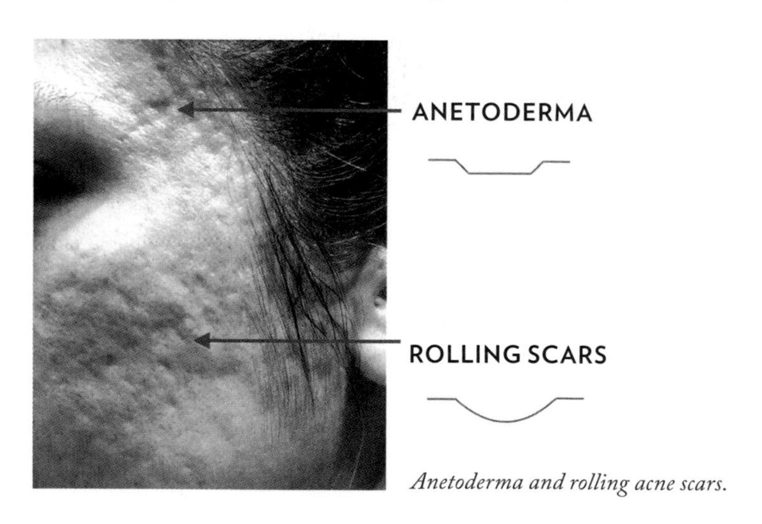

Anetoderma and rolling acne scars.

pressed (at a lower depth compared with surrounding skin) because the skin is noticeably thinner in the area. Anetoderma develop because acne and inflammation has led to a loss of collagen or tissue.

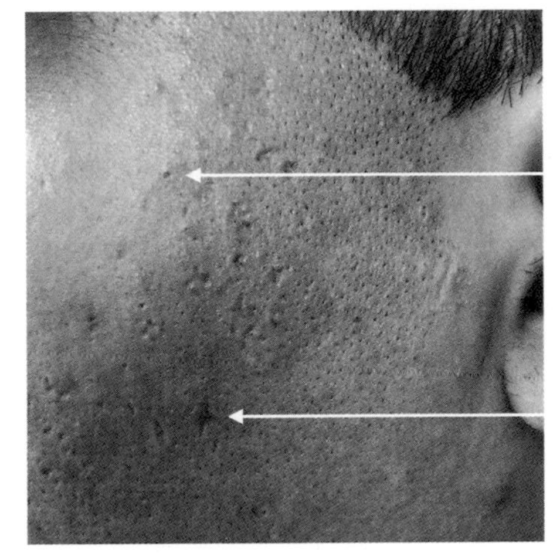

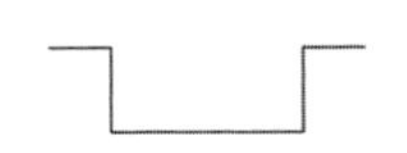

Ice pick and boxcar acne scars.

BOXCAR SCARS are broader scars whose edges slant up abruptly and steeply.

ICE PICK SCARS look like their name. Sharp, deep scars, they are also called pitted scars because they appear to come to a point deep under the skin.

ROLLING SCARS are like rolling hills in that the edges of the scar are more sloping as opposed to sharp and abrupt. These are best seen when light is shining from the side because rolling scars cast shadows across the skin, making it look very irregular and bumpy.

Treating acne scars is frustrating. No single treatment option effectively improves all types of acne scars and multiple treatments are often needed. Not every skin type and skin color will respond similarly to treatment, and some skin tones have a higher risk of side effects from certain treatments. I'll try to explain everything as well as I can here, but please schedule a personalized consultation with your cosmetic/laser dermatologist to see what treatment options are best for you. Remember too that new technologies come out all the time—some promising results that they simply cannot deliver.

The existence of acne scars is really the reason I feel so strongly that active acne, especially moderate to severe acne, should be treated! Some people think that it's unimportant to treat acne; after all, it's not life threatening, and many of us outgrow it eventually. As a dermatologist, I have seen many adults who no longer have acne but are still haunted by their acne scars because these are daily reminders of the way they felt when they suffered from terrible acne breakouts.

It's amazing to me how deeply it can affect people. I think it's similar to the emotions that surface after people lose a significant amount of weight—they say that they still feel like the "fat person" that they were, and they easily conjure the associated emotions of embarrassment and shame. You may not always have bad acne, but you will always remember how that acne made you feel, and your acne scars are a reminder of that terrible feeling.

I wish I had a magic wand to wave over some of my patients and—*poof!*—no more scars. But it's a long road with many treatments, some with downtime, and we're not even talking about the expense! And after all that time and money is spent, your acne scars may be only 50 percent improved. So, all this ranting by me is ultimately to make one statement: treat your acne when you have it because it's much harder to erase the emotional and physical reminders later in life.

TREATMENTS FOR ACNE SCARS

Anetoderma and rolling acne scars are probably the "easiest" to improve, with the least downtime and least up-front expense and risks. With these types of scars, a slight distension of the skin—heck, even pulling your skin up and back like you're simulating a facelift—will show an improvement. Ice pick and boxcar acne scars are more difficult to treat. You won't see these scars improve much when you stretch the skin. Fillers won't work, and facelifts don't improve much either. Instead, we try treatment options that "sand down the skin," or release the scar beneath the skin, as discussed here. And skin type and shade play a more important role here. I'll explain why after I tell you about the treatment options. Risks and benefits vary and should be discussed with your physician.

Dermabrasion

Dermabrasion lessens the appearance of scars by surgically sanding down the outer layer of skin where scars are present. There are some risks attached to dermabrasion, including further scarring, temporary redness and swelling, potential permanent loss of skin color and tissue damage, and infection, which can be treated with the appropriate antibiotic.

Excision and Punch Replacement Grafts

Your doctor surgically excises or uses a punch tool to surgically excise an acne scar and then closes the wound with stitches. Patients with deep icepick acne scarring are good candidates for excision and punch replacement grafting. These treatments can sometimes be combined with laser resurfacing. They can leave behind small, light scars.

For people who have large icepick scars, punch replacement grafting is a good solution. Sometimes laser resurfacing is used in conjunction with the technique to achieve a normal and "seamless" appearance where the scar once was.

Soft-Tissue Fillers

Fillers, including brand names such as Juvéderm, Radiesse, Belotero, Restylane, or Sculptra, are injected directly into or under acne scars with a very small needle to stretch and plump the skin in the area to minimize scars and also attempt to break up scar tissue and adhesions that could be pulling the skin.

Laser/Light Therapy

Laser/light therapy involves the use of an intense but gentle beam of light to minimize scar damage and destroy bacteria that causes acne.

CO_2 Laser Resurfacing

Ablative laser resurfacing uses a wandlike laser in a controlled way in an attempt to smooth the irregularities in the skin created by acne scars. At the same time that it's removing the top layer of skin, it's also heating it. This promotes collagen production.

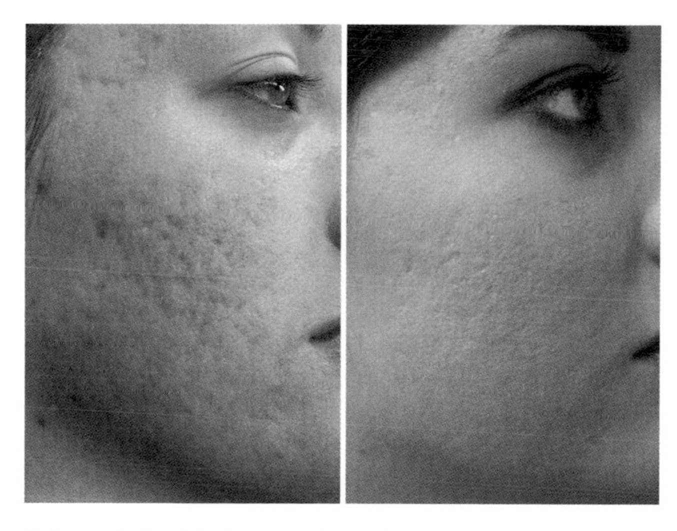

Before and after CO_2 laser resurfacing for acne scars.

Chapter 4

Time Won't Tell

YOU KNOW, WHEN WE ARE YOUNG, ADULTS GIVE US ADVICE (OR TRY, ANY-way) or share information, and we interpret it one way. But as we age, we begin to interpret those words of wisdom differently. Those of you in my age group (forties) and older understand. Those of you who are younger will find out soon enough. And I'm certainly not saying this because I'm a know-it-all. I cringe when I look back on my sixteen-year-old self, who had given my parents a run for their money, with nights of worry, and had told my dad, "You're not the boss of me!"

As a sixteen-year-old, I doubt I would have listened to this forty-five-plus-years-old self giving out advice about aging. But here goes, because I *know* I have young fans who are more mature than I was at their age and who may wonder what they can do now to help the aging process. In this era of social media pressure and technology that allows us to look perfect—no blemishes, no scars, straight teeth—you may think you are in trouble because your skin isn't flawless. Trust me, everyone's hiding something, showing themselves only in the best light possible. It is confusing and intimidating, and freakin' expensive to decide what to do about our skin.

But today we have more insight than ever for how to guide skin back to a more youthful appearance or at least slow down the ticking of the clock! Despite the infinite number of new anti-aging potions, lotions, serums, creams, and so on vying for our attention, true chemical advancements in the anti-aging field are relatively few. Basic, tried-and-true skincare strategies have worked to fight aging for decades. No one talks about this truth. Businesses capitalize on our desire to stay young. The skincare industry, especially anti-aging, is a worldwide multibillion-dollar industry. It's expected to total $191.7 billion in 2019 with an ever-rising ceiling. Changing basic lifestyle habits and amping up protective measures and education, however, *can* upend the effects of aging that unhealthy indulgences may have planted on our skin. We can reliably turn to these in our quest to have younger skin and achieve greater health.

In this chapter, I explain what we know so far about what happens to our body when we age, and what factors speed up this process the most. I mainly focus on the face, since this is how we present ourselves to the world. When I held my firstborn boy as a baby, cheek to cheek, and peered at us in the mirror, I was shocked to see how different my skin looked from his close up.

We divide the causes of aging into two broad categories: intrinsic (internal factors) and extrinsic (external factors). Intrinsic aging refers to the natural, internal process that occurs regardless of outside factors. Our genes largely control when intrinsic aging begins, but we can slow its progressing. Extrinsic or external agers are caused by environmental factors and habits including how much sun we get, whether or not we smoke, our exposure to air and other kinds of pollution, how many Zs we catch, our eating habits, and exercise.

INTRINSIC AGERS

As we age, new bone formation slows, and bone resorption is increased. The facial bones in general become less prominent, more flattened, which is probably most obvious in our cheekbones and around our eyes. Tooth loss also leads to a more sunken facial appearance. Depressing, isn't it?

Many of the wrinkles we develop on our face are due to repeated movements of our facial muscles, the muscles that make our expressions. Smiling so many times in our lifetimes and creating those crow's-feet creases repeatedly on the sides of our eyes eventually can cause those lines to stay there even when we are not smiling! Frowning creates permanent "11s" between our eyebrows, and raising our eyebrows in excitement and amazement can etch horizontal lines across our forehead.

Our skin and hair changes with age. There's a loss in elasticity and increased dryness and thinning of the skin, and brown spots appear, along with, of course, the dreaded wrinkles. I'm reminded this is happening when I wake up and have sleep lines from my pillow on my cheek, and an hour later, I *still* have those sleep lines! Intrinsic hair loss is happening too; no one's hair thickens as we age, although we do tend to get more errant hairs in areas we never had them before, like the chin, the nose, and the ears.

Gravity. I include the force of gravity as an intrinsic ager even though it's not really internal. However, it can't be avoided unless you get that ticket to live on Mars or the moon, or you spend most of your life standing on your head.

EXTRINSIC AGERS

Extrinsic agers are external, potentially more controllable factors such as our diet, how much we expose our skin to the sun, our lifestyle, whether we smoke or not, how much sleep we get, and how stressed we are on a daily or consistent basis. In general, our face appears as an upside-down triangle in youth, and as we age, the triangle inverts.

Extrinsic aging factors cause a thickening of the cornified layer of the skin, precancerous changes such as lesions called actinic keratoses, skin cancer (including basal cell carcinoma, squamous cell carcinoma, and melanoma), freckle and sun spot formation, and loss of collagen, elastin, and glycosaminoglycans. This results in skin that is rough, uneven, spotty, and wrinkled.

THE FOUR MAIN CULPRITS OF AGING SKIN

FREE RADICALS

Free radicals are electronically unstable and reactive molecules that intensify aging by damaging cells.[1] They are created as by-products of the normal burning of fuel that occurs in every cell. Your skin is also especially vulnerable to free radical damage from external sources such as ultraviolet light from the sun and the accumulation of pollutants, especially if you live in a big city. Stress and habits such as smoking and tanning (either from the sun or lying on a tanning bed) contribute to free radicals.

GLYCATION

Glycation leads to premature aging, along with a number of diseases. The process occurs on a cellular level when excess sugar molecules in our body bond with protein molecules. The new molecules are called advanced glycation end products (aka the extremely not-funny acronym AGEs).[2] AGEs are harmful compounds that create oxidative stress, which damages tissues.

AGEs prematurely age the body and wreak havoc on our health. The cross-linking chemical reaction causes permanent damage to the function and structure of the protein molecules, the majority of which are healthy collagen. Sugar consumes healthy collagen fibers and elastin, weakening them and reducing their elasticity, causing skin to look dull and dehydrated. Skin damage begins to accelerate, leading to wrinkles, deep lines, sagging skin, and loss of volume in the face. Combined with sun exposure, AGEs also cause sun spots; hyperpigmentation; dull, hard, uneven skin; inflammation; and tumors. AGEs make our skin more vulnerable to UV light and cigarette smoke.[3] That's another reason staying out of the sun as we age is the smart move. While compromised skin is a visible sign of AGEs' damage, it's also responsible for "invisible diseases" including heart disease, cancer, diabetes, and even Alzheimer's disease.

ULTRAVIOLET RADIATION

Too much sun exposure is a big deal—in case you haven't noticed by now, soaking up the sun for extended periods of time without protection is one of my pet peeves. It causes up to 90 percent of skin cancer. It's no accident that the major focus of the anti-aging skincare industry is to create products meant to counteract the sun's negative effects on the skin. We all know that the sun causes many of the visible signs of aging, but how, exactly?

Skin is made up of three layers: the epidermis (top layer), the dermis (middle layer), and the subcutis (bottom layer). Skin maintains a smooth, youthful appearance with help from the dermis. The dermis contains collagen, elastin, and fibers. Ultraviolet radiation (UV) damages these elements.

UV radiation is composed of two types of waves: UVA and UVB. UVB rays are the main culprit behind sunburn. But UVA rays cause the damage we associate with photoaging (wrinkles and spots). UVA rays penetrate deep enough to damage collagen fibers by forming high amounts of elastin and metalloproteinase production. Collagen malfunctions and decomposes, resulting in incorrectly rebuilt skin and wrinkles. This damage repeats with daily UVA exposure.

Repeated sun exposure can also cause brown spots, "wisdom" spots, or liver spots—small bits of pigmentation commonly found on places most often exposed to the sun such as the hands, arms, face, and chest.

According to the Skin Cancer Foundation, the best way to combat photoaging is through the proactive application of sunscreen to these and other areas exposed to the sun.[4] It may even help reverse existing damage, and it lowers your risk of developing skin cancers and precancers.

INFLAMMATION

Inflammation occurs when things like UV radiation, irritants (which can be anything from organic matter like certain kinds of plants to laundry detergent or perfume), or allergens attack a skin cell. The cells in turn become inflamed and produce cytokines and chemokines, hormones that bind to receptors on cells to produce more inflammatory signaling hormones. This can cause vasodilation, or nerve cell activation, which causes immune cells to migrate into the skin, where they produce *more* inflammatory hormones, as well as enzymes, free radicals, and chemicals that damage the skin. The result is the amplification of a large inflammatory response that can cause considerable damage to the skin.[5]

Inflammation can build up over time and result in numerous health issues. It can cause red, swollen skin, acne breakouts, rosacea, and even skin scarring, which can be costly and difficult to remove. It speeds up the aging process by inhibiting collagen production. Chronic inflammation can even lead to heart disease.

TIME-TESTED STRATEGIES TO COUNTER AGING

USE BROAD-SPECTRUM SUNSCREEN WITH SPF30 OR HIGHER

Wearing sunscreen is a must-do. I recommend choosing a broad-spectrum formula. Find one with zinc or titanium oxide! These are inert minerals that sit on top of the skin to block both UVA and UVB rays. Tip: zinc is a beneficial ingredient in makeup products as well. Micronized zinc has microscopic particles that reflect light (whereas sunscreen simply absorbs it).

In addition to wearing sunscreen, avoid sun-related aging by limiting the time you're exposed to its rays, which happen to be at their strongest between ten in the morning and four in the afternoon. When you're going to be outside, wear clothing that covers your skin. Many new clothing products are designed to cover you up and provide UV protection, but still keep you cool even in the heat of summer. Don't forget your broad-brimmed hat and UV-blocking sunglasses.

Acne, Sunscreen, and SPF

If you have oily skin and pimples, I tend to switch up my advice when it comes to sunscreen. Physical UV blockers like zinc and titanium dioxide are not as ideal for people with acne, because they tend to be thicker on the skin and cause acne breakouts. In the case of pimples, I recommend a lighter SPF but at least an SPF of 15. I also prefer chemical sunscreen ingredients like avobenzone and oxybenzone, because these ingredients don't give your skin a white hue like physical sunscreen blockers do. As a result, they sit better under our makeup, and most important, are less likely to promote more pimples.

GET CONSISTENTLY GOOD SLEEP

While we've long known that chronic sleep deprivation has been linked to obesity, diabetes, heart disease, and cancer, we now have scientific data detailing how lack of sleep causes our skin to age. Our skin is a critical barrier from external stressors such as pollution and UV radiation. A good night's sleep helps to renew our immune and physiological systems, and as a result, it can have a dramatic effect on how our skin looks, for better or worse.

Over time, insomnia, fitful sleeping, or just a chronic lack of sleep can give you wrinkles and make you look older. A landmark study conducted in 2013 at the Skin Study Center at University Hospitals Cleveland Medical Center found big differences in the skin between good- and poor-quality sleepers. It demonstrated that inadequate sleep accelerates skin aging.[6] The appearance of the poor-quality sleepers was determined to have aged twice as much as that of the good-quality sleepers. The researchers looked at increased signs of skin aging such as fine lines, uneven pigmentation, and slackening of skin/reduced elasticity.

Good-quality sleepers' skin recovered more successfully from stressors like sunburn, while recovery from a sunburn took longer in poor-quality sleepers. Something called a periodic transepidermal water loss (TEWL) test determined how effectively the skin served as a barrier against the loss of moisture. Good-quality sleepers recovered at a 30 percent higher rate than poor-quality sleepers, repairing damage more quickly.[7]

Self-esteem is affected too: the study found that poor-quality sleepers also had a worse assessment of their own skin and facial appearance. Good-quality sleepers rated themselves higher in attractiveness versus poor-quality sleepers.

This research paints a clear picture of the need for good-quality sleep on a nightly basis. Sleep quality is a powerful and determining factor in how we look and how we feel about ourselves. It is vital to the constant renewing of the fragile place where the skin meets the mind. The Sleep Foundation offers "Healthy Sleep Tips" that recommend how many hours a night we should be sleeping, along with healthy sleep habits. For more information, visit sleepfoundation.org.

TREAT THE SKIN AROUND YOUR EYES WITH TLC, BUT NOT WITH MORE MONEY!

While some face creams can irritate the delicate area around the eyes, honestly, in my opinion, special eye creams are a money-grab and just another way for cosmetic companies to convince you to buy more products. Yes, the skin around the eyes *is* the thinnest skin on our body, and yes, that skin can be more sensitive. However, I believe a good all-purpose facial moisturizer can be used safely and effectively around the eyes even if it's not marketed specifically for that purpose.

AVOID SMOKING

Truthfully, only one foolproof method can counter the negative effects of smoking—quitting if you smoke now, and not starting if you don't! More than anything else, I can often tell if someone is a chronic smoker just by looking at their skin. This is a big one. Smoking most definitely causes wrinkles!

How does smoking lead to wrinkles? According to the Mayo Clinic, the nicotine in cigarettes narrows blood vessels in the outermost layers of your skin, which impairs blood flow to your skin. Less blood flow means less oxygen and important nutrients for your skin. Moreover, many of the more than four thousand chemicals in tobacco smoke damage collagen and elastin, the fibers that give your skin its youthful appearance, strength, and elasticity. That means more sagging and wrinkling.[8] The heat from smoking and the motions of squinting your eyes and pursing your lips when you take a drag all conspire to add even more wrinkles to your face.

Finally, a single puff of cigarette smoke emits forty thousand free radicals, those unstable molecules that contribute to aging and disease. Studies show there are two types present in cigarette smoke, both of which deplete the body of vitamin C. Free radicals are also prevalent in the form of pollution, which occurs when molecules undergo a photodissociation process. Imagine the magnified synergistic consequences from one incident of smoking outside with pursed lips, in sun, traffic smog, or pollution!

REDUCE STRESS

Ha! Good luck avoiding stress; it's part of life. If you have ever wondered if stress makes one look older, try comparing photos taken of American presidents before their term begins and after they leave office. Every time. Am I right? And problems with stress aren't limited to those in power or high office. Between August 2016 and January 2017, Americans' overall stress level increased for the first time in ten years, according to a new study from the American Psychological Association.[9]

Chronic stress can change the regulation of hormones and chemicals in your body in a way that reduces immunity, leaving the body open to viruses. This can lead to cell damage—along with dull skin, stress lines, and other tissue damage. A recent study at Duke University Medical Center found that chronic stress ultimately led to DNA damage that ranged from aging of skin and hair to proliferation of diseases and malignancies.[10]

A small scientific study published in *The Lancet Oncology* showed that people who adopted stress modification techniques along with changes in diet and exercise could reverse the aging process at a cellular level.[11] Taking up yoga, meditating, and spending more time with family and friends are some of the best (and easiest!) ways to counter stress. We think, feel, and look better as a result within days. Changes from steady measures could be seen within twelve weeks.

HOW TO CHOOSE THE BEST ANTI-AGING SKINCARE PRODUCTS

With shimmering new anti-aging products entering the skincare market all the time, how do we know which ones are worthwhile? Effortlessly hip magazine editors report on the otherworldly qualities of ingredients with a hushed reverence usually reserved for the pope. You will be deeply curious about this magical potion, maybe even swayed. *The bottle is so pretty!* But don't jump on that bandwagon. Sit back and see what happens. Let other people be the guinea pigs.

START WITH SUNSCREEN AND MOISTURIZER: Sunscreen and moisturizer are the two most effective anti-aging products you can buy. You will notice a positive difference in your skin if you use both these products every day. You'll also be protecting it from further damage. Buy sunscreens that are broad spectrum (meaning that they protect against both UVA and UVB damage), SPF 30 (or higher), and water resistant, which helps cut down on reapplication throughout the day (although reapplication on exposed skin every two hours is still a good idea). Using a moisturizer with sunscreen is fine and it does double duty as long as it meets the criteria described here.

TREAT YOUR NUMBER ONE AGING-SKIN CONCERN: It could take a few weeks before you notice a difference in your skin with consistent sunscreen and moisturizer use. I also believe you get the best results when you use products to treat unique issues, like wrinkles or dark spots. Despite claims, no product can treat all signs of skin aging equally. That is, it's best to choose one product to treat wrinkles, and a different one to treat dark spots.

BUY PRODUCTS FORMULATED FOR YOUR SKIN TYPE: There is no one-size-fits-all skin product—so read labels and choose a product that meets the needs of your skin, whether it's oily, dry, sensitive, or combination.

READ PRODUCT LABELS AND SELECT A PRODUCT THAT OFFERS ALL OF THE FOLLOWING: Along with selecting a product that's right for your skin type, make sure the label also says the product is hypoallergenic to reduce the chance of an allergic reaction, and noncomedogenic or nonacnegenic to prevent acne.

AVOID THE FOLLOWING INGREDIENTS ON PRODUCT LABELS: Common irritants like alcohol and sodium lauryl sulfate. These can cause breakouts and are bad for your skin.

CHECK THE ORDER OF INGREDIENTS: The higher on a list an ingredient appears, the stronger its formulation. If the ingredient you seek is closer to the bottom, the product may not contain a potent amount or provide the effect you seek.

HAVE REALISTIC EXPECTATIONS: Be skeptical about dramatic claims like "look ten years younger in ten minutes." Anti-aging products can produce results, but they are much more modest and happen over time, sometimes weeks or months. Of course, if a product is $10 or $100 and you *truly enjoy* using it, it makes you feel good, and it's not doing any harm, use it—just know that you may not be getting a real medical benefit, but a psychological one (with maybe a little medical benefit).

BUY WHAT YOU CAN AFFORD: It simply isn't true that efficacy increases with the cost of a product. Beneficial and effective anti-aging products come at every price point.

THE BEST ANTI-AGING SKINCARE INGREDIENTS

No topical cream will do anything truly amazing for your skin, but here are the basic anti-aging ingredients that do have *some* proven benefits. This guide shows you the major categories of skincare ingredients, how they work, and if you're a good candidate to benefit from using them. My goal is to help you to be a smart consumer, and to look beautiful along the way.

ANTIOXIDANTS

Antioxidants are widely used anti-aging ingredients that are safe for all types of skin. They minimize fine lines and wrinkles by slowing the effects free radicals have on the body. You need ample amounts of antioxidants for effective absorption into your skin. Apply this ingredient at night—many antioxidants work like sunscreen, destroying UV-funded free radicals before they damage the skin. That means a morning dose of the potent anti-ager won't get absorbed into your skin cells to do its main job.

On the two-for-one front, research shows enhanced benefits can be derived from combining different antioxidants or using one antioxidant with another anti-aging ingredient. For example, combining certain retinoids with certain botanical antioxidants, like resveratrol or cherry extract, works beyond anti-aging benefits to prevent the irritation seen from vitamin A creams.

The anti-inflammatory properties of antioxidants work well for those with sensitive skin and rosacea, and those who benefit from the ingredient's minimizing of redness and peeling. While all antioxidants yield powerful benefits, below are the most effective ingredients to look for and why.

Green Tea

The ancient plant from which green tea is brewed is filled with nutrients that recharge the skin. Solid research proves that tea—green, black, or white—has numerous anti-aging benefits. The key compound that provides its antioxidant effects is epigallocatechin-3 gallate (EGCG). Applied topically, green tea protects skin from harmful environmental factors and repairs the damage done by oxidation. It calms and soothes the skin, making it especially good for reddish, sensitive skin or to help counter breakouts. Green tea works well to minimize dark circles when combined with caffeine in eye cream. Look for green tea in moisturizers.

Resveratrol

Resveratrol is a newer antioxidant that is present in red grapes, red wines, nuts, and fruits such as blueberries and cranberries. Research shows that resveratrol is an efficient antioxidant that, when applied topically, helps protect and brighten the skin, break up free radicals, and calm the skin. It also stimulates collagen. You'll find resveratrol in creams and moisturizers. Have a glass of red wine to double the results!

Vitamin E

Vitamin E is the secret service of antioxidants. It works to protect and defend the skin from dangerous foreign elements in the environment. Many sunscreens include it for its talent for fighting off the effects of UV exposure. Vitamin E is available in natural and synthetic forms, both of which offer distinct antioxidant benefits to the skin, though it lasts longer and is more effective in its natural form. Its skin-protective qualities combine well with rejuvenating skin creams. Pure vitamin E oil is popular for cracked cuticles, wound healing, and minimizing scars that range from mild to surgical. Vitamin E works synergistically with vitamin C for enhanced benefits, so finding an anti-aging product that contains both is smart. Look for vitamin E in moisturizers, creams, and serums.

Vitamin C

Vitamin C (ascorbic acid, tetrahexyldecyl ascorbate, and others) is a well-researched, super-effective antioxidant that all skin types can use. It's particularly effective in diffusing the look of fine lines, dullness, and uneven skin tone. Vitamin C is effective in concentrations from 0.5 percent to 20 percent. You'll get the most out of this antioxidant as an ingredient in skin-brightening products, as it decreases pigment production and inflammation. By neutralizing free radicals, it may even help protect the skin from precancerous changes due to UV light exposure. Store your product properly, as light degrades this potent antioxidant.

Coenzyme Q10

Coenzyme Q10 (Q10, vitamin Q10) is a naturally occurring substance similar to a vitamin that exists in our cells. Cells use it to produce energy our body needs to live and grow. It provides anti-aging properties by protecting elastic tissue and collagen. As we age, our bodies produce less natural coenzyme Q10 levels, slowing the skin's ability to protect itself and recover from damage. For enhanced results, try taking a dietary supplement along with using topical creams. Bonus! Some studies show that coenzyme Q10 supplements aid in preventing heart disease as well.

RETINOL AND OTHER RETINOIDS

Over-the-counter retinols and prescription-only retinoids like tretinoin (Retin-A) have been tested and proven successful more than any other ingredient in the anti-aging skincare world. Derivatives of vitamin A, they are clinically proven to speed up and stimulate healthy cell turnover and collagen. They also hinder acne lesions from forming and can prevent pigmentation. It's smart to start using a retinoid while you're in your thirties, when collagen and elastin usually start to decline. The ingredient can be listed in three variations of its name: retinol, retinaldehyde, or retinoic acid. Inexpensive yet still potent OTC topical retinols give you numerous options in your quest for younger skin.

PEPTIDES

The beneficiary of much glowing clinical research, peptides are widely considered to be top-tier anti-aging skincare ingredients. Peptides are derivatives of short chains of amino acids, the building blocks of the protein collagen. They signal the skin to stimulate the production of collagen, which as we know is key for wrinkle-free, healthy skin. Some peptides excel at smoothing skin, while others minimize wrinkles, restore firmness, and soften the look of expression lines.

These little powerhouses can be synthesized in untold combinations, and research tells us that *all* peptides restore skin, though some are better than others. We also know more about how to bring out their best benefits. For example, the formulation must support the type of peptide used and products must be packaged to prevent degrading from light and air exposure. That means you won't want to buy a product in a see-through container, like a glass jar.

Researchers have shown that naturally occurring peptides have certain vulnerabilities. They can lose stability in water-based formulas. Further, enzymes in skin can render peptides ineffective. With these weaknesses in mind, chemists work to engineer synthetic peptides that are more stable and that protect collagen. These überpeptides can survive easily on skin or swoop into their target areas.

Despite product claims, research shows that peptides cannot plump lips, stop skin from sagging, work like cosmetic procedures, or counter dark circles or puffy eyes.

Pentapeptides (Matrixyl)

Pentapeptides combine a lipopeptide (fatty acid) with five amino acids. The most well-known is palmitoyl pentapeptide-3, trademarked under the name Matrixyl. It stimulates the lower layers of skin to release both collagen and hyaluronic acid. One widely touted study from 2013 showed that Matrixyl can almost double the amount of collagen that the cells in our body produce, provided the concentration is high enough. The study defines high-enough levels as "1.7x if used 80 parts per million concentrations."[12] It's doubtful that any skin products on the market include the ingredient at this high a concentration, but watch for it: these stats aren't bad.

Copper Peptides

Copper peptides have nothing to do with pennies, but are tiny fragments of proteins combined with copper in our skin cells that are essential for collagen formation. They help to rejuvenate skin and heal wounds. Clinical studies have shown that copper aids in reconstructing fractured collagen, making it a helpful ingredient particularly for skin damaged by sun or scars. Copper peptides also work well for sensitive skin.

One important caveat: copper is a toxic metal and can be used on the skin only in a form that contains peptides that bind with the metal.

Hexapeptides (Argireline)

Hexapeptides are chains of six amino acids. A certain hexapeptide linked with acetic acid called acetyl hexapeptide-3, or Argireline, is often marketed as a replacement for Botox, and studies show that this is one time the hype might be real. Within reason, of course! This impressive synthetic peptide is proven to reduce the degree of facial wrinkles and protect against their development. Early studies have also shown that this ingredient can promote collagen and improve skin structure.

The truly amazing advantage of this potent peptide? You don't have to inject poison into your skin to decrease and soften wrinkles. This noninvasive ingredient can be applied everywhere on the face with your fingers.

HYALURONIC ACID: LOW MOLECULAR WEIGHT HYALURONIC ACID AND SODIUM HYALURONATE

Hyaluronic acid (HA) is a naturally occurring ingredient that hydrates and plumps up the skin, especially the face. It attracts water to fill up the spaces between the connective fibers collagen and elastin in the dermis. Problem is, adults have only one-twentieth the amount of HA that a baby has. HA depletion results in dry, flaky skin, and more obvious fine lines and wrinkles.

That's when we turn to the numerous HA products on the skincare market, which include creams, serums, numerous injectables (Juvéderm, Restylane, to name two), and even hyaluronic acid supplements. HA is an equal opportunity acid, working dutifully for all types of skin—oily, sensitive, or just skin prone to breakouts.

Truthfully, products containing traditional hyaluronic acid do a fine job of moisturizing, but they can't penetrate below the skin's surface. They'll plump up the skin for a good three hours, tops. That's because molecules of typical hyaluronic acid are too large to penetrate below the skin's outer surface.

Today's products are more innovative. Some companies use smaller molecules, or low molecular weight hyaluronic acid in addition to HA. Hyaluronic acid made with smaller molecules allows the acid to penetrate deeper into skin's uppermost layers, providing greater hydration for better results.

Still other products are enhanced with sodium hyaluronate, the sodium salt form of the acid that also has a smaller molecular size than HA, making it especially penetrative. Watch for this ingredients in HA products—it's worth it. Studies show that these two effectively work together to increase moisture and repair damage.

B VITAMINS (NIACINAMIDE, PANTHENOL, BIOTIN)

B vitamins appear so often and in so many products that we sometimes forget what they actually do, which is to convert food into energy to fuel vital body processes—in particular, those responsible for healthy skin, hair, and nails.

B vitamins in skincare products help to heal and regenerate damaged cells, moisturize skin, decease inflammation, and more. Deficiencies in this vitamin can lead to eczema or acne. Three vitamin B variations serve to glamour-up skincare. Vitamin B_3 or niacinamide is the hot new ticket in anti-aging skincare. Niacinamide is a multipurpose workhorse—a fine brightener, moisturizer, and pigment corrector. Niacinamide repairs and prevents sun damage by keeping melanin from reaching the surface of the skin. It also helps the skin retain moisture by increasing ceramide and free fatty acid levels in skin. You'll get quick results, too—simple overnight use provides complexion-boosting results. In addition, the anti-inflammatory benefits of niacinamide work well for people with acne and rosacea, melasma, and hyperpigmentation.

Vitamin B_5, commonly called panthenol, is a humectant that moisturizes dry, scaly, or rough skin; a 2002 study showed that B_5 decreases inflammation and helps to repair the skin's barrier. Then there's Vitamin B_7, known as biotin—while we don't know for sure how B_7 benefits those with normal levels of the vitamin, studies show that a B_7 deficiency can cause hair loss and dry, scaly skin.

LIPIDS, CERAMIDES, FATTY ACIDS

Lipids, ceramides, and fatty acids work together to improve skin texture and suppleness and reduce inflammation. Lipids are the natural fat in our outer skin. When our aging skin loses its luster, applying synthetic or botanical lipids plumps skin back up. They provide a needed buffer between your skin cells that helps maintain your skin barrier as you age.

Lipids are often listed as ceramides and fatty acids. Ceramides are skin barrier molecules deficient in dry skin. Our skin has nine different ceramides; a few are used in skincare products: look for ceramide AP, ceramide EOP, ceramide NG, ceramide

NP, ceramide NS, phytosphingosine, and sphingosine. Both synthetic and botanical ceramides are used in skincare products. Research has shown no preference.

Fatty acids help to produce cholesterol and ceramides. Look for fatty acid listed as sunflower or other oils in the ingredients of anti-aging products. Numerous studies show the effectiveness of ceramides in increasing moisture and repairing the skin barrier.

Chapter 5

Prescription for Beauty

SO I'M GONNA GIVE YOU THIS INFORMATION STRAIGHT. THERE IS A chronic low-lying war going on among different medical specialties, a competition for territory within the cosmetic fields, competition for *you* as our patients. As you may know, financial security has become a bigger struggle for physicians. I've heard of ob-gyns who consider leaving their specialty since their malpractice insurance is as high as their salary. Reimbursement from insurance companies has been reduced and scrutinized more and more every year, squeezing physicians a little tighter. It's like the airline business, slowly but gradually taking things from you that you have become used to having, such as legroom and the ability to bring more than one small carry-on bag with you on a trip. Many airlines now expect you to pay for any food served too.

Don't you get annoyed by the slowly decreasing legroom and the fact that you have no control over what rules the airlines impose on you? You can be stuck in a plane without air-conditioning on the tarmac for hours, and you have no control over the situation and no recourse. This is similar to what many people in the medical field are feeling. Physicians are fed up. The "golden years" (those years when my father was a physician) are over. Many physicians are actually fleeing medicine altogether, frustrated with the increased restrictions on their ability to practice medicine. That's because your medical insurance company creates incentives for a doctor to manage patient's medical problems that would be better served by a specialist. In addition, many health insurance companies are now significantly cutting the amount they will reimburse a physician for a procedure.

Besides leaving medicine, another option for physicians is to search for work that is not controlled or dictated by health insurance companies—and is not covered by insurance—such as those procedures within the realm of cosmetics. This is why many physicians in other medical specialties—emergency medicine, obstetrics and gynecology, internal medicine, dentistry—have decided to jump into the cosmetic, fee-for-service, cash-based medical world. And this is a world that many specialties fight over. There are plastic surgeons, cosmetic surgeons, dermatologists, ENT docs, emergency room docs, and dentists doing Botox injections and fillers, breast implants, rhinoplasty, liposuction. What specialty has *true* rights to such procedures? Well, this is something that can be argued from every direction, and unfortunately, it is.

I think the appropriateness of a certain type of physician practicing cosmetic medicine and surgery has a lot to do with the ability of the physician, no matter the specialty. And this is why social media and YouTube can help you to determine who is best qualified. But you still must be careful; people can still filter and manipulate reviews. Sneaky physicians can certainly do this.

And then there are medical providers who aren't actually physicians at all. Mid-level providers (MLPs), including physician assistants, nurse practitioners, and nurses, are practicing medicine and doing cosmetic procedures independently. Social media is flush with people who are misrepresenting themselves or sort of bending the truth. Is that woman doing cosmetic procedures and posting on Instagram with ten thousand followers really board certified in dermatology, or is she board certified in family practice or . . . not board certified at all? And is she using descriptive words in her bio to make the true facts intentionally vague?

Don't get me wrong, an MLP can be *very* good in their medical specialty, but as is true in any other field (including physicians), some are not. It is my strong belief that MLPs serve our community best when they are part of a medical team run by a physician. By team, I mean that the physician is on site working side by side with the MLP the majority of the time. In doing so, the physician assistant or nurse practitioner has the ability to "curb side" their supervising physician and ask questions, show him or her complicated cases, and get advice, while the physician can observe the MLP at work and develop boundaries and confidence in abilities.

What I strongly disagree with is when MLPs are out on an "island" and are the only provider seeing patients at a particular location the majority of the time. Of course, sometimes this is necessary in areas where there are no physicians available. The worst instances are those MLPs that go into business for themselves and have some shady arrangement with a "sponsoring" or "collaborating" physician who provides no oversight to the business other than to lend their name, medical license, and malpractice insurance to comply with state laws.

My advice is this: I think midlevel providers can be a fantastic addition to a medical practice and provide excellent care for patients most of the time. In my private practice, we employ several, and put effort and care into making sure they are qualified to do what is being asked of them. They are an asset and an extension of me and the way I want to practice medicine. As a patient, you need to ensure that the medical provider you are seeing works closely with a qualified physician. Otherwise you may find yourself in a compromised position when things don't go so smoothly, which unfortunately is always a real risk when doing cosmetic procedures.

Is a physician assistant or nurse wearing a long white coat and introducing him- or herself as a "doctor" when they have actually had only two or three years of postgraduate training (compared to a dermatologist, who is required to have at least eight years of training after university) to get where they are? It truly makes me angry and frustrated that there is so much misinformation out there. I think it's important the general public understands and remembers that just as we can add filters to photographs on social media and magazines, so too do people filter their true credentials to make themselves appear more impressive than they really may be.

What I'm getting at is that many specialties and even nonphysicians may practice soft cosmetic treatments or cosmetic surgery. And specialties argue over territory all the time. What do you do? Don't be fooled. But I can't say that an ER doc may not be amazing at administering fillers or doing breast implant surgery. It has a lot to do with experience, and their surgical prowess and education. Heck, someone who went to the top plastic surgery residency and graduated top of their class isn't necessarily better at doing breast implants. Maybe they are just not that good at surgery. Maybe they are just too damn cocky. Great surgical technique, education, and experience are extremely important, but some people are just born with better hands and an innate ability. I hope that all doctors are drawn to the best specialty for them.

I'm sure this may stress you out because I'm not telling you how to find the best medical provider for you—that is difficult. In fact, people often ask me to refer them to a plastic surgeon, a hand surgeon, an orthopedic surgeon, a pediatrician, or a primary care doc. And, yes, I can refer you to one I know in the community, but for me it's difficult because I haven't seen their work. The people to ask are the nurses who work side by side with doctors in hospitals and see how they work. Ask your friends who look like they have had great work done who did it. If you're lucky, they will share the names of the people they are devoted to and trust.

My medical training is mainly in dermatology, learning how to identify and treat diseases of the skin, hair, and nails. My subspecialty *within* the specialty of dermatology is surgical, cosmetic, and laser dermatology. This won't be a complete list of cosmetic procedures because I don't do all cosmetic procedures. I'll discuss here the procedures that I am familiar with in the hopes that this knowledge will be useful for you. If you are interested in one of these procedures or a variant of it, I recommend getting a personalized evaluation from your surgical dermatologist, your cosmetic surgeon, or your plastic surgeon. Just like bakers who specialize in baking cupcakes or artists who only work in granite, we physicians all have our specialties: things we are particularly familiar with and things we know we do well.

If you are expecting a textbook chapter here, a reference chapter for all things cosmetic surgery, that's not what you're going to get. But I *will* include little tips and tricks that I use in the office to determine whether someone is a candidate for a certain procedure. So maybe this will help you in assessing whether a particular procedure is the right one for you, and maybe it will save you a trip to your doctor—or at least give you some knowledge beforehand so you can ask the right questions and understand better why you may or may not be a good candidate.

I'm going to include here mainly the things that I do or used to do, as I have personal knowledge in these areas. These are tricks I've learned from mentors but also figured out on my own, after being in practice for well over a decade. For completeness, I may sometimes include procedures that are popular, but I will state upfront in that section that I don't actually do that procedure, so I can't accurately or with confidence give you the real scoop. If I don't include something that you may be interested in, see your local dermatologist or plastic surgeon to get the most accurate and sound advice.

Not all dermatologists are the same. Some like to see youngsters, so they become pediatric dermatologists. Some really like research, and maybe they go on for further training, doing a fellowship in immunology and becoming an expert at immunology in dermatology. Some people are fascinated with seeing what the skin looks like under the microscope, and they become dermatopathologists. I like performing procedures, and I really love the relationships I create with my patients. I'm interested in beauty and fashion and love working with my hands, so my business now concentrates mainly on skin cancer surgery, soft cosmetic treatments, and cosmetic and laser surgery. If I just did Mohs surgery, my life would get boring. If I only poked people with Botox and fillers all day, I think I would go bonkers. If I did liposuction day in and day out, my right arm would fall off and I would go cross-eyed! It's the mix that I love, the variety.

Oh, and how can I forget: I can say with confidence that I have become a true expert at popping blackheads, milia, cysts, and lipomas. That wasn't really by choice, but because of all you popaholics out in the world. The strengths I have in dermatology really lend to being successful with popping procedures, though, so I guess all the planets really aligned and that's why I'm here writing this book for you!

Several factors determine the cost for most cosmetic procedures and surgeries, and there are so many variables that determine costs that I cannot talk about them here with any accuracy. The type of surgery you choose, the amount of time involved to complete the treatment, the geographic location of your surgeon, and your surgeon's experience are all taken into consideration. In general, fees don't include anesthesia, operating room facilities, or other expenses. Most insurance doesn't cover cosmetic surgery, although some practices may offer finance plans. Discuss all these details in advance of the surgery so that there are no surprises on your bill.

THINNING HAIR

Many men are mentally prepared to lose their hair. Some of them embrace it and shave their head bald, some men deny it with a major comb-over, and some fight it every step of the way. But across the board it can be utterly devastating for a woman to find that she is losing her hair. We women know that childbirth changes our bodies forever, that it gets harder and harder to lose weight as we age, that one day we'll look in the mirror and see our mothers looking back at us (which is not always a bad thing), and that menopause sucks, but losing our *hair*? This was not part of the deal!

Female pattern hair loss, which is different from telogen effluvium (discussed on page 232), is the most common kind of hair loss in women. Every strand of hair sits in a follicle, a small hole in the skin. Baldness happens when the hair follicle shrinks (aging again!), making hair finer and shorter. Over time, the follicle stops generating new hair. Yet the follicles remain alive, meaning it might be possible for them to grow new hair. Hormonal changes in menopause can also lead to baldness or severe hair loss in women. Family history of pattern baldness can also be a factor.

Hair thinning differs in women as opposed to men in that it starts at the top and crown of the scalp, and there can be a widening of the center hair part. The front hairline can stay the same, aside from normal recession, which unfortunately happens to all of us as we age. Woman rarely experience total baldness, as men do. Most of the time hair loss is moderate and doesn't require treatment unless you are bothered by it and it is affecting your quality of life and self-esteem.

Only one medicine, minoxidil, is approved by the US Food and Drug Administration to treat female pattern baldness. This topical treatment is applied directly to the scalp. Most doctors recommend a 2 percent solution or 5 percent foam. Minoxidil has been shown to help hair grow in about one in four or five women. In most women, it slows or stops hair loss. Once you're in, though, you're in: you have to use it for a long time to see a difference and maintain the results. Hair loss will start again after you stop using it. If minoxidil isn't effective, other medicines, including spironolactone, cimetidine, ketoconazole, finasteride, and some birth control pills, have been shown to be effective in some women.

Hair transplant is an option because it involves removing tiny plugs of hair from areas where your hair is thicker and then transplanting them into areas where hair is thin or absent. You could see minor scarring in the areas where hair was removed and there is a low risk of infection. To be truly effective, numerous transplanted plugs may be necessary, so that can add up; hair transplants are expensive. But they are also permanent and they make a dramatic difference in the appearance of your hair. Less expensive alternatives (that are not permanent) include hair weaving or a wig or hairpiece, and even those sprays that deposit tiny fake hairs to the scalp to disguise bald spots.

Hair Loss on Scalp

You probably didn't know that I have been trained to do hair transplants. I chose to not include this in my practice, although I strongly considered it. I think it's a job better suited to a male dermatologist. Just like I think women choose me, a fellow woman, to advise them on their liposuction or filler placement, so too do I believe men feel more comfortable relating to a male dermatologist for advice on a possible hair transplant.

COSMETIC INJECTABLES AND FILLING IN THE LINES

The facial aesthetic industry is enormous and growing quickly. The most popular cosmetic injectables are neuromodulators, followed by injectable fillers. When I was in my residency just fifteen years ago, we were using Botox in limited areas, and the filler we used then (bovine collagen) is one we no longer use now. Just as I was completing my residency, the new extremely popular hyaluronic acid fillers, Restylane and Juvéderm, were coming out. I remember how excited my fellow dermatology mentors were to be getting these products! And now looking back, I can see how techniques have changed so dramatically. We have learned how to use these products well as a group. Presently, they are extremely safe and very forgiving and "easy" to use. Which is why so many physicians are getting into this business! However, they are *not* without risk, so please find an injector with experience.

Many of the techniques and treatments for line filling are off-label, and may vary from physician to physician, even from country to country because different variations of the following products are available in different parts of the world. In fact, my own technique is not like it was ten years ago, since the more we use these products, the more we learn how to use them well. So this is not meant as the gold standard review, but as a guide for you so you are well informed when you see someone for your own personal issues. The key is finding an experienced physician, no matter if they are a dermatologist, plastic surgeon, emergency medicine doc, nurse practitioner, or physician assistant.

There is really a lot of negative press and misunderstanding when it comes to the use of these products. It's shocking to me how many people don't know the difference between Botox and fillers (which are really apples and oranges). Also, it is sad to me that so many people have preconceived notions about the products and insist they would "never do Botox because it is a poison!" or never use filler in their lips "because I'll look like Goldie Hawn in that movie, or did you see that crazy OC housewife?" and so on. Just like anything, some people can take things to the extreme. My personal opinion: less is more.

You would not believe how many people actually get filler and Botox and go undetected. These are wonderful products that can enhance and improve our appearance, and make us feel more confident and happy with a relatively small monetary investment, low risk, and little downtime. With hyaluronic acid fillers, for example, there is a get-out-of-jail-free card. There is a product called hyaluronidase that can break down a hyaluronic acid filler immediately, so if you don't like it you can make it disappear. Botox is not permanent, in fact its effects wane in three to five months. First, I'll explain what Botox and fillers are and what they do. I know you will have questions about what type of product or treatment is the best for you! Then I'll cover treatment options according to the area of complaint so that you can make the right decision.

What's in a Name?

I use *Botox* generically here like you use *Kleenex* or *Xerox* because it is the first and most recognizable term. Currently, there are two other FDA-approved forms of botulinum toxin that can be used for cosmetic use: Dysport and Xeomin.

BOTOX

You know, a few years ago, I got this crazy idea that I should try to get into the *Guinness Book of World Records* by treating the highest number of people with Botox during a four-hour period. I thought of this because at my office we have a yearly cosmetic event called the Envy Party, which is really a thank-you to our devoted patients, a gift to them in the form of heavy discounts on many of the cosmetic treatments we do in my office. During the four hours of this event, people line up for me to treat them with Botox, and I thought, "*Wow*, I could get into the *Guinness Book of World Records* for this!" I set my alarm for three in the morning so I could call Guinness's headquarters in the United Kingdom and spoke to a nice man who was reviewing my application. I wish I had been connected with a woman! "This is a ridiculous application, because Botox is a *poison*. Did you know it is already in the *Guinness Book of World Records* as the most poisonous product in the world?!?!" I guess that was a no. It made me angry, though! Let me explain why. And let me also state that I've got dibs on this world record when this goes to press and Guinness comes calling!

What It Does

Botox is the leading cosmetic aesthetic procedure in the world. It is an injectable neuromodulator and has the effect of temporarily preventing a muscle from moving. Yes, it is technically called botulinum toxin, but I don't like to use the word *toxin* because it is a scary term—I don't want a toxin in myself, either! In actuality, Botox is a spectacular cosmetic treatment option because it is so quick and easy to administer, there is no downtime, and it is *temporary*. Yes, being temporary is actually a good thing, because if you don't like it (which is rare), it goes away. Also, our faces and bodies naturally change over time as we age, and it's great to change the way you get Botox to accommodate for these natural changes. It is injected directly into the muscle, not into the skin like some people think. Acetylcholine (ACh) is a neurotransmitter, or chemical messenger, that makes our muscles move, and Botox inhibits the release of ACh from the presynaptic motor neuron, so if the connection is not made, the muscle the nerve innervates won't respond.

Botox helps temporarily soften the muscles of expression. For example, it's most commonly used to treat the glabella, what we call the "11s"—the grooves we can develop between our eyebrows after frowning, scowling, and squinting for so many years. If you use Botox to prevent the muscles that create these lines from moving (the muscles are the procerus and part of the corrugator muscle), then you won't be able to furrow your brow, and many of us like this because when we make that face, it makes us look angry and older. How great is it that we can specifically prevent certain muscles from moving to prevent this scowling face? Better yet, if you treat these muscles before you ever develop a line at rest, then you will *never* get such lines.

It's important to understand that Botox doesn't directly erase wrinkles; it eliminates them because the muscles can't move in the same repetitive pattern that creates the wrinkles. Remember, less is more. It's important not to get a frozen face, because that is not attractive, either. You can always add a little more, but you can't take it away—you have to wait until it wears off.

If you're still freaked out that Botox is a "poison," consider this: Botox is the by-product of a *Clostridium botulinum* bacterium, and this by-product happens to temporarily prevent muscles from moving. Similarly, penicillin is also the by-product of a mold called *Penicillium notatum*. Penicillin happens to kill certain bacteria, and that is how it is used to our benefit. Botox has a different function: it can temporarily prevent muscles that it comes into contact with from moving, so we can use it to our advantage to look younger and more rested. Botox has to get into our body in a high dose, *much* higher than what we inject carefully and directly into specific muscles (try 40,000 units, compared with the mere 40 units that is commonly injected to minimize crow's-feet and frown lines), in order to be dangerous. I swear I don't have stock in Botox, but I sure wish I did, because it does something that no other type of product can do, and the results can truly be amazing.

Results

Patients can return to most everyday activities right after the procedure, which can be performed during a fifteen-minute office visit, and will see initial results within three to seven days. The improvements last about three to five months—and sometimes longer.

SOFT-TISSUE FILLERS

The most common fillers used today are hyaluronic acid (HA) fillers, with major name brands being Juvéderm and Restylane, and therefore these are the ones I'll discuss in some detail. Please speak to your dermatologist or plastic surgeon about the best treatment option for *you*. HA is actually a normal substance found in our skin that helps keep it soft, plump, and well moisturized. An HA filler is a clear, malleable gel that is easily injected either superficially or more deeply under the skin's surface to help lessen the appearance of fine lines and wrinkles, plump the lips, and even change some of the general contours of the face, giving it more fullness and lift.

SIDE EFFECTS FROM INJECTABLES

Botox has mild immediate side effects including redness, bruising, pain/soreness, and swelling. Fillers do require a little bit more planning comparatively because there can be more swelling and bruising immediately posttreatment compared to Botox, but sometimes treatment is undetectable and there is no downtime at all. To be on the safe side, I recommend that fillers not be administered right before you're getting your holiday photos taken or you're going on a blind date! Ideally, I like to tell my patients if you want to plan well, do these types of procedures two to six weeks before a big event where you want to look your best. That way, you can decide if you want to fine-tune your results at a follow-up treatment, and it will give any bruising and swelling time to subside.

Stay away from aspirin for ten days before any injectable procedure to minimize your chances for bleeding and bruising. Avoid drinking alcohol for twenty-four hours before and after treatment to minimize its ability to increase your chance of bleeding. If a filler is injected too superficially, you can get a slight bluish-gray discoloration to the skin which is called the Tyndall effect. Also, this can happen more often if you are getting aggressive treatment to the area under the eyes because this skin is very thin and more translucent. Hyaluronic acid fillers are hydrophilic, meaning they attract water, so they can draw more fluid to the area and, especially in a thin-skinned area, it can manifest as swelling.

Allergic reactions with hyaluronic acids are extremely uncommon. Complications that can come up later and not immediately within the first week or treatment, such as infection, persistent redness and swelling, and scarring, are extremely uncommon. Intravascular occlusion is always something we physicians who treat with this product look out for, and it is scary when this happens as it can lead to ulcers, scarring, and even blindness. Also, if you are at risk for developing herpes breakouts, you may want to ask your physician for treatment beforehand to decrease this risk.

A Cautionary Tale

Some people feel like they are wasting their money on fillers that are temporary (although they can be pretty long lasting) and look into using permanent fillers.

Overall, this is a bad idea. Permanent fillers, such as silicone, can lead to permanent changes that you may not like, and worse, permanent side effects. Don't do it. There is certainly some "permanence" with these temporary fillers, because any time there is introduction of a needle under the skin, this triggers our own collagen to thicken and lessen the wrinkle or fold we are trying to correct. In other words, I definitely can report that people who have been treating a stubborn wrinkle successfully for years with fillers find that they need less filler over time and that the results last longer. All this because the skin has likely thickened on its own and helped to improve the wrinkle permanently to some degree.

FOREHEAD

Forehead lines are those horizontal lines that can span the width of the forehead and can be quite deep in many people. The trouble is that they still stick around even when you're not actively creating them by looking surprised or looking up at the sky, two movements that definitely elicit these lines. In many people, over the years, these lines can become etched in the skin, and even if you stretch the skin, the lines remain carved there. People hate them and they often ask me if Botox can erase them.

It's true that Botox can greatly diminish, perhaps completely erase your forehead lines. But this is not for everyone and let me explain why. The frontalis muscle covers the span of your forehead like a thin sheet. You contract this muscle when you raise your eyebrows, and as you know, this then produces those horizontal lines. In other words, that's why you get those annoying lines: because you are lifting your brows. The question is, do you like to lift your eyebrows, or rather do you "need" to lift your brows?

There are two observations I make in my patients to see whether they are indeed candidates for this specific treatment. First, I ask my patient to close their eyes, and once they do, I ask them to open them. When they open their eyes, do they actually lift their brows at the same time? Also, I "stalk" them during our consultation. I really watch their expressions while they speak to me. Do they use their eyebrows to express themselves? Do they have heavy brows?

If you are very expressive with your eyebrows, if you raise them incessantly every time you have an animated conversation, if you have your dad's eyes, and his brows have dropped down closer to his eyes as he has aged, then you probably want very little Botox in your forehead, if any. Sure, your lines may lessen with Botox, but if you have heavy brows to begin with and use them when you communicate, then you won't be able to lift your brows up away from your eyes much or at all. You will hate that if you apply eye shadow, the eye shadow seems to disappear, that your eyes feel heavy, that you can't look up to the sky without bending back at the neck.

I speak from personal experience here, though I love Botox. But when I had my forehead treated once because I hate my forehead lines, I also absolutely hated that I couldn't look upward, and I especially detested that I had to use my nondominant hand to physically pull up my brow to apply mascara. It changed the shape of my eyes, made them feel heavy, and made me feel tired. It wasn't worth it for me. Thank goodness it fades away in three to five months. And remember, this is why having an evaluation done by an experienced doctor is so important. Everyone is not treated in the same fashion because everyone has unique facial movements and features.

Filler can also be used to soften the horizontal lines but not completely if they are actually etched in your skin (meaning when you stretch your skin you still see the lines). Chemical peels and laser resurfacing can "sand" down etched lines that are carved into the forehead. However, Botox is really the first-line treatment, because you need to prevent the movement that creates the lines in the first place. I compare it to ironing a crisp cotton shirt. If you just iron the creases with filler and/or peels or laser, sure, the lines diminish, but if you don't get Botox, you are just re-creating those creases and wrinkles again right away because the muscles are still able to move.

TEMPLES

Temporal atrophy is most often seen in people who have a low body fat percentage. However, anyone can have a hollowing of their temple area, which is that area on the side of your face between your eyes and the tops of your ears. This makes us look gaunt, scrawny, tired, sick, and older. Although you may not readily notice this in others, when it is improved upon, you *do* notice that a person looks younger and healthier, you just may not be able to figure out specifically why. And this is what makes this kind of aesthetics so amazing. Any hyaluronic acid filler can be used, depending on how thick the skin is in the area. Can you see a theme starting in this section? It's all about sculpting! Subtle and specifically undetectable treatments give you an overall better result, one that is of effortless youthfulness.

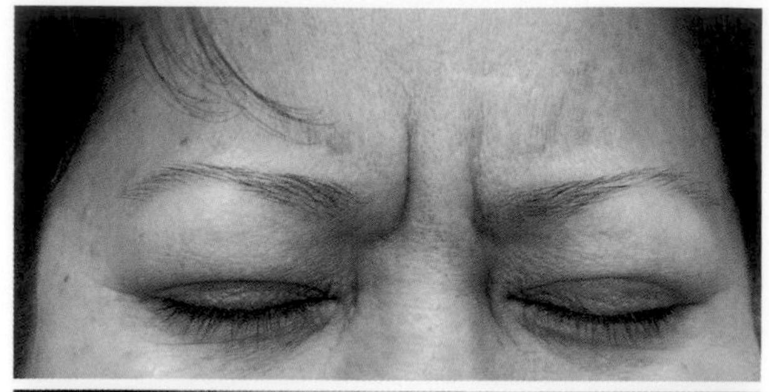

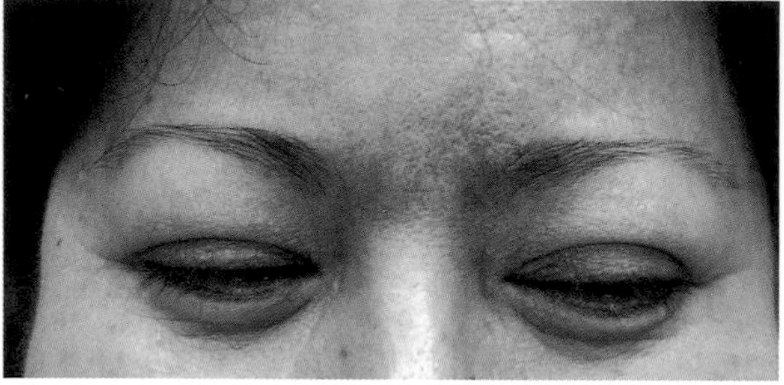

Before and after Botox and filler to glabellar lines.

GLABELLA

The 11s, or glabellar frowns, are most often treated with Botox. Here we target specific small muscles, the procerus and the corrugator muscle. Essentially these two muscles have one function alone: to make us scowl, frown, and help us squint in the sun—*that* movement! And that is nothing but an angry expression. Our kids or friends know when we are upset; we don't have to look it too, right? And you know how your momma told you to quit making that face because one day it will freeze like that? Well, she was right! For many people, years of frowning and squinting has led to furrows in this area, which we call lines or furrows "at rest" (meaning without flexing the muscles). Although this is an area that yields a lot of satisfaction when treated skillfully, poor injection technique (an injection too close to the eye) in this area can cause ptosis, which is when you have heaviness of the eyelid. Now, there is a difference between ptosis and just a heaviness of the eyebrows.

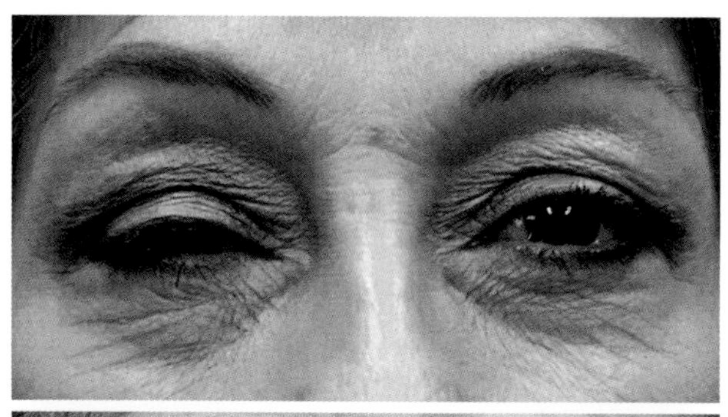

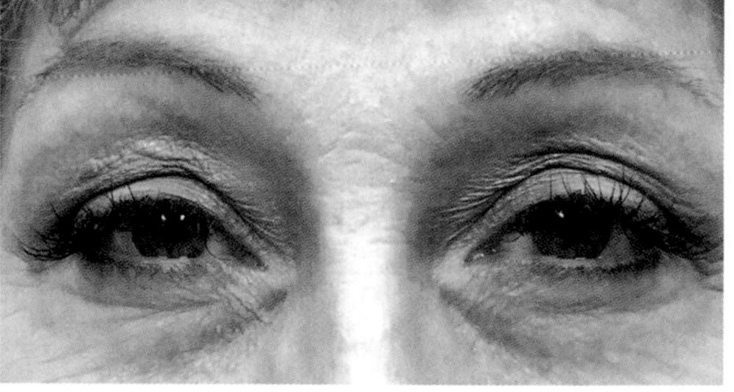

Ptosis of the right eye due to Botox being placed too close to the eye. As you can see in the bottom picture, it does *resolve eventually.*

Botox on Me

Yes, I get Botox! I get very little, though, maybe twelve units or so every three to four months. Partly this is because I don't want to turn into the lion lady! (Sometimes it's a slippery slope, in this beauty business, and we all have a pact in my office between providers and staff that we won't let one another take the cosmetics thing too far!) Partly it is because I want to show my patients that if used conservatively, it's not very expensive, and it can actually prevent lines and wrinkles from forming in the first place! And of course I neeeed Botox now, he-he. I joke that it is the "gateway" cosmetic drug. It's the first cosmetic treatment that many people try, and once you go Botox, you usually don't go back, if it's done right!

I remember the first time I got Botox. It was a dark and stormy Monday back in 2002. Just kidding, but it was back in 2002, when I was in my early thirties (which is actually kinda late to the game). I thought, "Okay, I'll just have my glabella treated, so I can't frown. No big deal!" And it wasn't a big deal, and just like my patients tell me about their first time, I kept thinking: "Is it working, is it working? Hmm, I don't think it's working. . ." Then a few days later, I stepped out of my car into the sunlight and squinted. Or at least, *tried* to squint. So weird: I was literally trying to scrunch my eyes together to shield them from the sun, and I *couldn't*. That's when I knew that the Botox was working; I could no longer create those creases between my brows that also allow me to squint. And actually, I said, "Okay, no big deal. Not sure if it's really doing anything significant. Botox? I can take it or leave it." However, let me tell you, it was a *whole* different story when the Botox began to wear off in three to four months. That's when I realized (and when most people realize) that Botox is amazing. And yes, I needed it.

Did You Know

Botox may help improve depression. Doctors who study the relationship between the injectable and mood say that our facial expressions are part of the circuit of the brain related to our emotions. Botox subdues the muscles that can make frowns and grimaces, and so it makes it harder to feel emotions not being expressed on the face![1] In other words, if you can't physically frown, maybe this means you feel less angry, concerned, and depressed.

EYEBROWS

Our eyebrows change both shape and position as we age, and many people notice this because they slowly change the way they pluck their brows to accommodate it. Botox and filler can elevate the brow in a natural way. Botox in small amounts can affect the muscle that pulls down slightly on our inner brows, so if that muscle is hindered, the outer brow can lift somewhat. Also, filler can be placed under the eyebrow to lift up from underneath, elevating the brow somewhat. However, Botox and filler can do only so much, and sometimes too much of a good thing is too much. I mean, you don't want your eyebrows so lifted you look like Spock from *Star Trek*.

Most women in the United States like an arched brow (brow lifted higher on the outer edges), and Botox can actually achieve this in many people. And this preference is geographical. For example, many women in Asian countries prefer a flatter or just gently curved eyebrow. Men, though, do not usually want this look because it is feminizing. Botox is great for both men and women but generally should be placed differently depending on the gender of the patient, and also the geographical preference. Communicating what you are looking for with your doctor is key to getting what you want.

If Botox and filler do not give enough lift for you, then you may want to speak to a cosmetic or plastic surgeon about a surgical brow lift.

EYES

Crow's-feet are those smile lines that radiate from the outside edge of our eyes, and Botox can really soften these lines. I find that you can't eliminate these expressive lines completely in many people, and this is an important point I explain because I don't want a dissatisfied or disappointed patient. When you smile, your cheeks rise up as well and this movement can also create smile lines. We don't want to prevent ourselves from smiling, right?

This can best be explained to people by having them make particular movements. To minimize crow's-feet, Botox is injected into the lateral edge of the orbicularis oculi muscle, which is a muscle that circles our eyes. To try to isolate the movement of this muscle alone, I ask my patients to purse their lips and keep that position while smiling with their eyes. In doing so, I want to eliminate as best I can any crow's-feet that develop because our cheeks lift when we smile—those can't be treated with Botox, while the other lines can.

You can also slightly round or widen the shape of the eye by placing a tiny amount of Botox just under the center of the lower eyelid.

Less Is More

I personally use only a very small amount of Botox around my own eyes. I have very strong smile lines that are quite deep and noticeable, but I feel they are happy lines (for now anyway; I may change my mind in five or ten years!). And when I did get a full treatment of Botox in the area, I liked the way it looked but didn't like the way I felt. It's so interesting to me how closely our facial movements are tied with our emotions! Smiling is so tightly linked to when we are happy that if we can't physically smile like we are accustomed to doing when we are happy or laughing, does this actually make us *feel* less happy? Well, it did to me. I actually felt compelled to apologize to people who said something witty and funny to me, because I felt like I was "fake smiling" when I had Botox in my crow's-feet. And this certainly doesn't happen to everyone—after all, this is the second most popular area to treat with Botox. But for now I'll stick with just a little bit to treat my crow's-feet, thank you very much. I need my smile to be happy!

UNDER THE EYES: DARK CIRCLES AND BAGS

Okay, this is a big topic and an area of concern for many people. There are many reasons for dark circles or bags under the eyes. I'll explain the four most common and their treatments so you can hopefully figure out what type of "baggage" you have.

1. Pigmentation of the Skin

Quite literally, you have dark circles under your eyes.

Get under a really good light—preferably natural sunlight—close to a mirror. If you stretch your skin under your eye and you see the dark spots or circles move as you stretch, that's because the discoloration is *on* the skin, and the eye baggage is due to skin pigmentation. Treatment options include skin-lightening creams and camouflage with makeup concealer. Possibly some laser treatments can help improve this pigment on the surface of the skin. However, it depends on what level of your skin this pigment resides in, and what color the pigment is. Speak to your dermatologist to get treatment options based on what you personally have.

2. Blood Vessels Under the Eyes

Okay, you stretch the skin under your eyes gently, but you're sure that the darkness is not coming from the skin itself, because even as you stretch the skin, the dark color doesn't move or change much. In fact, sometimes it gets more prominent. Well, this discoloration can come from color *under* the skin. Under-eye skin is the thinnest skin we have on our bodies. The thinner your skin, the more translucent it is. Like with a dark balloon, the more you fill it with air, the thinner the walls of the balloon become, the lighter in color it gets, and the more easily you can see through it. We have blood vessels just under the skin, and the thinner your skin, the more likely you can see these vessels. Sometimes you can even see veins underneath this thin skin. Veins often give off a purplish hue, and this appears as dark circles under the eyes.

Sometimes these vessels under the skin can be treated with injections, called sclerotherapy, and possibly even lasers that treat blood vessels can help to eliminate some of these vessels. A short-term fix can be achieved with topical products that constrict superficial blood vessels, making them temporarily less visible. These products include prescriptions such as Rhofade and Mirvaso. Over-the-counter products such as Afrin, which contains oxymetazoline, may even help. Makeup concealers that have a green tint are a great option to disguise redness under the eyes. Yellow-tinted concealer can help cancel out purple discoloration.

Color Me Beautiful

Do you know what a color wheel is? Artists and designers use it to decide on color schemes and to see the relationship between colors. *You* can use it to help make discolorations on your skin less visible! All you need to know is that colors opposite from each other on the color wheel cancel each other out. If you apply red color over green, it neutralizes that color. Makeup artists take advantage of this knowledge and this is why concealers are made in all these strange colors, such as red, orange, yellow, and green.

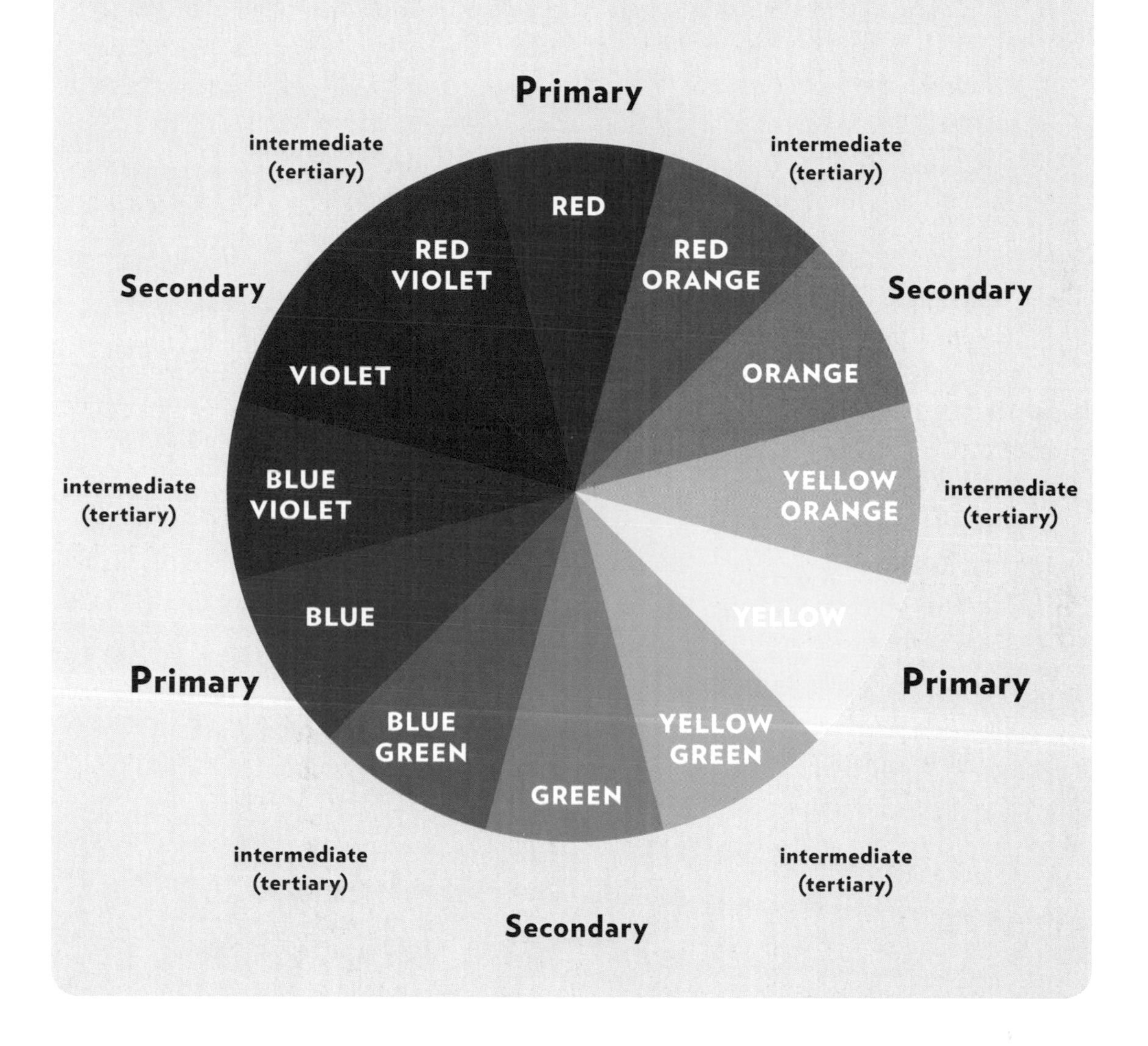

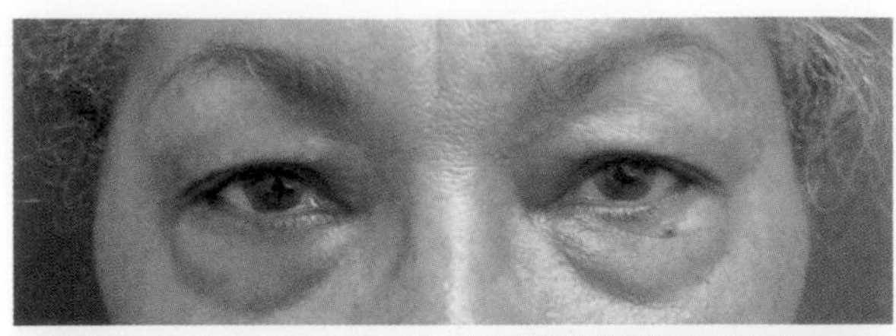

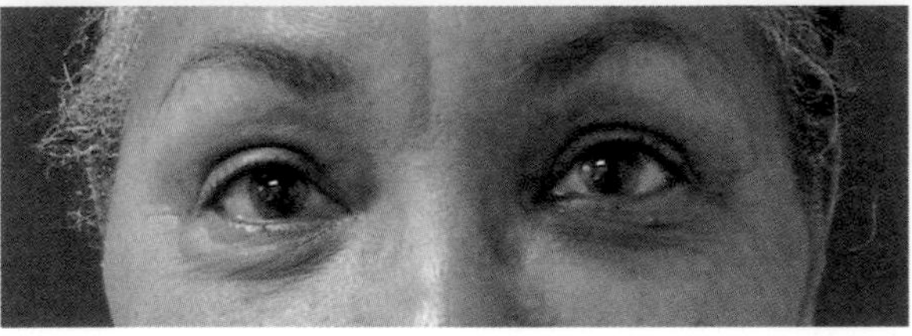

Fat pockets under the eyes before and after lower eyelift (upper eyelift also done).

3. Fat Deposits or Fluid Accumulation

This is true "baggage" under the eyes. It's a bulging under the eye, from either fat or fluid, or both. This is often a hereditary trait. Truly, the most definitive treatment is to surgically remove these little pockets of fat, a procedure called a lower blepharoplasty. However, you can sometimes disguise this somewhat with filler in the surrounding tissue to try to narrow the height difference.

4. Tear Troughs

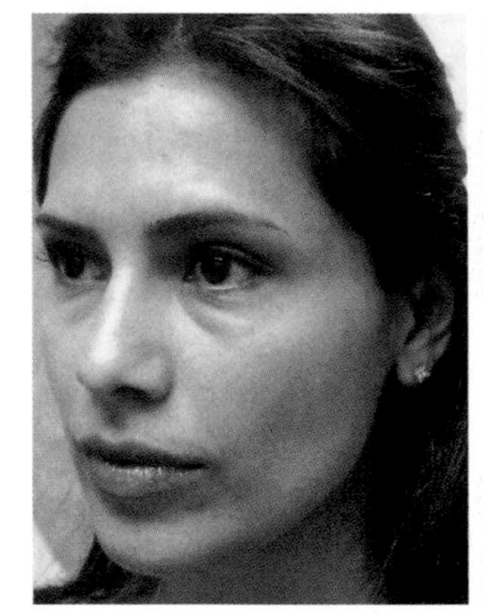

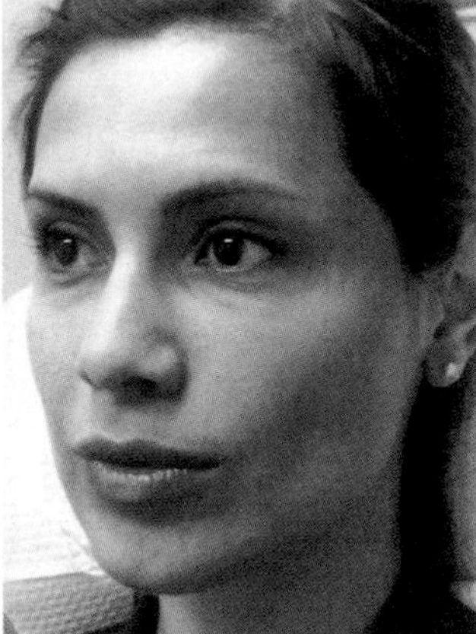

Tear trough before and after treatment with filler.

These we call by a truly memorable name, sorry: "tear troughs." They are the depression between your undereye area and your cheek, which can be hereditary and most often appears in your twenties. You can see them better if light is cast on your face from the side, since they create shadows. Tear troughs can usually be improved with a hyaluronic acid filler, but don't let your doc overtreat you! It's a very thin-skinned area, and if you overdo it, you can actually get the opposite effect—too much fullness in the area, which frankly doesn't look good.

Remember that you can be unlucky enough to have more than one of the above issues, as many people do. So you may need to undergo multiple treatments to see improvement.

NOSE

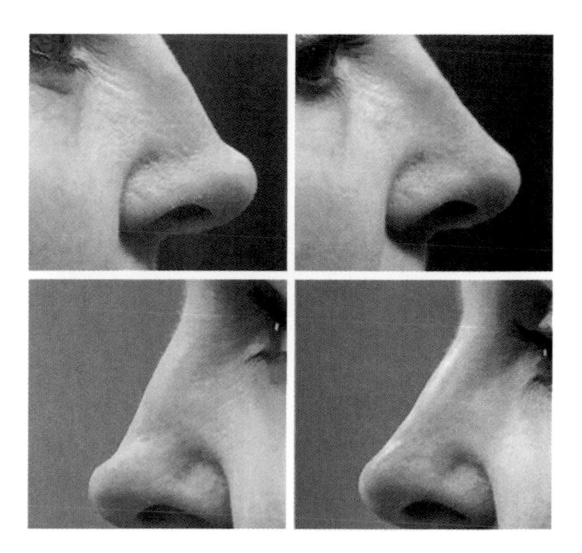

Hyaluronic acid filler to smooth a bumpy nose.

Many people think the only way their nose can be properly straightened or smoothed out is to undergo a rhinoplasty, a surgery with small hammers and chisels to reshape the center of your face. Well, you don't need to do that in all cases! There *is* something that can be done that doesn't require a knife or surgery at all, just a hyaluronic acid filler. We can now smooth a nose hump, straighten the appearance of a deviated septum, or lift the tip of a downturned nose, and all within ten to fifteen minutes. Results aren't permanent, but they are long lasting, about one to two years.

Bunny Lines

Scrunch your nose up like you're smelling something bad. See those creases that appear at the base of your nose near your eyes? We call those bunny lines, to be cute, I guess. Botox can be injected in small amounts into the muscle that creates these lines, called the dorsal nasalis muscle, to minimize them.

CHEEKS, PARENTHESES LINES, AND JOWLING

Interestingly, many people don't think about their cheeks. They are usually much more concerned that their jowls are becoming more prominent, or that those parentheses-shaped lines that connect the corner of our nose to our mouth are deepening. Think about it, though. When you look at yourself in the mirror and you try to fix that jowling or those deep lines, what do you do? You pull up on your cheeks, directing the lift toward the tips of your ears, right?

Have you seen people with strange-looking faces, seeming like they are always trying to smile a little too hard? Well, when you have filler continually placed *only* in your nasolabial fold to lessen that parenthesis groove, it *can* lessen the depth of the fold, but at the expense of making your face look false or plastic. But the point of all this for most of us is to make us look like our younger selves, not like a completely different person!

We've gotten smarter about the way we use filler to make us look more youthful.

Instead of treating the actual area that we complain about, we treat the cause. The deepening of the parentheses lines and the increase in jowling is due to gravity pulling down on our cheeks. So putting volume back into our cheeks with HA filler lifts the cheeks up and lessens any sagging downstream.

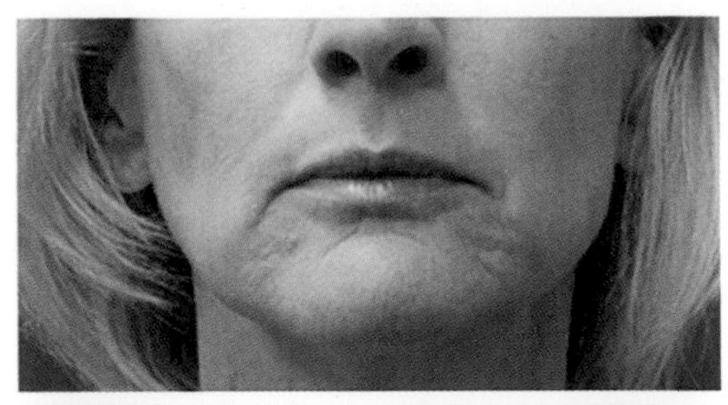

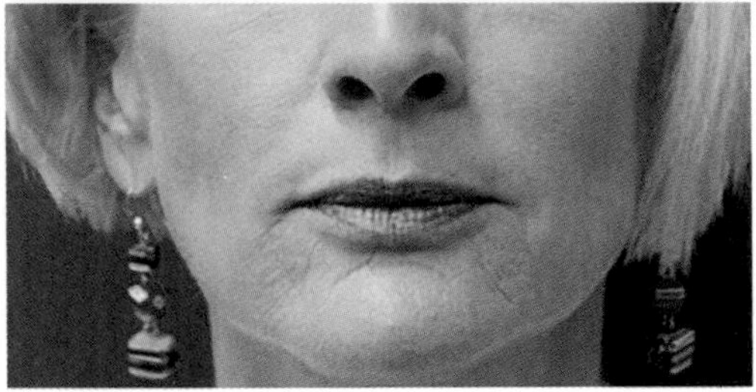

Example of turning up the edges of the mouth with Botox and filler.

LIPS

It's true that our lips shrink as we get older. Partly this is due to the natural loss of collagen and elastin—expression lines are created from kissing, speaking, and pursing the lips, and in many cases the lines start to "stick" even without making any movement at all. Smoking, genetics, and excess sun exposure certainly play large roles as well. Our bones shrink with age too, which is part of the reason why many of us notice that our lips appear to be turning inward, and less of the actual lip can be seen over time.

Right now the big trend is to get injections to create very full lips. It's the millennials, influenced by social media, who are getting their lips very inflated and full. It's great that there is a safe (and reversible) way to do this, using hyaluronic acid filler. No, plumping your lips won't stretch them out so they will be all loose and floppy later in your life. However, putting filler in your lips is done not just to inflate their size, so don't doubt this may be a good option for you. There are more people who don't want full lips, but just want to reduce the lines around their mouth or who want to lift the outside edges of their mouth so that they are not downturned, to return their lips to how they used to be ten to twenty years ago. The fuller lip trend really scares off these people from trying this anti-aging technique. But yes, doing too much filler too fast in the area can make the lips look quite ridiculous. Duck lips. Beaver tail lips. Balloon lips. Many people say *no.* Just *no.*

BEFORE

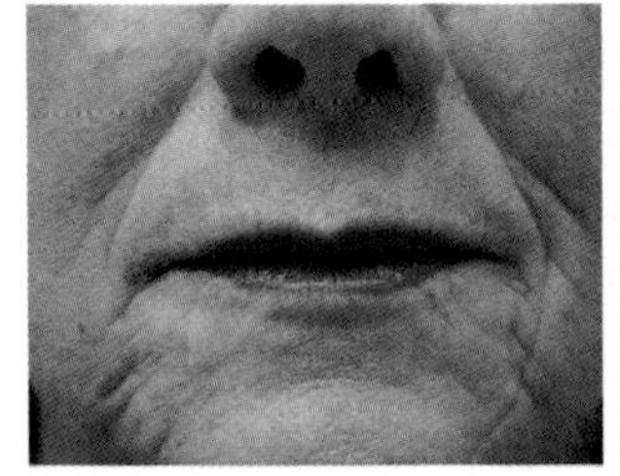

AFTER

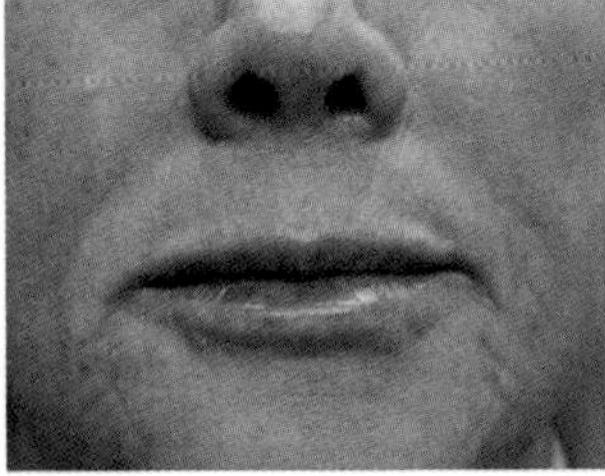

Hyaluronic acid filler to nasolabial fold, lips, and mandibular folds.

There are a few other important things for you to know if you want to plump your lips. It is much easier to make already full lips look even fuller naturally. If you are born with thin lips, it's not easy to make them much fuller without their looking ridiculous and fake; if you have thin lips and bring in a picture of Angelina Jolie's lips and ask if you can have those, well, good luck. This is nearly impossible with filler alone, and usually cosmetic surgery is needed to attain this. Find an injector with experience, who looks carefully at your lips and discusses the options with you at length before treatment. The goal is to enhance the natural contours of the lips and use little "tricks" to make them appear as big but as natural as you can.

You may look with some jealousy at certain celebrities' lips and want their fullness and plumpness. Let's take one of the most famous lips to be injected: Kylie Jenner's lips. Before she had filler (and she has admitted to this treatment), she had very thin lips and now she has very full lips, lips that many people are jealous of and wish to emulate. But if you look really closely at her lips now, she still has a pretty thin upper lip, and it's her *lower* lip that is much larger. She actually overlines her upper lip with lip liner and matching lipstick to increase the size of her upper lip more.

In general, the beauty ideal is for the lower lip to be slightly larger to one and a half times the size of the upper lip. But who decides on this "beauty ideal," anyway? And, hey, there are certainly cultural differences! A Caucasian usually has a smaller upper lip or tends to have thinner lips in general. Asian, Hispanic, and African Americans tend to have naturally fuller lips, with the upper and lower lips about the same size.

But let's get back to the main reasons most people seek out improvement of their lips: they feel like their lips are shrinking and the tips are turning downward, which are really natural occurrences as most of us age, and complain of smoker's lines (you don't have to actually smoke to have these). The latter are the lines that radiate from your lips, deepening in appearance when you purse your lips or move them like you're drinking out of a straw. These are also lines of expression, which is normal! We can use filler to subtly but effectively turn up the edges of the lip, and Botox can be injected into the depressor anguli oris muscles, the muscles that pull down on the outer edges of your lips, so you no longer have a continuous frown.

Gummy Smile

Can you imagine actually hating your smile? Well, I suspect that some of you reading can—we are so darn critical of ourselves. Remember that smiling is contagious, that smiling should be because you're happy and should never cause you distress. Some people, though, show off their gums of their upper bite too much when they smile broadly, and this is source of embarrassment. But just a little Botox, just a couple of units here and there under the nose, can soften a broad, gummy grin. Speak to your cosmetic physician if you're interested in seeing if you're a candidate.

CHIN

One of the parts of the face that many people are concerned with is the chin area. Many of us hate the irregular and bumpy look that can develop on the chin over time, which we call "chinulite," or better yet, "chimples," as well as the lines and grooves that often form along the outer edges of the chin to the outer edges of the lips, aka marionette or puppet lines. Lovely, aren't they? Well, there are some easy, no-downtime methods for slowing the aging process here. Botox in pretty small portions can be injected into the mentalis muscle in the chin, which is the muscle that you use when you pout with your mouth, and this can decrease this bumpiness and minimize lines.

Weak Chin

You may not be weak of heart or mind, but you may be weak of chin. This is best seen in profile—if your chin doesn't project that much and instead leans in toward the body, you have this condition, which is very often inherited or genetic. Many people may not even realize that they have it, but actually supporting this weak chin with a chin implant or even a simple office procedure like filler placement into the chin can project the area forward and really make your face appear more balanced. It can even minimize the appearance of loose neck skin or a double chin! Filler is such a simple in-office procedure and can really yield long-lasting results.

Double Chin

We all know the worst angle to take a photo from is when you're looking down at the camera lens! Most of us have a double chin when in that position. There *is* help for a double chin and it's not always surgery! I do chin/neck liposuction under local anesthesia alone, and this can help a more dramatic double chin. Those of you who have some extra fullness right under your chin and don't have much looseness of the tissue there can really benefit from a simple office procedure with an injectable called Kybella. Kybella is a synthetic form of deoxycholic acid, an enzyme that is found in our gut that helps to break down fat. If injected into the area under your chin, it specifically targets the fat cells there.

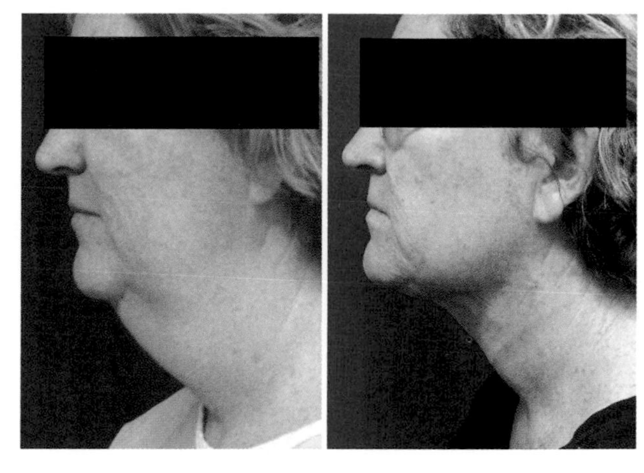

Liposuction, under local anesthesia, of the neck.

People usually need two to four treatments to achieve their desired results, and there can be temporary bruising, numbness, swelling, discomfort, and firmness or hardening in the area for a week or so posttreatment. Serious side effects are not common but include nerve damage in the area, causing a crooked smile, trouble swallowing, infection, and cell damage and death (skin necrosis). This treatment is not for everyone with a double chin. If you have a lot of loose skin in the area you are better off with a neck lift, a surgery to pull the skin tighter, because Kybella can only minimize the fat in the area and doesn't do much to tighten the skin.

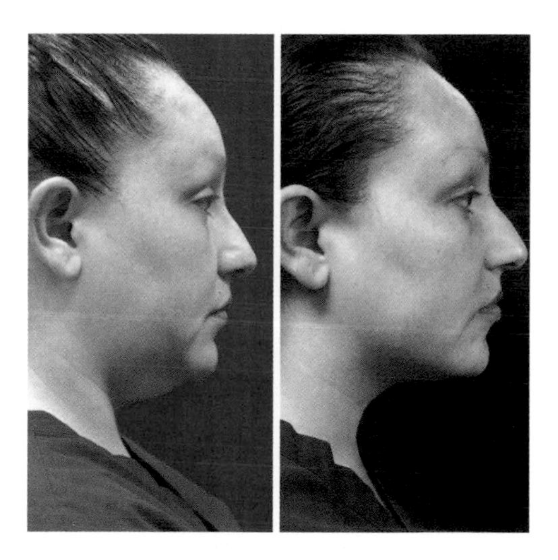

Before and after treatment of double chin with Kybella.

JAWLINE

Some women have a strong jawline, which gives their facial shape a more masculine appearance. This can be caused by a strong bite muscle. Place two fingers on one of your cheeks as you bite down. There is a muscle there that lifts up your cheek when you bite, called the masseter muscle. It's also the muscle that gets overused if you have TMJ (temporomandibular joint dysfunction) caused by teeth grinding when you sleep. This muscle can be built up from overuse or it may just be a hereditary trait that you have a stronger muscle here than most.

Either way, if you don't like it, you can lessen that strong jaw and give your cheeks and jawline a softer, more feminine contour with a little Botox to this muscle. Just don't overdo it, and I wouldn't recommend it if you're a circus performer who has to hang in the air doing stunts clenching your teeth on a rope to save your life! Softening this muscle with Botox may make your bite weaker, but if it makes you feel much better about your appearance, this may be worth it for you.

NECK

Yes, I'm with you. I hate my neck too! And I think I look pretty good, until I catch sight of myself in the mirror while animatedly speaking on my phone. What is that neck of mine *doing*? Why is it so loose in this area, and so tight in the other? Why do those bands pop out when I'm excited about something? They make me look *too* excited, like my head could pop from my neck or something. When we were young, our neck was so neglected by us, forgotten when we applied sunscreen, ignored when we tended to our face, our eyebrows, our hair, and suddenly we wake up one day and all we can focus on is our neck.

There are many treatment options for our neck, but of course, not all of them work as well as we'd like them to. Laser treatments can remove superficial blood vessels and redness, lighten brown spots, and tighten the skin to lessen fine lines and grooves. There are even thread lifts, which involve using needles and cannulas to insert dissolvable barbed sutures in the area that are then pulled, grabbing tissue with the hope of suspending that tissue and tightening the skin.

I have a little looseness of the skin under my neck, but what bothers me more are the bands that pop from my neck when I tighten the muscles there, called the platysmal muscles. These muscles wrap around our neck like a scarf, and flexing them makes them more prominent; I don't know if it makes me feel older or just look scary. When I see them pop like that, it certainly draws my attention, and then all I can do is stare at those muscles if I watch myself in a video. Botox to the rescue again! Small amounts injected along the prominent parts of this muscle can lessen their appearance. I've had it done myself and haven't had any problems, though I warn patients it may make you feel like you have a little difficulty swallowing if too much is injected and too deeply.

SURGICAL PROCEDURES

Surgical procedures are less invasive than in the past, and recovery times have also improved. Good candidates for the procedures here are healthy nonsmokers who do not have medical conditions that impair healing, and those people who have a positive outlook and realistic expectations. Smoking is a big no-no here and anytime an extensive flap or fancy graft (like I might do in Mohs surgery) is needed, because nicotine actually constricts superficial blood vessels, decreasing blood flow in the skin.

EARLOBE RECONSTRUCTION

I would say people most often request earlobe repair because of a stretched earring hole or a torn earlobe. Heavy earrings are usually the cause. Or maybe, as happened to Beyoncé, a patient's earring hoop got caught on something and, with one quick movement, suddenly the earring was gone and blood was everywhere. Yes, it can be a scary scene, but don't worry, you won't bleed out; a little pressure on the ear will stop the bleeding.

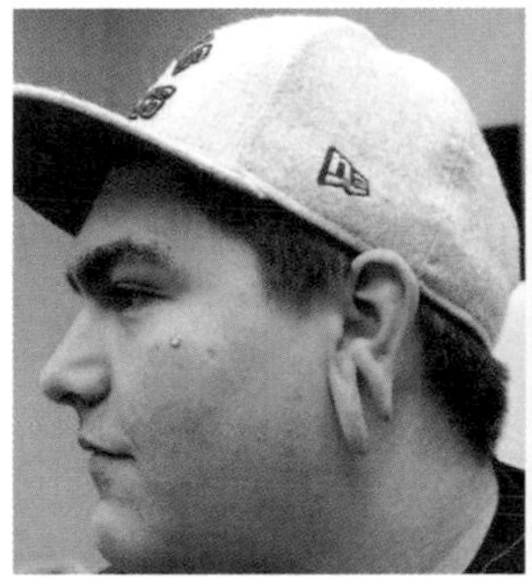

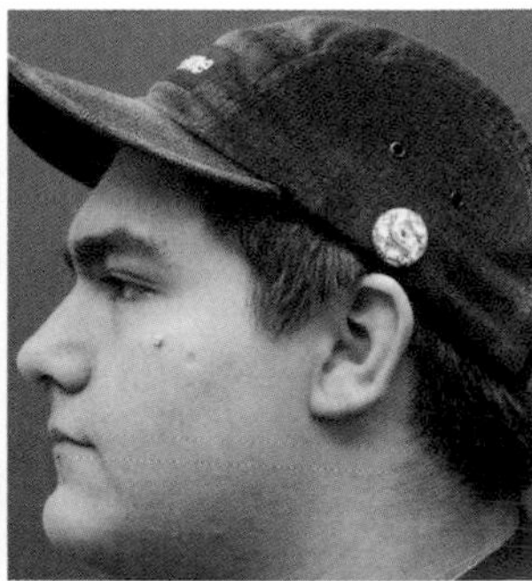

A stretched and torn earlobe before and after repair.

Women who have a history of wearing large, heavy earrings also come in to have their earlobes "tightened"—maybe the earring hole is not torn but has been stretched over time, and often the earlobe gets thinner and sags more as we age.

If you're older and feel like your earlobes have just lost volume and have more wrinkles or don't seem to support your earrings anymore, leaving your earring studs to point downward, you may want to consider adding a hyaluronic acid filler to your earlobe to make it a little fuller and thicker.

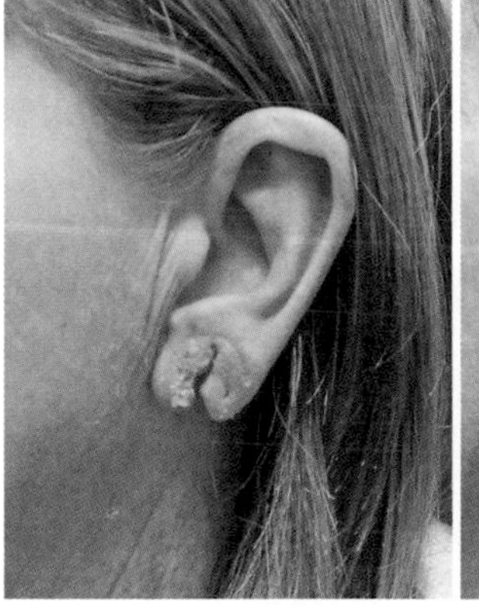

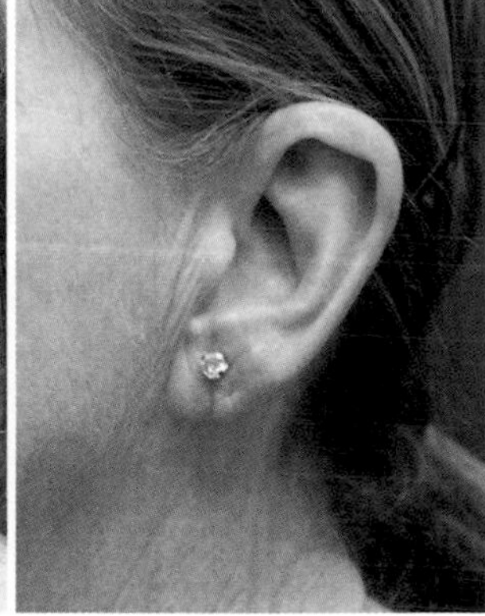

A torn earlobe repaired.

I've also seen an increase in people seeking closure of earlobes that have been stretched by gauges, which dilate the earlobe to create a hole of increasing size. This is still a popular trend but it seems to be on a decline (though this is just my opinion). In this case, people with really stretched lobes may want them closed up because they are perhaps finding it hard to secure certain jobs, are maybe just tired of explaining their lobes to their friends, acquaintances, and loved ones, or have merely grown tired of the way they look.

Sometimes people just don't like their earlobes they were born with. They think they are too big (in my opinion, a big earlobe is good luck; I have big earlobes). But as with most cosmetic treatments, beauty is indeed in the eye of the beholder.

Earlobe reconstruction takes between fifteen minutes and an hour, depending on the complexity of the surgical repair. Essentially, to close a hole or repair a tear, you have to refresh the edges of skin so that they stick back together again. These are simple surgeries and are usually completed in under an hour using just local anesthesia. Yet for the surgeon they can also be complicated and challenging because they need to make the earlobe look as close in appearance to the original earlobes. If the earlobe has been significantly stretched, the surgeon has to be a bit creative in order to devise a way to stick cut edges back together to look totally natural. I enjoy doing these because they require concentration and creativity, but they almost always take a little longer to do than I anticipate. The procedure is like a little puzzle that needs to be solved in my head before it all comes together, but it always seems to come together in the end.

FACELIFT

A facelift (rhytidectomy) is a surgical procedure that corrects the signs of aging on the face by essentially tightening the muscles under the skin and then removing any excess skin after this tightening process. In 2016, 131,106 facelifts were performed in the United States, making this the fifth most frequently performed cosmetic surgery. The surgery varies from the minimally invasive "lunchtime lift" or "mini-facelift" to the more extensive full facelift. It can lift heavy brows and correct midface sagging, marionette lines, jowls, and a double chin. I don't perform full facelifts, but I do lower face facelifts, called demi-lifts, mainly lifting and tightening the neck and the jawline.

This surgery can be done under general or local anesthesia, depending on the extensiveness of the procedure, and recovery time can vary as well. While most people feel comfortable going out in public within ten to fourteen days, it will take two to three months for the face to look "back to normal."

NECK LIFT

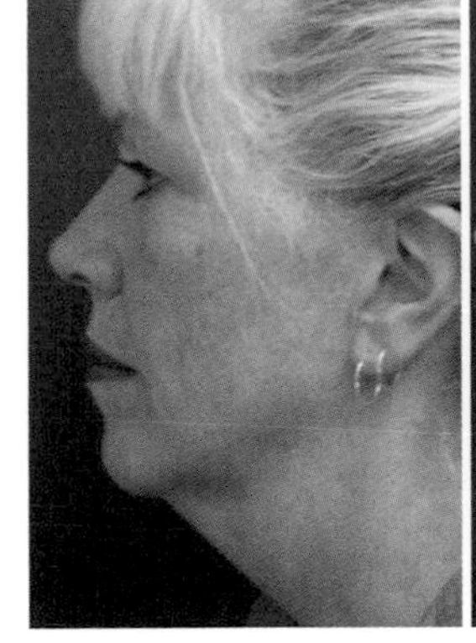
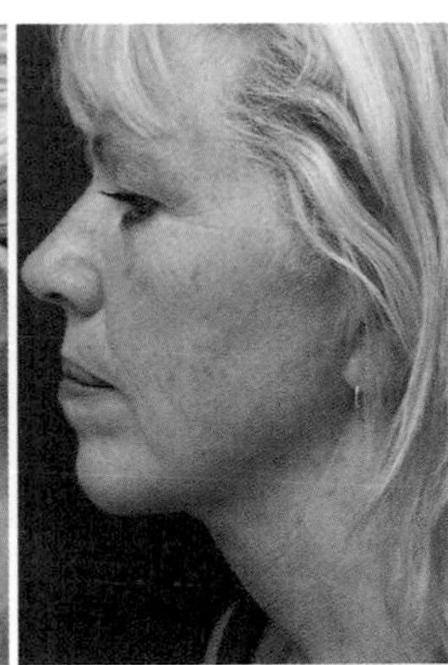

Neck lift before and after.

A neck lift surgically improves signs of aging in the neck and jawline. A neck lift treats the excess sagging fat in the lower face that creates jowls, fatty deposits under the chin (double chin), loose neck skin ("turkey wattle"), and muscle banding. The neck lift incision usually starts in front of the earlobe, wraps around behind the ear, and ends in the posterior hair behind the ear.

Surgeons often perform two procedures during neck lifts:

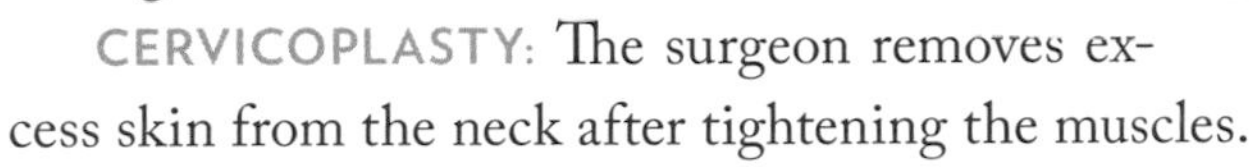

CERVICOPLASTY: The surgeon removes excess skin from the neck after tightening the muscles.

PLATYSMAPLASTY: This word means "reconstruction of the neck muscles." The surgeon reduces neck folds by removing, tightening, or realigning the neck muscles, especially those underneath the chin, by winding the suture along and cinching the muscles tighter together, kind of like how corset lacing works. People can generally resume their daily activities, including returning to work, within two weeks after their neck surgery.

EYELIFT

Eyelift surgery corrects wrinkles, sagging skin, and puffiness around the upper and lower eyelids. This surgery also corrects sagging eyelid skin that obstructs the ability to see. In 2016, there were 209,020 eyelift procedures; this is an increase of 2 percent from 2015.

Upper eyelid surgery helps to remove sagging excess skin and to restore a naturally youthful shape to the eyelids and a more open, refreshed appearance to the

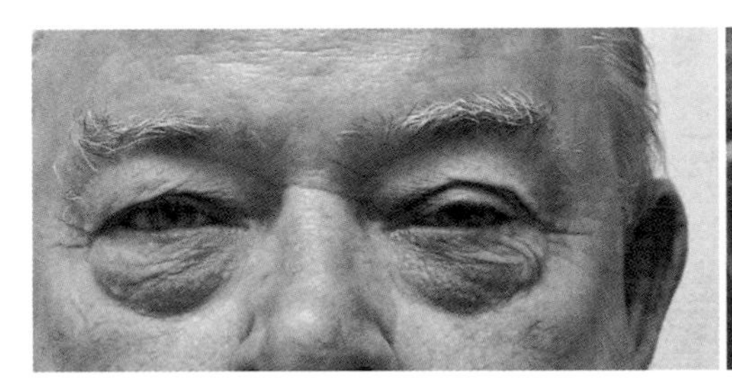
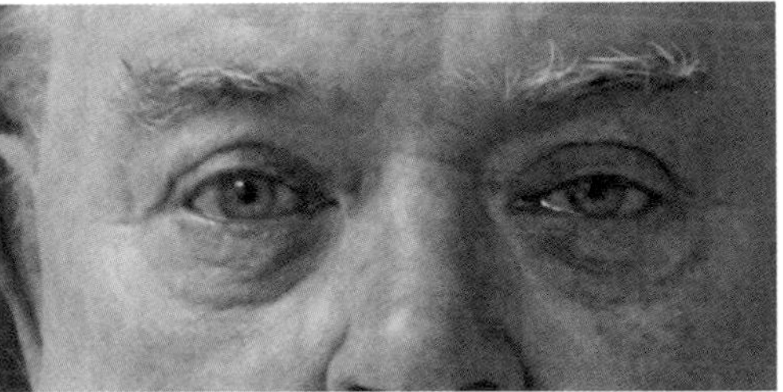

Upper and lower eyelift.

eyes. A surgeon makes an incision in the crease above the eye, then removes excess skin and fat and/or adjusts the surrounding muscles.

Lower eyelid surgery corrects puffy, sagging bags under the eye, which are caused by fat that collects beneath the eyes and protrudes up from the skin's surface. Through incisions made on the inner portion of your lower eyelid, or on the outside just below your lash line, your cosmetic surgeon removes fat and excess skin and tightens muscles to create a smooth look.

TRUE TUMESCENT LIPOSUCTION

Liposuction removes excess body fat with special surgical equipment that suctions out the fat. It can contour anywhere that you have excess fat that is above muscle, including the chin, neck, cheeks, upper arms, breasts, abdomen, buttocks, hips, thighs, knees, calves, and ankle areas.

Remember, liposuction is *not* a weight loss procedure; it is a body sculpting procedure. It is ideal for individuals who maintain their weight at a steady level and don't yo-yo dramatically in weight. This includes healthy adults within 30 percent of their ideal weight who also have firm, elastic skin and good muscle tone, and who are nonsmokers without a life-threatening illness or medical conditions that can impair healing. Positive people with specific goals in mind for body contouring are also good candidates. The patients who get the best results and the most out of this procedure are those who have a trouble area that is genetic, like a family propensity to develop saddle bags, or "cankles," or a double chin. These areas of fat are usually the first areas to increase in size if you gain fat and the last areas to decrease in size if you diet and lose weight. Or else the fat just won't budge from that area no matter what you do.

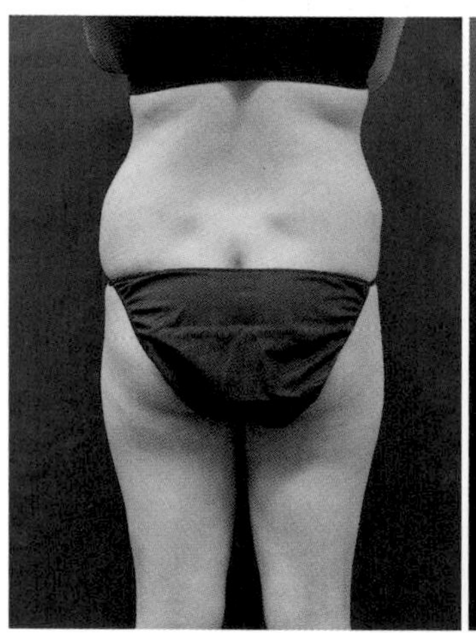

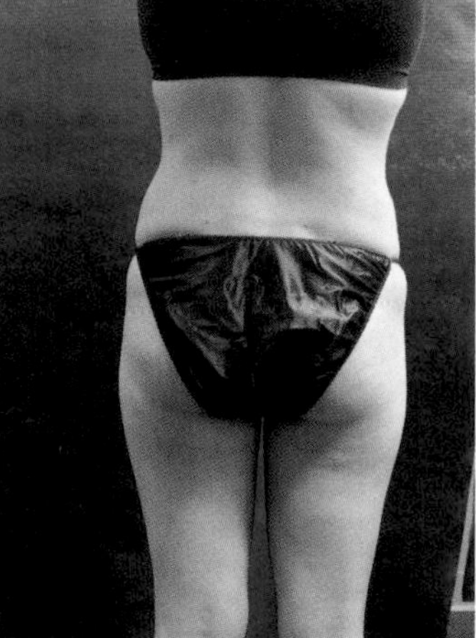

True tumescent liposuction of the hips.

Liposuction changes your contours and shape. It is a time-consuming procedure for me to perform, and sometimes it's a workout for *me* to do this procedure, but I would never give it up in my medical practice because it is just too rewarding for the patients and this makes all the hard work worth it.

Many people criticize liposuction and make people who are interested in it feel guilty or embarrassed about considering this type of procedure. They say things such as: "Why don't you just eat better and exercise?! You'll be able to do the same thing!" Well, in my opinion, that's incorrect. Tumescent liposuction is specific, targeted fat loss, focusing on areas that are genetically predetermined to hold more fat cells, and that really cannot be removed without a surgery like this. In other words, no healthy diet and exercise program can rid someone of the cankles that run in their family. But liposuction can.

Tumescent liposuction is the most common type of liposuction and is carried out even by surgeons who work with general anesthesia. But we dermatologic surgeons who do "true tumescence" don't use general anesthesia at all. Instead, we rely on the tumescence, or swelling created with numbing fluid, itself to provide local anesthesia. Before fat removal, a surgeon infiltrates a large amount of medicated solution into an area. The fluid is a mixture of local anesthetic (lidocaine) and a drug that contracts the blood vessels (epinephrine, to reduce blood loss, bruising, and swelling), diluted in normal saline, which is a salt solution. This numbs the area and makes it easier to suction out the fat. The surgeon suctions out this salt solution and the fat simultaneously. Remember, I do this procedure under local anesthesia, so my patients are awake. Sometimes they may take some medications that relax them, but for the most part they are alert and comfortable, joining in on our conversations in the operating room as we remove their fat.

Your surgeon will likely have you wear a compression garment or elastic bandages over treated areas to control swelling and contour the skin to your new shape. I have my patients wear their special garments for one week only, but some docs may have you wear them for longer. The very next day after your surgery, you will see the amazing results (my favorite part of the procedure), but then as you heal, the area will swell a little and may be bruised. Your swelling and fluid retention

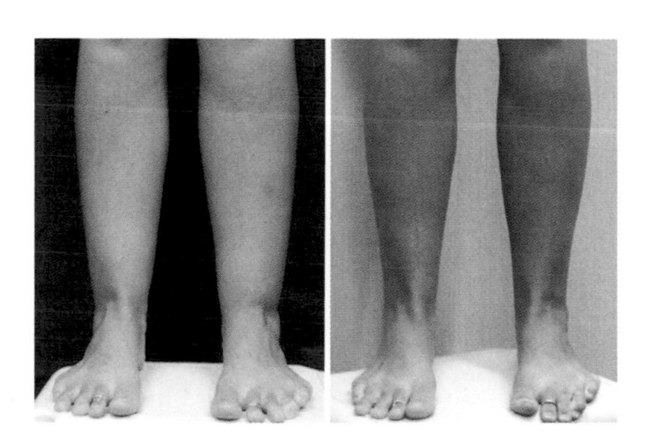

Liposuction under local anesthesia to the calves and ankles.

will go down over the next few months. Make sure to handle the surgical incisions with care and to follow your surgeon's instructions. The results should be long lasting as long as you generally stay fit and maintain a steady weight.

Fat Chance

There are other noninvasive methods to minimize fat in focused areas. Some were popular for a season and didn't really work, and the attention petered out, while others have been advertised widely, and there seem to be some benefits. CoolSculpting is one current favorite, using cooling of the fat to eliminate it. However, liposuction remains the superior procedure to remove fat permanently. You can also "recycle" the fat that was removed and place it back into your body in other areas, most popularly into concave scars from previous surgeries or procedures, to fill in lines and grooves in the face (instead of fillers), add more fullness to the breasts, and the currently trendy BBL (Brazilian butt lift).

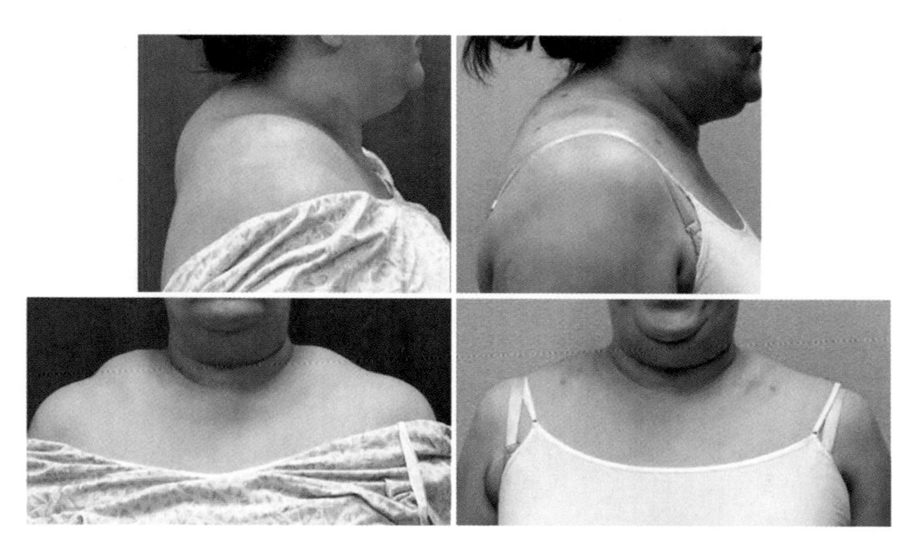

Liposuction of the upper back and shoulders.

Liposuction Is Not a License to Eat

There is misinformation out there that if you get liposuction you are destined to gain that weight back and probably more. Well, let me explain why this can happen, and it goes back to the fact that liposuction is *not* really a weight loss procedure. Think of weight loss as an added benefit to this procedure, not the primary reason for it. We all have a general set weight that our body sticks with and gravitates toward, and unfortunately most of us generally pack on a couple of extra pounds every couple of years as we age. If you overeat and don't exercise regularly, this means you will retain more fat on your body. If you have liposuction to get rid of that spare tire around your midriff or those love handles near your hips and you gain weight after such a procedure you *are* less likely to gain this weight back *where you have had liposuction,* because this procedure has permanently removed fat cells from that area of your body. But, as always, if you gain weight, this weight has to come back somewhere! Remember, liposuction does not give you the ability to overeat.

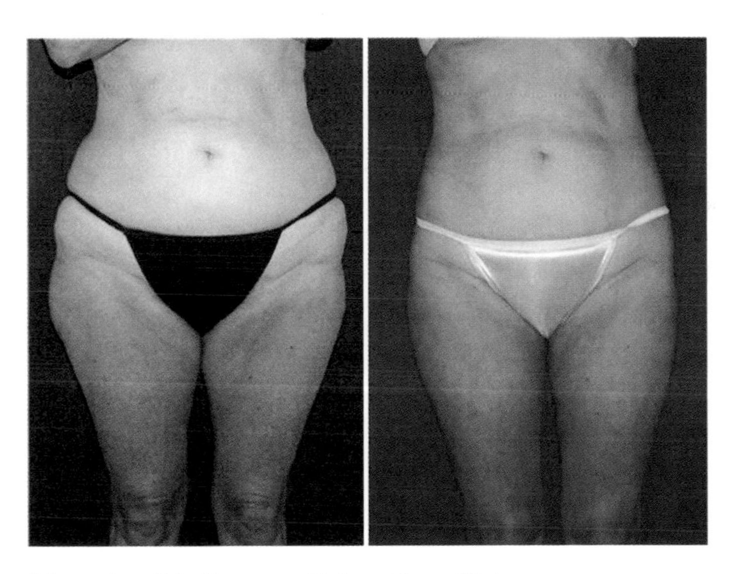

Liposuction of the hips, outer thigh, and inner thigh.

MINIMALLY INVASIVE PROCEDURES

Let's talk about some of the minimally invasive procedures that we do as cosmetic dermatologists and surgeons. By definition, these are office-based procedures that have little to no downtime and include things we've discussed previously in the book, such as wrinkle treatment injections like Botox and hyaluronic acid fillers, chemical peels, and laser and light treatments.

These procedures have gained in popularity because they are available at lower costs and due to the ease of the procedures themselves relative to their surgical counterparts. Still, that doesn't mean that providers shouldn't have the same expertise or rigorous training as board-certified surgeons. As consumers, we must check out the credentials of a potential provider before undergoing any procedure to make sure we're under the care of a highly trained, experienced, and qualified expert. Even though these procedures aren't actual surgeries, we still need to take them seriously. There can certainly be adverse effects with all of these procedures that can leave you with permanent changes to your body and skin that you may not want or didn't expect.

Below is a roundup of the most common minimally invasive procedures available that I haven't discussed yet, what they do, who they can help, and how long the results last.

LASER HAIR REMOVAL

Laser hair removal involves using a laser to permanently remove hair. The pigment or color in your hair follicles absorbs the wavelength emitted by the laser, and this obliterates the pigment (and therefore the hair). Burns, scars, and changes in skin color are potential unwanted side effects that can result from laser hair removal, so the American Academy of Dermatology recommends choosing a board-certified dermatologist to perform laser treatments. Keep in mind that it is best *not* to wax or pluck your hairs before treatment, since you need at least the root of the hair to still be present if you want the laser to target it and destroy it. To prepare for treatment, shave your hair closely instead. Also avoid sun exposure and tanning for six weeks before treatment.

The ideal candidate for laser hair removal is someone who has pale skin and dark, coarse hair. This is because the laser wavelength targets *color,* not the hair itself. The laser doesn't actually know it's treating hair per se, but different wavelengths target different colors in the ultraviolet spectrum (you know, the colors of the rainbow). The lasers we use in laser hair removal target the darker colors of the spectrum, as close to black as you can get!

Unwanted effects like burns and scars to the skin happen because the skin is too close in color to the hair you're trying to target and/or the laser power is dialed up too high—remember, the laser doesn't know whether it's treating hair or not, so if the power is up too high and the laser detects and targets the color in your skin, this leads to a burn, which can possibly lead to permanent scarring or lightening of the skin.

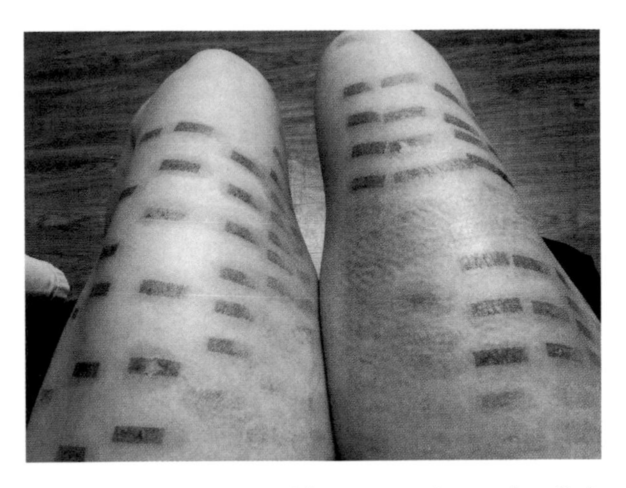

Burns from laser hair removal (patient treated at another office).

After the first treatment, people see a 10 percent to 25 percent reduction in hair. Most patients need between two and seven treatments to remove all of the unwanted hair. Each treatment should be spaced four to six weeks apart. Results last for several months or years. If some hair regrows, it tends to be thinner, finer, and lighter. Treatment can be time consuming depending on the area you want covered. It's quicker to treat armpit hair than it is to treat all the hair on your back, for example. If your skin color is closer to the color of your hair, the laser energy will need to be dialed down to avoid burns. This means more treatments at lower energy to get the desired effect.

TATTOO REMOVAL

Roughly 40 percent of Americans ages twenty-five to forty have a tattoo, and this has certainly been on the increase. Interestingly, as many as 17 percent of people who bear a tattoo say they regret their decision to get one. More than 10 percent have or will get them removed. Tattoo removal involves the use of lasers that break up the tattoo's pigment with a high-intensity wavelength beam. The age, size, color, and depth of the tattoo dictates the number of treatments and the technique needed to remove it.

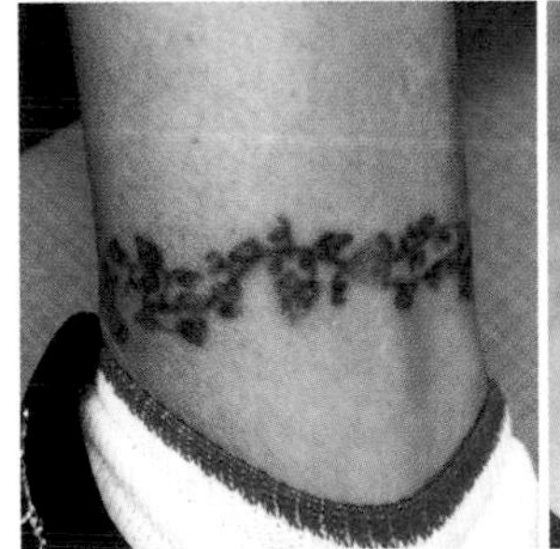

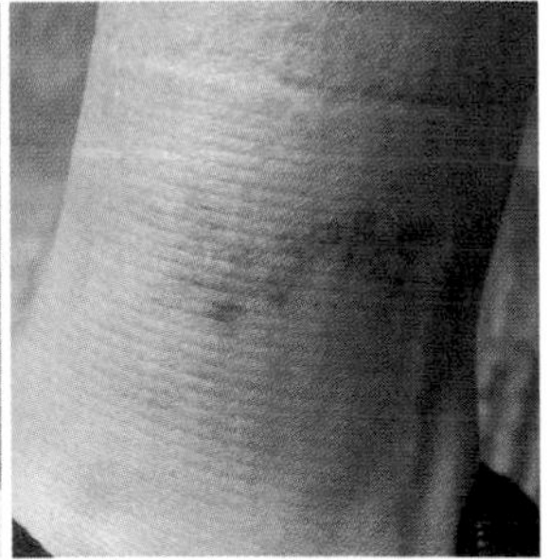

Tattoo removal with residual pigment.

A laser tattoo removal session is a simple three-step process:

1. You will wear a pair of protective eye shields.
2. The doctor or care provider tests your skin's reaction to the laser to determine the best energy level for treatment.
3. A laser passes pulses of intense light through the top layers of your skin that are absorbed only by the tattoo pigment.

Because laser tattoo removal depends on a person's immune system to eliminate broken-down ink particles, the most successful laser tattoo removal is performed on the healthiest people. Tattoo removal from those with fair skin is faster and easier than from those with dark skin because there is a greater difference between the tattoo ink pigments and the skin. More caution and time is taken on dark skin to make sure that the skin surrounding the tattoo doesn't lighten or darken.

Keep in mind that most tattoos won't be removed completely, especially if they are professional tattoos and have a lot of colors and an intricate design. Each session removes the tattoo bit by bit, and every tattoo removal requires several sessions. Sometimes different lasers are needed to target different tattoo pigments better. Some colors such as green are more difficult to treat and often won't disappear completely.

CHEMICAL PEEL

This is the procedure dermatologists use to improve the way your skin looks by removing the most superficial, outermost layers of the skin in a controlled manner. A chemical solution applied to the face, neck, or hands causes skin to exfoliate, sometimes even to blister and peel off depending on the strength and depth of the peel. The goal is to leave you with new, regenerated skin that has a smoother look and feel, and a more even tone. The new skin will be more sensitive to the sun, so be sure to wear sunscreen. Peels work well for people who have acne, scars, sun damage, wisdom and liver spots, fine lines and wrinkles, uneven skin tone, freckles, and rough skin.

There are in general three levels of chemical peels: light, medium, and heavy. Light peels can be done by estheticians (nonphysicians) in general, but the rules vary from state to state and country to country. Medium and heavy peels are usually performed by physicians, and, in fact, heavy peels are sometimes done under local or even general anesthesia. The deeper the peel, the longer the recovery time and the higher the risk of side effects, but also the greater the improvement to the skin.

Three types of chemical peels treat different levels of skin issues:

SUPERFICIAL (LUNCHTIME) PEEL: A low percentage strength of acid (such as a single or combination of alpha hydroxy acid and beta hydroxy acid) is applied to the outer layer of skin (epidermis), which gently exfoliates it, getting rid of the superficial dry, dull, and dead skin to refresh and rejuvenate the face, neck, hands, or chest. This peel also improves mild skin discoloration and rough skin. Minor side effects include stinging, red skin, irritation, and local skin allergic reaction. Hyperpigmentation and infection can happen too, but these risks tend to be low and increase with the increased depth of the peel, and this type of peel is the mildest, most superficial type. Apply topical creams or lotions as recommended by your provider during the healing process, which may be minimal or take up to one week. Use sunscreen daily.

MEDIUM PEEL: A higher percentage of glycolic acid and/or up to 35 percent trichloroacetic (TCA) acid is applied, which penetrates the middle (dermis) and outer layers of skin to remove damaged skin cells. This peel is more effective at improving age/wisdom spots, fine lines, wrinkles, freckles, acne scars, and moderate skin discoloration. In addition, it treats some precancerous skin growths such as actinic keratosis. The medium peel heals in one to two weeks. The skin may redden, swell, and blister for the first forty-eight hours and you can have social downtime of about a week or so. Avoid sun exposure until healing is complete, and then continue to avoid sun exposure! You don't want to just reverse all the hard work of the chemical peel. Results last several months to even years.

DEEP PEEL: This deepest peel provides the most noticeable results but has the longest recovery. It is usually done with a high percentage of TCA, or another chemical called phenol. Phenol penetrates through to the middle layer of skin to remove damaged skin cells. The treatment is designed as a onetime treatment because it is pretty aggressive; it removes moderate lines, dark spots (including freckles), and moderate scars. Essentially, it's getting to the very edge of safely removing the thickest amount of skin without causing permanent scarring or changes in pigmentation. A bandage usually covers the targeted skin during the one- to two-week healing process.

Higher maintenance is needed for the skin after a deep chemical peel, so follow your doctor's postoperative instructions closely. Often, skin must be soaked multiple times daily. Ointment has to be applied daily for the first two weeks after treatment to prevent drying out and scabbing. Your dermatologist will frequently prescribe antiviral medication to prevent a cold sore breakout, and will sometimes also prescribe antibacterial and antifungal medications to avoid local skin infections. Protect your skin from sun exposure for three to six months after treatment. Although greater care and longer downtime are needed for a deep chemical peel, patients will see a dramatic improvement in skin appearance. Results last up to a year or more.

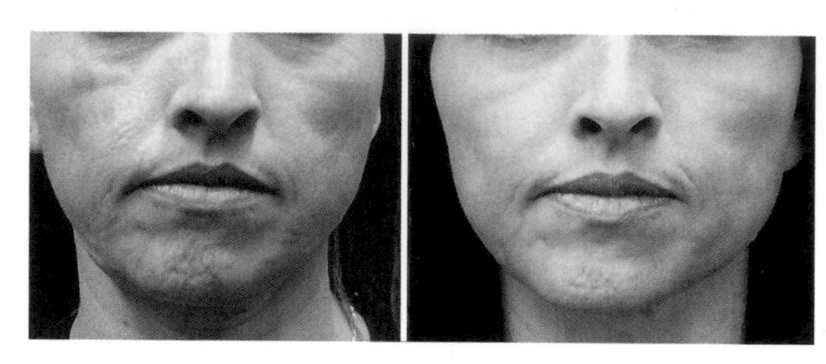

Fractionated CO_2 laser treatment for brown spots and fine lines.

CO_2 LASER RESURFACING

CO_2 lasers treat numerous skin conditions. These lasers deliver very short, pulsed light energy to remove thin layers of skin. Fractional CO_2 and erbium lasers treat a "fraction" of the skin's surface, thereby getting very close to the same effectiveness as the traditional lasers but with less risk of side effects, and more patient comfort and tolerability.

ERBIUM LASER RESURFACING

This laser treats superficial and moderately deep lines and wrinkles on the face, neck, chest, or hands. It does not treat as deeply as a CO_2 laser can.

NONABLATIVE LASER RESURFACING TREATMENTS

Fractional lasers use heat to deliver thousands of tiny, deep columns known as microthermal treatment zones through the skin (ablative methods actually remove the outer layer of the skin). Old epidermal pigmented cells are eliminated, and the heat tightens skin and stimulates collagen growth. Treating only a fraction of the skin, sometimes as little as 5 percent but often closer to 20 to 60 percent, at any one time allows for quicker recovery, shorter healing time, and less discomfort and pain, and potentially avoids many adverse effects, such as permanent unwanted scarring or changes in pigmentation.

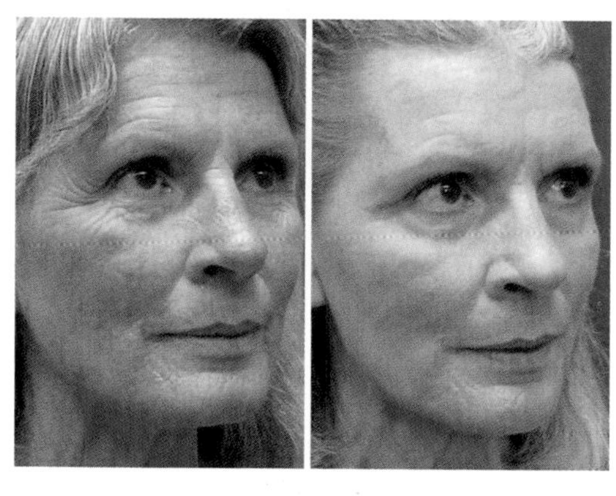

Heavy fractionated CO_2 treatment for fine lines and wrinkles.

In laser skin resurfacing, the surrounding tissue is unaffected, and the skin heals much faster than if the entire area was treated. Treatment usually takes less than one hour, and recovery time is usually under a week. In some cases, multiple sessions are needed depending on the laser used, the depth of treatment, and the reasons for treatment.

MICRODERMABRASION

Microdermabrasion is considered a spa treatment, often done by estheticians along with facials and superficial chemical peels. It should be a painless procedure that treats superficial skin issues. A special machine gently sprays fine particles of sand on the skin of the face, chest, or hands to gently abrade and remove the uppermost layer of dead skin, then sucks this dead skin and sand up and away to discard. This treatment is safe for all skin types and shades, with only minor risks such as infection and skin irritation. Microdermabrasion recovery time is minimal but results for the large part are temporary. Dramatic changes to your skin will not be seen with this type of treatment, but it is still a great treatment option, and people who do this on a regular basis over time do keep their skin in great shape.

DERMABRASION/DERMAPLANING

Dermabrasion and dermaplaning are methods that resurface the outer layers of skin by using a rapidly rotating device much like an electric rotary tool is used to sand down the surface of wood. If used by an experienced physician in a controlled manner, treatment can lead to "new" skin that is smoother; more even in texture, tone, and pigment; and younger looking. Fine lines and scars can be diminished with dermabrasion. Your provider will numb your skin with a local anesthetic. It's also possible to take a sedative or even have general anesthesia administered if the extent of your treatment requires it.

People of all ages can benefit from dermabrasion. Important factors are your skin type, coloring, and medical history. Black, Asian, and other dark-skinned people are not the best candidates for this procedure because dark skin can be permanently discolored or blotchy after treatment. People who have a history of cold sores may experience a flare-up after treatment. Freckles could disappear in the treated area. Keep in mind if you have active acne or a very bad sunburn, or if you have had a chemical peel in the past, many practitioners will decline this service.

This procedure has become less popular because of the availability of lasers, which can do the same thing and are less operator dependent. Also, dermabrasion is a messy procedure; a full splash guard is usually used, since it can be bloody.

After dermabrasion, you will notice some swelling and redness in the treated areas. Depending on the individual, this can last a week or more, but sometimes it can last several months. I recommend protecting your skin from the sun for six to twelve months to prevent permanent changes in skin color. You can see dermabrasion results for a fairly long time, perhaps many years, but they aren't permanent because the face continues its natural aging process. New sun damage can reverse results.

TISSUE TIGHTENING DEVICES AND CELLULITE REDUCTION MACHINES

Skin tightening can help the skin on your body look more youthful, smoother, and less bumpy overall. To accomplish this, radiofrequency devices use energy to heat the tissue beneath the surface of the skin, resulting in some shrinkage of the tissue treated, which can translate into visible tightening of the skin itself. These devices are used to try to tighten droopy, saggy, loose skin, such as that seen on the jowls and the neck, and even the eyebrows, arms, legs, breasts, and buttocks. Ultrasound technology can also be used to bypass disruption of the skin's surface and instead work under the skin, causing "thermal injury" to stimulate new collagen production and even destroy fat cells. There are many types of ultrasound devices on the market to rejuvenate the skin without affecting the skin's surface, and because of this, they may be safer for those with darker skin tones.

For cellulite, there are machines that try to break up the fibrous bands that cause the dimpling that we detest (for example, Cellfina), and there are massaging machines and machines that heat up the skin, cool the skin, introduce microcurrent—the list goes on, all to try to tap into the beauty industry and rid you of your cellulite. However, that's not so easy to do, and no one device is exceptionally effective. In the case of cosmetic procedures such as this, if it sounds too much like a good thing, it's probably not a very good thing.

THIS IS NOT A COMPLETE AND COMPREHENSIVE LIST OF ALL THE WAYS TO SLOW down the aging process and make us happier with the skin we're in. And I don't think it could ever be complete, since there are new devices, new techniques, and new ideas being developed all the time. Anti-aging is a multibillion-dollar business, and this is why many businesses and companies have their hands in it, seeking to profit from our desire to look healthy and younger and feel good about ourselves. I believe it is done with great intentions, but unfortunately many times promises cannot be fulfilled.

How do you know what to spend your hard-earned money on? We all want something that has little to no downtime, is very cost manageable, and produces dramatic but natural results. My best advice to you is to eat healthy, get your exercise, have hobbies that give you enjoyment and satisfaction, surround yourself with family and friends who love you as you love them and who make you happy and encourage your self-confidence and self-worth, and . . . use your sunscreen!

Anti-aging treatment is truly an inexact science. Do your research, look on the internet for as much information as you can, interview multiple doctors to get the most opinions you can, and don't be one of the first in line to try a brand-new treatment modality. Wait a couple of years for the kinks to be ironed out, and either it will be a great treatment option that may yield impressive results, or it will be unsuccessful and become obsolete in the coming years. The good thing about all of this is that technology continues to progress, and amazing new and effective discoveries continue to be made.

In regard to the many advertisements that tell you this treatment will shrink your pores, this other device will take you down three dress sizes overnight, another treatment will erase all your signs of aging in a single instant treatment—well, please look upon these things with a skeptical eye. There *are* amazing treatments out there, but there are more that promise you the world and can't deliver.

BODY DYSMORPHIC DISORDER

I was twelve years old in seventh grade science class, and there was a boy I had a serious crush on. It turned out he had a crush on me too, and maybe this was why he said some words that truly crushed me: "Why do you have a pie face?" He was joking, I suppose, and my face was pretty round and, yes, I don't have much of a nasal bridge. Nowadays I joke that I don't really have a nose, just two holes in my face (it's a joke that I make of myself!). But his comment devastated me. I remember it to this day, though there's a 100 percent chance that *he* doesn't remember that he said it.

The point here is that something you might say to another person thinking that it's tongue in cheek or just an off-the-cuff observation can be felt deeply and burn a hole in another person's memory, and actually be a source of self-doubt and self-consciousness that the other person will carry throughout their life. And this is something I think physicians in particular should be conscious of when we speak to our patients, especially those coming to us asking for our help because they want to look better and feel better about themselves.

You probably feel self-conscious about a certain part of your body—some of us don't like our ears or our nose, or we wish our muscles were different or our thighs were smaller. Unfortunately for some people, worry over their body's imperfections affects them all day, every day. This condition is called body dysmorphic disorder, or BDD for short. When people have BDD, they obsess over perceived flaws in their bodies, often for several hours a day, every day. That's because they find it impossible to control the self-hating thoughts that are constantly running through their minds, and this causes extreme emotional distress. Even when people tell them they look fine, they won't believe them. BDD interferes with people's daily lives—they can't get themselves to work or school, they won't go out with friends or see their family, and they isolate themselves because they're worried other people will notice their imperfections. In extreme cases, they'll even undergo surgery and cosmetic procedures to "fix" these flaws, but they will never find happiness in the results.

BDD affects people of all ages, races, and genders, but the American Psychiatric Association has identified that BDD most often develops in adolescents and teens, usually around the ages of twelve or thirteen, and research shows that it affects men and women almost equally. In the United States, BDD occurs in about 2.5 percent of males, and in 2.2 percent of females. What causes BDD is unclear, but both biological and environmental factors can contribute. The biological factors include genetic predisposition, neurobiological factors (like the malfunctioning of serotonin in our brains), or personality traits; the environmental ones are usually life experiences, such as bullying, abuse, or trauma.[2]

BDD episodes and thoughts can last for a few hours or an entire day, and people with the disorder are often obsessed with their body's muscle mass or definition. They may have suicidal thoughts and/or develop compulsive, repetitive behaviors that help them deal with their BDD. Some examples of those behaviors include camouflaging their body (with clothing, makeup, hair, hats, and so on), seeking surgery, constantly checking *or* avoiding mirrors, skin picking, excessive grooming, excessive exercise, or changing clothes numerous times a day.

If you know anything about eating disorders (anorexia or bulimia are two of the most common), you may wonder if BDD and eating disorders are the same. A study from the Department of Psychiatry and Human Behavior at Brown Medical School and the Butler Hospital, in Providence, Rhode Island, looked at exactly that and determined that there are some important differences. The study does note that even though anorexia and BDD should be differentiated clinically, "these disorders overlap in intriguing ways, and in some cases are hard to differentiate. When BDD and anorexia co-occur, it's important to diagnose both of them because women with both disorders are, it appears, more severely ill than those with anorexia alone."[3]

In fact, when people have BDD, it's not just eating disorders that they may suffer from simultaneously—they could also have depression, anxiety, social anxiety, and/or obsessive-compulsive disorder (OCD). In some cases, people who are suffering from BDD can be misdiagnosed as having one of these other mental conditions because the symptoms can be so similar. According to the Anxiety and Depression Association of America, an international organization that works to better the lives of people living with certain mental disorders, "The intrusive thoughts and repetitive behaviors exhibited in BDD are similar to the obsessions and compulsions of OCD. Avoiding social situations is similar to the behavior of some people with social anxiety disorder."[4]

For some people, BDD can also coincide with a body-focused repetitive behavior (BFRB). This is an umbrella term for a behavior that causes people to repeatedly touch, pull, or pick at their skin or hair, sometimes causing themselves physical harm. The most common types of BFRB are hair pulling disorder (trichotillomania), skin picking disorder (excoriation disorder), and nail biting (onychophagia). Some people confuse their habit or "need" to pick their pimples or scabs as BFRB, but those with BFRB have a serious disorder and compulsion. I have heard from lots of popaholics that BFRBs affect many of you, and that's part of the reason this issue is so important to me.

WHY DO PEOPLE GET BDD?

As awareness about BDD continues to increase, researchers are beginning to study *why* people feel so compelled to hate, and change, their appearance. Both BDD and BFRB are multifaceted and can occur for a huge range of reasons. For some, these disorders coexist; for others, they're entirely separate. That said, studies over the last few decades have proven that for those with BDD specifically, their disorder is rooted in poor body image.

I found it very interesting that half of adults who seek plastic surgery report a history of bullying. A May 2017 study showed that teenagers who were involved in bullying—both those who were bullied and those who *were bullying*—were more likely to seek cosmetic surgery to change their appearance. The study explains that bullied teens have "poor psychological functioning," which can lead to an increased desire to seek plastic surgery—a desire that turns out to be long lasting. Those who do the bullying seek cosmetic surgery in order to look better and therefore become more popular and gain social dominance.[5]

This study also showed that girls, older teens, and those in low education households are more interested in plastic surgery. There are a lot of ways to help this population increase their self-esteem—more research suggests that cosmetic and plastic surgeons can (and should!) increase psychological testing and screen for a history of bullying in teenagers and adults before they accept potential patients. Of course, providing mental health for adolescents involved in bullying can certainly help to decrease the desire to seek cosmetic surgery in the first place.

THE IMPORTANCE OF RAISING AWARENESS ABOUT BDD AND BFRB

Jumping back to BDD *and* BFRB, I think it's very important that we raise awareness about these mental issues and their physical manifestation. That's why I wanted to take the opportunity to voice something to my fans. According to the statistics on my social media, three-quarters of my fans are female, and most of you are between eighteen and thirty-four years old. So this next section is directed to you. Sometimes I wonder: What would I tell my younger self, the Sandra in her twenties? When I think about it, I really wish I could tell my younger self not to be catty to others, not to be so competitive.

I'm not talking about the competitiveness of getting the highest grade on your organic chemistry test, or taking first place in the long jump or the hundred-meter race. I'm talking about supporting and really loving your girlfriends. Build your friends up—remind them of how unique and beautiful they all are. Nobody in this world is perfect, and we all have things about our body we don't love. It's okay to be aware of those flaws, but as a friend, remind your friend that the flaws she may think are a big deal really aren't—you probably don't even notice them!

Unfortunately, your kind words and positivity toward your friends can't fix everything, and sadly there are going to be people who find themselves suffering from BDD or BFRB. And for those people, make sure you support them in the best way possible: Help them get help. Join in #BFRBWeek, a campaign to help end the shame and isolation associated with BFRB. Part of that effort is helping people become aware of what body-focused repetitive behaviors are. It's often held in October, and is an annual event.

That's also why I've included this section here—to spread awareness about these serious mental and physical disorders, to help teach people that skin picking and BDD aren't just myths, they're real issues that people battle every day. Many of my popaholics are touched by these disorders, and I want you to know you're not alone—there are resources available for you, and communities where you don't have to feel embarrassed, isolated, or lonely. I have listed several in the back of this book, on page 259.

Chapter 6

Sack the Lies, Hack the Truth

WHEN PATIENTS OR FRIENDS SAY SOMETHING THAT I BELIEVE TO BE COMpletely false about skin health and care, I often want to take them by their shoulders and shake them. Of course, I wouldn't do that to my dear friends; I just try to explain nicely that no, it's not true that eating pizza gives you pimples or that a base tan will protect you from skin cancer. Ugh! There are *so* many untruths people swear by, and while some could be harmless (so you don't eat much pizza, big deal), others can be dangerous—like convincing people not to protect themselves from exposure to the sun. In this section I tackle the big lies that are pervasive and passed from generation to generation, like a good urban legend or scary ghost story. Only this is about real life, so it's important to set the record straight. Ask yourself, are you *speaking truths* or just *popping off* when you talk about your skin? Once you know fact from fiction, tune in to some of my favorite easy skin hacks and fun facts that are interspersed in sidebars through this section.

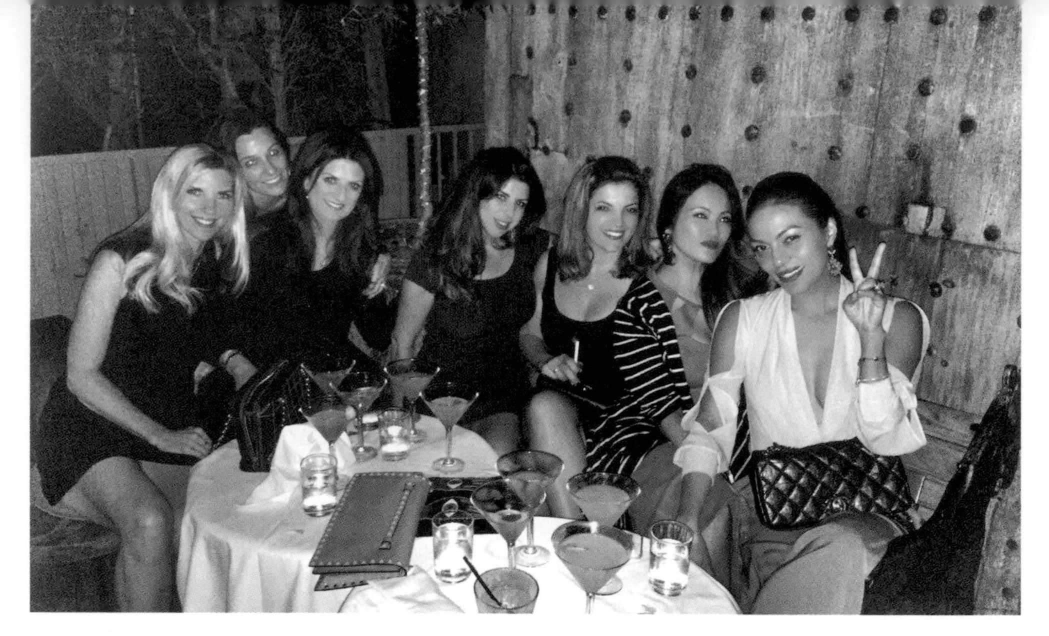

My clique bonding over drinks and wonderful conversation.

Your hair will grow longer much more quickly if you cut it often.
FALSE

I have the *most* wonderful girlfriends, who love me and support me, always raising me up and never breaking me down. Remember this, young women, because that's what life is about! Great friends and great family. Quit the cattiness and hating. When you have a friend who has your back under any and all circumstances, who you know will defend you when you're not around to defend yourself, this means the *world*. However, sometimes I have to bite my tongue when I hear some "truths" that my good friends swear by.

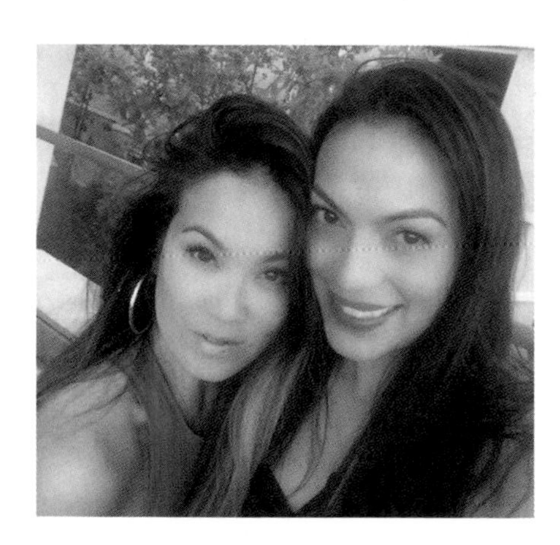

Me and my BFF, Raquel.

It just goes to show that there are many myths out there that perfectly intelligent people believe about our skin, our hair, and our nails. For example, I've overheard my friend tell another that if you cut your hair often, it will grow longer much faster. Sorry to throw you under the bus, bestie, but this is not exactly true. To understand why, let me explain how hair grows. As many of you know, hair and nails are "dead" cells, which is why it doesn't physically pain you to cut them (maybe it just emotionally scars you sometimes). New hair cells are created within the scalp. You know that white/gray bulb you see when you pull out a hair from the root? Well, the bulb is actually where new hair cells are created.

Scalp hair grows an average of half an inch per month, which translates into about six inches a year, but of course this differs somewhat from person to person. So if you have hair that is long enough to brush your shoulders, the hair cells at the tips have likely been by your side for at least a year! (Incidentally, if you are getting a hair sample drug test and they take a lock of your hair clippings from the end, that sample will test what was in your body perhaps a year ago or maybe more!)

So does frequently trimming your hair encourage faster growth? No, your hair would not grow any faster . . . *but* trimming your hair can get rid of split ends or other external damage that your hair has incurred (most commonly from styling products that heat the hair, or strip or weaken it). Split ends are damage to the ends of your hair, and trimming these split ends off will prevent the damage from extending up along the length of your hair shaft toward your scalp. In this way, trimming your hair does at least prevent your hair from getting shorter through breakage, but it has no effect whatsoever on how quickly your hair grows. Besides, if it was true that cutting your hair often leads to faster and thicker regrowth, then I would think that the "prescription" for balding men (and women) would be to cut their hair as often as they can!

DPP Hack: Nailed It!

Do you know that our hair and nails can tell a little story about how we may have lived our most recent months and years, or may give the first indication that you have something unusual going on inside you? Did you have a baby, or have surgery recently? Do you have heart disease or kidney disease? Your hair and nails can provide important and sometimes lifesaving clues. Have you ever noticed a horizontal indentation or white band going across all your fingernails, with the bands seeming to all be at the same position on all of your nails? If you do, you may have a Beau's line. When a dermatologist sees this, they are sneaking a peek into your previous life (insert evil laugh here). In fact, sometimes after I examine a patient's nails, I can accurately predict that they had a significant event in their life recently, such as a surgery, accident, even the birth of a baby, about, oh, let's say, six months ago. Sorcery? Nope, that would be freaky. It's just science. As your hair and nails grow, they can reflect changes going on internally in your body, both physical and emotional, and this can disrupt nail growth, putting a hitch in your nails.

My hair seems to be suddenly falling out! I find a clump of hair covering the drain of my shower. I must be quickly losing all of my hair.

PROBABLY FALSE

First, I need to explain the typical hair growth cycle. There are three phases of hair growth: anagen, catagen, and telogen. Anagen is the growth phase and lasts about three to five years. Catagen is called the involution phase (sort of like the "pause" phase where nothing much goes on), and it lasts about two weeks. It's when the hair follicle shrinks and detaches from its blood supply and moves upward. Telogen is the resting or death phase, which lasts about three to six months. On the scalp at any given moment in time, 80 percent to 90 percent of the hairs are in the anagen phase. Do you know why the hairs that grow on your body don't get as long

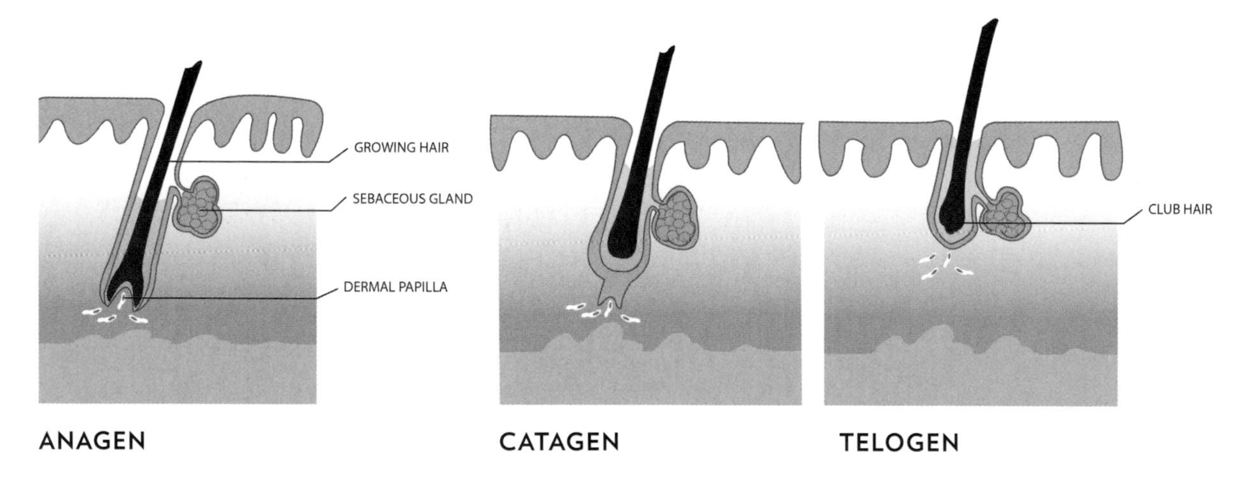

The three stages of hair growth.

as your scalp hair? Well, it's because in these areas the anagen phase is much shorter and the telogen phase is much longer, so hairs stay in place for longer periods of time but don't grow as long.

Hairy Situation

Some people will get hair transplants to other areas, like their eyebrows, and this is a great permanent option if you have thin brows. Just know that you will have to trim those hairs, because those transplanted hairs will still grow as long as they would have where they originated. Imagine: you could have eyebrow hairs that reach your shoulders!

Other animals shed their hair or fur seasonally, and human hair growth is cyclical too, but the difference is that each hair follicle cycles independently. Your hair gets lusher during pregnancy because pregnancy triggers more of the hair to stay in the anagen phase and prolongs the telogen phase as well.

Now getting back to the question: I'm freaking out because I'm noticing that my hair is thinning and there is so much hair in my hairbrush and my shower drain! Is all my hair falling out? This is a question I get often, and honestly, I quietly dread seeing female patients who complain of hair loss because finding the answer is rarely simple. Losing hair, especially in women, can be quite terrifying. I mean, it can be just as difficult for men to endure, but it is more socially acceptable for men to experience hair loss. The reason I dread discussing this issue with women is that it's difficult to give someone a firm diagnosis that they have the equivalent to "balding" in men.

Female pattern androgenic hair loss is what is called a diagnosis of exclusion. In other words, no blood test or skin biopsy can confirm the diagnosis that you may be losing your hair; it's happening just because it's a part of life. It's hard to hear that there may not be an answer to your hair loss. We try to rule out causes that we can treat. We check blood thyroid and ferritin levels because we know that a decrease in either of these may promote a treatable cause of hair loss. Many people try biotin, which can increase the strength of hair and nails. However, this helps only if we have a deficiency in biotin in our diet, and most of us do not.

However, I am pleased and a little relieved when I can tell a woman stressed out about hair loss that it is a temporary phenomenon called telogen effluvium (the medical term for hair loss is alopecia). When a woman comes to my office complaining of hair loss, the first question I ask is "Did you experience a physically or emotionally stressful event about six months ago?" If she says yes, I mentally breathe a little sigh of relief because I can tell her she likely has telogen effluvium. Her hair will grow back!

When we experience something that causes stress to our body, such as childbirth, this triggers more of our hairs than usual to go into the death phase. Okay, you say, then why do we notice hair loss not right after the stressful event but six months later? This is because, yes, your hairs go into the death phase immediately, but the hair doesn't actually fall out until your *new* hairs grow enough to push out the dead hair. The reassuring finding that I point out is: Don't you notice the preponderance of short hairs that stick straight up as they grow from the scalp? Don't you notice these short hairs especially when your hair is wet? Well, those are all the new hairs growing out! If you have more of these then usual, that's a sign that your hair is growing back!

I know I have an allergy to penicillin because I got a rash from it when I was a kid.

FALSE

A study that was recently published made me say under my breath with a mental fist pump, "Yes, that's right! I knew it!" Many of us *don't* have an allergy to penicillin when we think we do! Those of us who have been told we have a penicillin allergy are often foggy about the details that led our doctors or us to this conclusion. My suspicions about this being a myth were confirmed in a new study that found many people are often misdiagnosed with a penicillin allergy. The study confirmed that 90 percent of people who believe they have a penicillin allergy actually do not. This misdiagnosis has a lot to do with the fact that many youngsters are given amoxicillin for an upper respiratory infection and can subsequently develop a rash. This rash is not technically an allergy. When someone tells me they are allergic to penicillin, I will often follow this up with another question: What happened to you when you took penicillin?

DPP Hack: Crack-Up

Isn't it annoying when you get a crack or split in the corner of your lip? This is called *perleche* and it's caused by saliva becoming stuck in the area of skin between your upper lip and its transition to the lower lip. Your lips have a different kind of "skin," called mucous membranes, and it's designed to withstand the acidity of our saliva. But if you continually lick an area of "regular" skin, like the skin between our upper and lower lips, the acidity of our saliva will actually irritate and damage it. The area stings when you eat acidic food and it's difficult for it to heal because every time you open your mouth widely to speak or eat, it cracks open again.

Well, I have a little trick for you. Take a small bottle or tube of cream that is about one inch in diameter and stick it in the corner of your mouth to stretch that area open. Do this at home so you don't get stares from strangers, because you will look a little silly. Walk around like this for thirty minutes or so, allowing the split in the skin to heal in the open, stretched position. To prevent this from happening again, don't let saliva just sit on your skin and keep moisture away from the area. If you tend to drool when you sleep (we have all done this before, don't deny it!), apply a little Vaseline/petroleum jelly to the skin you want to protect before bed.

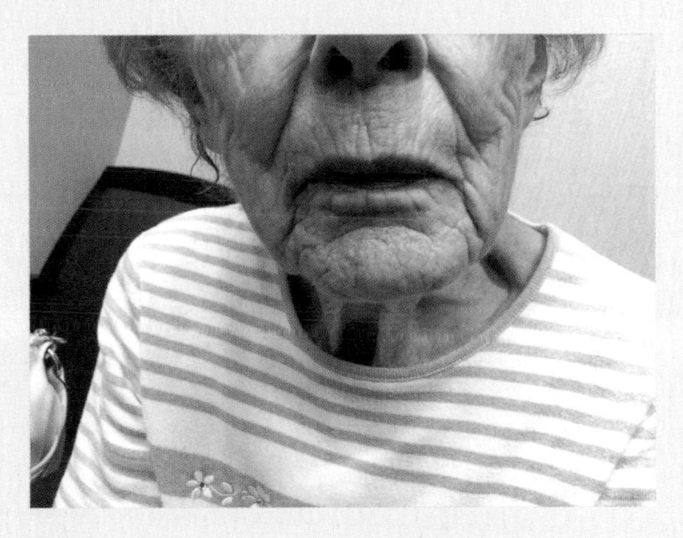

Perleche.

If they say, "I got hives" or "My lips and throat swelled," yes! I will definitely stay away from penicillin. However, if they say, "I got a rash," then I know this is not a true allergy. Penicillin is a great antibiotic with a long record of accomplishment and safety, and people who mistakenly think they are allergic to penicillin are instead opting for other medications that may be reserved for more significant and complicated infections, or that have more side effects and risks. A common solution is a simple two-step test, followed, if needed, by low-dose oral penicillin. The process takes about three hours, and then we can say a patient is free to take penicillin going forward.

I can get rid of my hair permanently with a hair removal laser.
MAYBE

Do you know how a laser that removes hair *really* works? Many people ask about laser hair removal, and it's tantalizing to think you will never have to shave your upper lip, your armpits, or your legs ever again. Remember that the laser doesn't know that it is treating hair; it's really just treating a *color*: the darkest color possible. So if you don't have pale skin and dark hair, laser removal will not permanently remove your hairs. Treatment can temporarily pulverize the hair above the surface of the skin but it won't destroy the entire hair follicle, so ultimately it would be equivalent to a really expensive wax job.

It's Not Easy Being Green

If you want to get a tattoo and guarantee that you will *never* be able to erase it with any laser (at least in the year 2018), be sure to choose the color green. With current laser tattoo removal technology, the color green can't be eliminated completely. So if you want a real commitment from someone, insist that they tattoo your name in green.

You need to wait fifteen to twenty minutes after applying sunscreen before going out in the sun.
FALSE

Have you gotten sunburned despite wearing sunscreen, and decided that this may be because you didn't apply the sunscreen fifteen to thirty minutes before you went out into the sun, as described in the instructions? It's more likely that you needed to apply *more* sunscreen *more* often. This is because that rule is not law, just like the rule that you have to wait fifteen minutes after you eat before you jump into the pool. Are these statements really true? While I'm not certain about getting cramps after eating, I do know where the timing precaution comes from in terms of sunscreen application, and the reason for it may surprise you. When sunscreen studies were first conducted, parameters were put in place to try to eliminate variables and to make the study as accurate as possible. For consistency, they told all participants to apply sunscreen thirty minutes before sun exposure. This helped ensure that the study subjects were actually wearing sunscreen. The timing has *nothing* to do with increasing sunscreen effectiveness. It has everything to do with how they designed the sunscreen studies. Go ahead and apply your sunscreen right before you go out in the sun, and don't worry that you're timing it wrong! You aren't.

You need some daily sun exposure to get enough vitamin D.
FALSE

I hear this myth a lot: that we need "fifteen minutes of unprotected sunshine a day" to make enough vitamin D. First of all, if you live in certain parts of the country, especially northern areas of the United States, you could lay out naked on a sunny January day and still not make enough vitamin D to help you! Plus, you'd get sun damage and frostbite! This myth is so pervasive that the bigwigs at the American Academy of Dermatology have spoken up. They recommend getting vitamin D from a healthy diet that includes foods naturally rich in vitamin D, such as sockeye salmon, herring, sardines, tuna, and eggs; foods/beverages fortified with vitamin D, such as whole grain breads, dairy, and nut milks; and/or vitamin D supplements. The organization definitively states that vitamin D should *not* be obtained from unprotected exposure to ultraviolet (UV) radiation because such exposure, including that from both the sun and indoor tanning devices, is a known risk factor for the development of skin cancer.

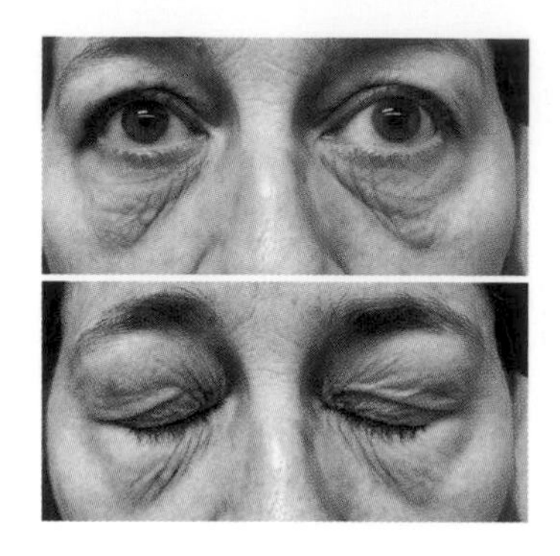

Allergic contact dermatitis around the eyes.

My eyes are red, itchy, and irritated because I am allergic to my makeup, face creams, and so on.

FALSE

When you get an itchy red rash around your eyes, it's a major bummer, isn't it? Your skin flakes from the upper lids and the corner of the eyes and thickens slightly, which accentuates skin lines—in other words, it makes us look older . . . and none of us want that! And we all immediately blame our contact lens solution, or our eye shadow, or our mascara, or something, anything, that we may have put on and around our eyes. Well, do you know that the most common cause of eyelid dermatitis (rash around the eyes) is *acrylic nails*? When we develop an allergic contact dermatitis rash on the eyelids, it's caused most commonly by touching something with our *hands* and inadvertently bringing them up to our eyes. The skin on our hands is thick and less likely to get irritated by something we come in contact with, but the skin around our eyes, which is the thinnest skin on our body, will respond. If you develop an irritating rash around your eyes, don't automatically point the finger at products you put on your eyes, but take a close look at what you touch with your fingers.

A Quick Fix for a Broken Fingernail

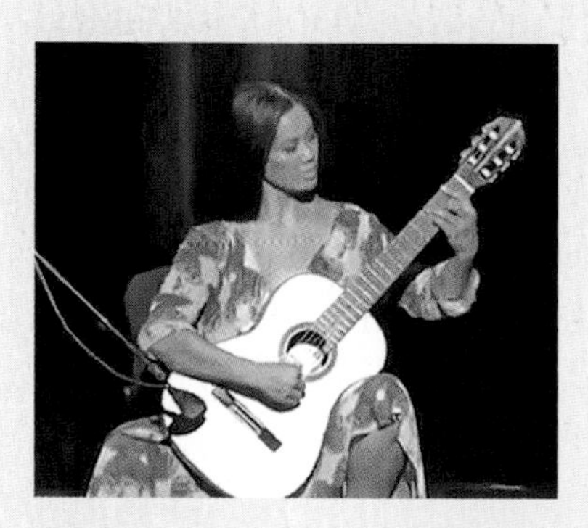

Me plucking the strings of my classical guitar.

I learned this trick not from a manicurist, but from my dear classical guitar teacher, Jack Sanders! If you play classical guitar, you know that you live and die by your fingernails. Your left hand needs fingernails cut very short, and your right hand needs nails smoothed and shaped a particular way so that you can pluck those guitar strings. If you break a nail, it essentially paralyzes your ability to pluck the strings and perform. So this solution is for when you have a nail that has split down within the nail bed, and you can't clip it short to fix it. You have to temporarily bind the nail back together to support the nail as it grows out. All you need is a regular tea bag, superglue, and nail varnish. Tea bag paper is pretty strong, yet thin and sheer. Cut a piece big enough to cover the split in your nail, apply superglue atop it and let it soak in, then place it over the split. Top with nail varnish. That will give that nail some added strength and protect it from snagging and splitting more.

Washing your hair less frequently makes it less flaky.

FALSE

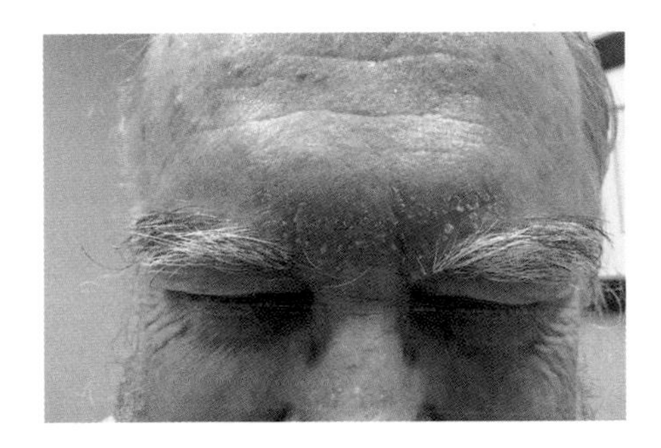

Seborrheic dermatitis (aka dandruff) along and between the eyebrows.

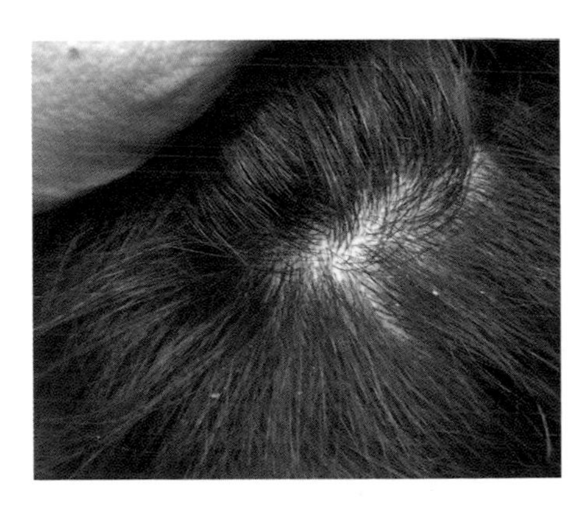

Mild dandruff of the scalp.

Do you have an itchy, scaly scalp? Did you think washing your hair *less* frequently would make this better? Well, this is usually incorrect, but you're not alone in this thinking. This is a common decision people make. They believe that this itchiness and flaking is due to a dry scalp, and that if they wash the hair less, the scalp stays more moisturized and less itchy and scaly. But this is incorrect. Some people also mistakenly believe that they have psoriasis, not the much more common seborrheic dermatitis, aka dandruff. However, psoriasis looks different, usually with really thick white scales/flaking over a red scalp, while seborrheic dermatitis/dandruff is usually a finer, flaky scale overlying a greasy scalp that is only pink or mildly red. People also commonly get seborrheic dermatitis on the ear opening. In addition, seborrheic dermatitis can affect other hair-bearing parts of

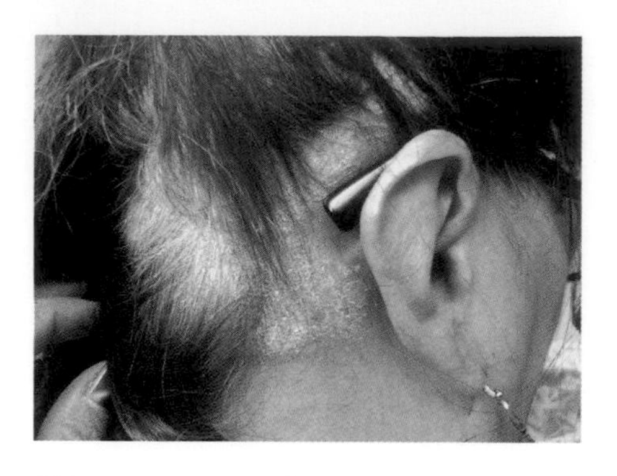

This is psoriasis, not seborrheic dermatitis.

the body, most commonly the skin around the eyebrows and the hairy mid-chest, seen as greasy scale usually overlying a red base. Those areas will be itchy, a little scaly, and maybe red from rubbing.

One mistake that people make when they buy an over-the-counter dandruff shampoo is to use it like other hair shampoos to clean their hair, not really placing the product on their scalp. When you are treating dandruff, you need to treat the *scalp,* not the hair. You should massage the dandruff shampoo into the scalp and let it sit there for a good five minutes. I recommend that you even apply the shampoo before you get into the shower and let it sit a little while you do other bathroom-type things. If you prefer the scent of your regular shampoo, you can certainly use that shampoo on your hair and reserve the medicated shampoo for your scalp. And if you have seborrheic dermatitis on areas other than your scalp, rub a little of this dandruff shampoo on those areas too.

But my BFF swears by this *product. . . .*
MAYBE

Products your BFF swears by . . . may just make you swear! Just because your bestie swears by a cream or serum that she insists has transformed her skin and taken a decade off her appearance or erased all of her age spots, that doesn't mean that this may be the best product for *you.* Remember that our skin type is largely dependent on our genetics, our ethnicity, and our environment, and your best pal may not share very similar qualities and experiences as you.

I can't be allergic to my hair dye; I've been using the same product for years!
FALSE

Say you have an itchy rash that you strongly suspect is due to some product you are putting on your skin. A common example of a product that causes skin reactions is hair dye. Does your scalp get itchy after you get your hair colored? Worse, do your scalp and even your face swell afterward? Well, this very likely means you have an allergy to hair dye, and the common allergen within hair dye is paraphenylenediamine. You may counter this diagnosis by saying, "I've been using the same hairdresser and the same hair dye all my life!" Actually, you can develop a skin allergy to a product that you have been using on your skin for years. Suddenly, your own immune system becomes attuned to this product and decides that it is the enemy and that it must mount an immune response and declare war against that product. The results of this reaction can literally look like a war is being waged on your skin.

Let's say you develop a skin reaction to a product that has been recommended to you, but you've tried a bunch of new things and don't know what's causing it. Or you just think you may have developed an allergy to your hair dye. Dab a bit of product—one at a time—behind your ear or on your inner arm and leave it for a couple of days per product to see if you have a reaction.

A weird growth on my ear is likely skin cancer or an infection.
MAYBE

You may have chondrodermatitis nodularis helicis. My patients always widen their eyes and back up ever so slightly when I spout this term. Yes, it's pretty impressive sounding. It's also a somewhat common condition that creates noticeable and often painful bumps on the edges of our ears, the helices of our ears, or any part of the ear that projects the farthest from our head. It's so common, in fact, that products are available to help alleviate the discomfort it causes. The bumps are caused by chronic pressure placed on the ear; when you sleep, or even if you often wear a motorcycle or football helmet or headphones, pressure is applied on the part of your ear that juts out the most, and this compresses the skin and causes constriction of blood vessels locally, decreasing blood supply, which leads to localized necrosis of the cartilage.

There are actually sleeping pillows made to accommodate this condition—they have a hole cut out of them so that when you sleep you avoid placing pressure on this part of your ear. If you see a dermatologist, we can often try to shrink the bump with a corticosteroid injection (and we will make sure it's not a squamous cell carcinoma, a type of skin cancer I discussed more on page 123, which can look very similar). In the foot care aisle of your local drugstore, you may find corn pads, which are thick foam stickers with a hole in the middle meant to be placed on corns on your feet. You can use these corn cushions on the bumps on your ears to alleviate the pressure placed on them while you're sleeping and make your life a lot better.

DPP Hack: Get the Red Out

Afrin nasal spray is an over-the-counter treatment option for nasal congestion, but it can be used for other purposes if you understand what the active ingredient, oxymetazoline, does. When sprayed into the nose, it narrows the caliber of our superficial blood vessels, thereby decreasing congestion and swelling. Oxymetazoline can do the same thing to any superficial blood vessels you have, so if you have tiny but noticeable superficial blood vessels on your face, you can apply it to your skin to temporarily decrease this redness. Be forewarned, though, that you can develop a dependence on this, and so it shouldn't be used all the time. Save it for special occasions, when you want to look your best.

My laptop is hurting me.

TRUE

Erythema ab igne is an interesting skin condition, which could also be called laptop-on-thigh disease. It creates this grayish blue discoloration of the skin in a reticulated, or netlike pattern. In the past, we saw this very recognizable condition most often on the front of the lower legs or on the back. If I saw it on the shins, I would ask if that person often sat very close to a portable heater. If I saw it on another area of the body, I would ask the patient if she often applied a hot water bottle or other warm compresses there. Now we are seeing an increase in this condition on the front of the thighs. Why? The increase in the popularity of laptop computers! People who set their laptop directly on their thighs and allow the heat to be felt on the skin are at risk of this condition. And this can possibly be a permanent change in the appearance of your skin, so please take heed! Always place a blanket or pillow between your laptop and your thighs to avoid this condition.

DPP Hack: Leave Your Baggage Behind

Do you look tired in the morning, even after you have had a very restful sleep, and you feel it has everything to do with increased baggage under the eyes? Well, this happens to many people, and although dark circles under the eyes are due to many causes (as I reviewed on page 198), if you notice that your undereye area looks the worst in the morning and improves throughout the day, then at least a part of your issue has to do with fluid retention.

If this is a problem for you, I suggest a little preparation to look your best before an important event. Fluid retention occurs while we sleep because when we lie flat, fluid pools, often most noticeably around the eyes, as the skin there is the thinnest on the body. You see an improvement over the course of the day because you are upright and gravity is helping to drain this fluid. So when sleeping, try to prop your head up higher and get up earlier than usual to allow gravity to take more effect. Also, avoid excess salt intake, which can cause you to retain more fluids.

Moisturizer is best applied when you're still damp after a bath or shower.

TRUE

Do you know that your regular shower or bath may clean your skin, but also really strip your skin of its natural oils? Those of us prone to rashes such as atopic dermatitis, xerotic eczema, or ichthyosis (all these rashes and many more are essentially exacerbated by dry skin) know this, because we can often feel the tightness and increased itchiness of our skin after we bathe. Bathing dries us out! There are some simple ways to avoid this, though. When you finish bathing and your skin is still damp, *this* is the time to apply your moisturizer. I personally grew up with atopic dermatitis, and because of this I always keep a tub of moisturizer stored in my shower stall to make sure I seal as much moisture into my skin as I can. When the residual water on your skin evaporates, it pulls moisture with it, drying you out more. Applying moisturizer to damp skin locks in the moisture efficiently. It's good to know that "lotions" are water based and therefore less moisturizing than "creams," which are oil based. Remember from the acne section that creams can sometimes make acne worse, especially if you have oily skin.

My mom was right when she told me to stay away from greasy foods like French fries because they cause acne.

FALSE

I tell my patients, "The only way greasy foods like pizza give you acne is if you rub that pizza all over your face." There are very few foods that trigger acne, aside from foods that contain hormones, such as cow's milk and cheese. In short: be mindful of dairy if you are breakout prone, but other than that, foods don't promote acne breakouts. This is a big myth!

DPP Hack: Back Up Beauty

Did you know that a lot of the fine lines and wrinkles we get on our face occur while we are sleeping? Well, actually, more like *because* we are sleeping. The wrinkles we get are due to aging, the expressions we repeatedly make, and also the position our face is pushed and prodded into when we sleep. This is actually one of the issues that I personally find hardest to avoid because I like to sleep on my stomach, which leaves my face smooshed into my pillow. You know when your mom told you not to make that face because it will eventually stay like that? Well, I try to remind myself of this, but to no avail. I see this causing wrinkles most often on people's cheeks and foreheads. In this case, do as I say, not as I do: try to sleep on your back!

A "base tan" will actually protect you from the sun, sun damage, and skin cancer.

FALSE

I had to tape my mouth shut (figuratively, of course) the other day when I heard a friend state that he got a base tan recently to "protect [himself] from the sun." No, no, no, just . . . *no*! You may feel lucky that you get tanned easily (or at all) with sun exposure, but a tan is *not* protective in any way. If you are getting any color at all after sun exposure, then you are actually not doing a very good job with your sunscreen, because you're not avoiding premature aging or protecting yourself from skin cancer. Think of it this way: your skin tans as a protective mechanism; it's scrambling to create an umbrella of pigment to protect itself from the sun. Once you get a little color, though, some damage is already done. Not as much damage as if you were to get a sunburn, but a tan still means that your skin is recognizing that it is getting too much sun and going into protective mode.

Makeup makes acne worse.
MAYBE

Be ingredient savvy when it comes to anything you're putting on your skin, including makeup. Look for ingredients such as titanium dioxide, zinc oxide, mica, bismuth oxychloride, and iron oxides (normally found in mineral makeup), which will offer coverage and won't clog pores—which in turn will not aggravate acne. Products that you put on your skin that are more "occlusive" are thicker and can clog your pores. If you think your makeup promotes pimples, look for lotions and serums rather than creams, because lotions and serums are water or alcohol based, whereas creams are oil based and are more likely to make acne worse.

Sunscreen clogs the pores.
MAYBE

The "wrong" kind of sunscreen *can* cause a chemical reaction on the skin, which can lead to acne. There are two different kinds of sunscreens: chemical sunscreens and physical sunscreens. There's a better kind of sunscreen for you depending on the circumstances that you are in. Chemical sunscreens are organic compounds that actually absorb the sun's rays and convert them to energy that is not damaging to the skin, and in the process, produce heat. Examples are para-aminobenzoic acid (PABA), oxybenzone, avobenzone, and octisalate. Physical sunscreens are opaque inorganic compounds that reflect or scatter the sun's rays, preventing them from penetrating the skin. Examples of physical sunscreen ingredients are titanium dioxide and zinc oxide. This is what you see people in old movies or pictures wearing when they paint their noses white.

DPP Hack: Ring Barer

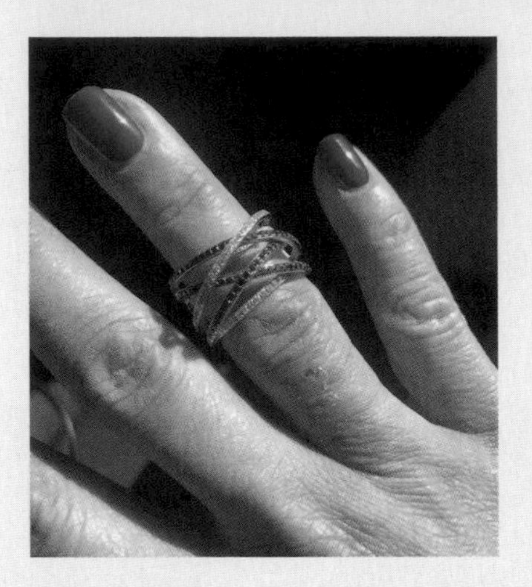

My own ring finger, with irritant contact dermatitis.

Do you always get rashes under your rings, and you think that you are allergic to the metal in your jewelry? Well, this is likely *not* the case, and I will guess that you are washing your hands without removing your rings. Am I right? You should keep a jewelry holder next to the sink where you wash your hands to help prevent this rash, which is not an allergy but an irritation. Soap gets trapped under your jewelry when you wash your hands, and if you don't completely remove this soap, it can really cause a bad rash. If you forget to take your ring off, at least spend more time cleansing the soap from under your ring and make sure there is no moisture trapped under your ring, and ta-dah, like magic, you won't get any more rashes there!

Chemical sunscreens are superior for applying to your face if you are wearing makeup because they don't leave a whitish residue that can clash with your makeup foundation. However, certain skin conditions like rosacea can be exacerbated by heat, so in this case, consider using a physical sunscreen instead. Luckily, many physical sunscreens have micronized their active ingredients and slightly tinted their products, so that the particles are much smaller and don't create such a stark whitish tinge to the skin. I like the *idea* of a physical sunscreen better because, if used correctly and often enough, you are guaranteed that it blocks *all* of the harmful UVA and UVB rays. In addition, physical sunscreens are less likely to clog your pores and therefore less likely to lead to acne outbreaks. However, if you have a skin condition that you are trying to disguise with makeup, you may prefer a chemical sunscreen because it won't change the color of your skin.

Oil-based cleansers actually make your skin oilier and therefore cause acne.

MAYBE

If you have oily skin and you know increased oil on the skin promotes acne, why would you use more oil to cleanse your face? Just because oil-based cleansers are popular doesn't mean that they are more useful or more beneficial. I prefer salicylic acid–based cleansers, since chemical peel ingredients such as this will encourage exfoliation of the skin, remove skin debris from within our pores, and help to clear up acne as well as prevent new acne from forming. I recommend my SLMD Salicylic Acid Cleanser. It's safe for all skin types and can help minimize brown spots.

DPP Hack: Cocktail Time

Wash your hands after you fix yourself a margarita at the beach or pool. Why?

Have you ever been at a pool party and the next day developed a strange streaky rash that leads to darkening of the skin in an area across your forearm or your chest or abdomen, or even your thigh, and you have no idea where it came from? You might have phytophotodermatitis. Don't call the ambulance, but just stay away from the limes you used to garnish your margaritas yesterday. Lime juice dripped or dropped onto your skin, and with the proper wavelength exposure from the sun, it caused a reaction.

The biggest culprit in America is the rind of the Persian lime, *Citrus latifolia,* but you can get the same reaction from other citrus fruits and even other noncitrus liquids, like perfume (in this case it's called berloque dermatitis). When you squeeze a lime into your drink, and some of that lime juice drips onto your arm, and this area is exposed to sunlight, you can get a reaction that leads to noticeable redness, then darkening in that same bizarre shape that the lime juice dripped onto your skin. Keep an eye out for this, and you may impress your friends when you explain what is happening to their skin. (And, more important, you can avoid it on your own skin.)

People get acne breakouts because their face is dirty.

MAYBE

Sure, if your face is dirty, pores are more likely to fill with debris and this can promote pimples. However, most people with acne don't have it because their skin is dirty, and in fact, I *do* know that many people with acne may be too aggressive about washing their skin. If you have pimples, you can't scrub them away, and washing your face too often and too roughly can irritate your skin and even make your acne worse. Use common sense. Wash away makeup, dirt, and sweat before you go to bed, and if you feel your skin is greasy in the morning, wash it again! But don't overdo it. Be gentle.

Body acne is totally different from face acne.

FALSE

Body acne is the same as face acne is the same as shoulder acne is the same as butt acne, but they can occur for different reasons. For example, football players may notice more acne breakouts on the back, shoulders, and chest because of the heavy protective body pads in their uniforms and the sweat accumulating underneath. Wearing tight jeans and sitting for long durations can promote more acne breakouts on the buttock area because of all the occlusion to the area. Chin acne can be predominant in wrestlers who wear chin straps and in violinists who rest their chin on their instrument. Essentially you can get acne anywhere that hair can grow, and occlusion plays an important role.

ChapStick/Blistex/Carmex can make the lips even drier.

TRUE

Are you addicted to your ChapStick or Carmex? Well, you're not alone. Do you notice that the more you use it, the more you seem to need it? We can often get dependent on these products, and without them, we feel our lips shriveling up. If they contain fragrances or menthol, these are actually drying agents that can temporarily make our lips feel or look better, but lead to *more* dryness, flaking, and peeling. Avoid lip licking—your saliva will evaporate on your lips and dry them out more—and use plain petrolatum jelly instead of lip balm if you really need something.

Fragranced moisturizers and cleansers are more drying.

TRUE

You may like a moisturizer or body cleanser because of its pleasing smell, but if you have issues with dry skin, it's best to avoid fragrance altogether, because added fragrances tend to dry out the skin more.

DPP Hack: Be Gentle with Your Nails

I'm with everyone else in that I don't like dirty fingernails and toenails. As a result, we clean under the nails and so do our manicurists. However, it's better to wash your hands well instead of picking under your nails to clean them out. Don't clean under your nails too aggressively, because you don't want to lift your nail up from its nail plate (the part it's stuck to underneath). The medical term for this is onycholysis. If the nail separates from the nail plate underneath, moisture can become trapped under there (a little water or sweat will do the trick!) and this will prevent the area from "reattaching." In fact, you have to wait for it to grow out, which can take many months depending on how wide of a separation was created. If this happens, keep the area dry. You may want to get a Q-tip, dip it in nail polish remover with acetone, and gently rub it against the area that is lifted up on your nail. But don't force anything under that nail, and calm your compulsions to clean under that area even more because that will make the problem worse!

Although you're unhappy with your saddlebags, your cankles, or your stomach pooch, the only solution is diet and exercise. Liposuction is "cheating," and the fat will return.

FALSE

Liposuction is one of my favorite cosmetic surgeries to perform. It's so rewarding to see something so many of us wrestle with for so many years be improved within a few hours, without the risk of general anesthesia, and with very little downtime.

I hate the stigma that is associated with this procedure, though—that the patient is taking the "easy way out" and that they just don't have the commitment to sticking to a healthy diet and exercise because "they could do it themselves if they weren't so lazy and just tried harder."

As I said earlier, liposuction is *not* a weight loss strategy. If you want to lose weight, you *should* stick to a healthy diet and exercise program. Liposuction is a *body sculpting* procedure. In fact, the ideal patient who will have the most long-lasting results is someone who has low body fat percentage, eats a healthy diet, and has maintained the same weight for many years. The perfect patient is someone who is in great shape but has cankles—excess fat deposition in the space between the calves and the ankles that makes them self-conscious because they feel that their legs are shaped like tree trunks. Or a patient with a hereditary predisposition for saddlebags—a trait passed on and shared by her mother, uncles, and even her grandma. You can actually permanently *change* the contours of your body to a shape that is more pleasing to you, and that's what this is all about. These are stubborn areas of fat. They are almost always the first places you gain weight and the last places you lose fat from.

The reason that liposuction is truly not a mode of weight loss is that if you use it to lose weight or debulk your body of fat, you will very likely gain that weight back, since most of us hover around the same body fat percentage throughout our lives, or at least our bodies tend to gravitate toward a comfortable level of body fat. Liposuction does not grant you permission to eat with abandon afterward. If you consume excess calories, no matter if you've had lipo or not, you will gain weight. If you've had liposuction, you will be less likely to gain weight in those areas that have been treated. This is why when someone who gets liposuction around their abdomen overeats, they may notice when they gain weight it settles in their rear end or their arms or their upper back—it will be less likely to accumulate in the area that was previously treated with liposuction.

Cosmetic products have inferior sunscreens.

TRUE SOMETIMES

Cosmetic products such as makeup foundations, moisturizer, and anti-aging creams are not regulated by the FDA in the United States and therefore don't have to abide by the same strict rules that govern true sunscreens. In other words, a makeup or other cosmetic product can advertise that it contains sunscreen, but treat this with some skepticism.

I watch Dr. Lee's videos on YouTube, and she has a tremor! Her hands shake a lot when she uses a needle and syringe to anesthetize her patients!

FALSE

New viewers to my YouTube videos often ask if I'm nervous or have a tremor. Why else would my hands shake sometimes? Well, I purposely shake my left hand, vibrating the patient's skin, when I inject local anesthetic and I keep my right hand, which is my injecting hand, still. This all has to do with the gate control theory of pain. What do you do when you slam your finger in a car door or accidently kick your baby toe against your bed? One of your first responses is to shake your fingers or to rub your toes. Well, you are doing exactly what I am doing when I shake while administering anesthesia. It is a method of distraction. The gate control theory explains that there are nerves in our skin that transmit the sensation of pain to our brains that are separate and distinct from the nerves that tell our brain that we are experiencing vibration. So if we activate the vibration nerves at the same time that pain nerves are activated, all these nerves are competing with each other for attention from your brain. Therefore, not as many nerves that transmit the sensation of pain get to your brain; your brain is being "distracted" by the vibration nerves simultaneously.

Oh, that bump on my leg, arm, back, shoulder—that's from a spider bite!

FALSE

In more than a decade as a private practice dermatologist, I've seen only about three true spider bites. Maybe it's because someone with a spider bite goes to urgent care or even to the emergency room or their primary care doctor, and not to their dermatologist? So that mark on your skin is probably *not* a spider bite. People often blame spiders for odd bumps. They recount the story of how they woke up at night, felt a spider bite, and saw a spider scurry from their bed, and ever since that day a decade ago, they have had this growth on their arm. But I know it's not caused by a spider but by chronic sun exposure, since it's a skin cancer. Now, there is one type of spider that I do truly fear, and that is the brown recluse, because it causes a dramatic and horror-movie-type reaction in our skin.

I'm allergic to lidocaine.
PROBABLY FALSE

I'll often hear this from a patient: that they can't tolerate the local anesthetic lidocaine, that they have an allergy. A true lidocaine allergy is extremely rare. In fact, I personally have never seen it, nor have any of my close colleagues. Most people claim that they experienced this allergy at their dentist's office when they got a shot to numb them before a procedure. Likely this reaction was not due to lidocaine but to the epinephrine that we add to lidocaine. Epinephrine in high doses, or if you are more sensitive to it, can increase your heart rate, and this can make you feel like you're having a panic attack. If this happens to you in the doctor's or dentist's office, make sure to let them know right away. This will go away in five to ten minutes and you will feel back to normal, but it is *not* a nice feeling and makes people leery of getting into the same situation again.

If I get a cold sore, I just use one of those over-the-counter cold sore creams, because that's the best treatment.
FALSE

A cold sore is caused by the herpesvirus. Yes, it's herpes, and you've heard people say, "Herpes is forever." When people hear that they could have herpes, many tend to freak out. But don't freak out. Okay, it *is* considered a sexually transmitted disease (STD), but did you know that 90 percent of the human population in the United States has been exposed to the virus? Some people just don't get breakouts so easily.

There are great prescription oral medications that can decrease the intensity and the duration of your cold sore breakout. Over-the-counter and prescription topical antiviral medications are really not that effective. Oral medications that require a doctor's prescription are actually very safe to take! It's most important to know that timing is key. You must take the med during the prodrome, or the moment when you feel that tingling sensation that heralds a breakout of blisters on the horizon.

*If I wear rubber gloves when I do housework,
I will protect my hands from developing a rash.*

FALSE

Wearing rubber gloves can actually make your hand eczema and/or rash *worse*. People who work with chemicals, for example, including those of us who have to clean around our house using harsh cleaning chemicals, will often wear gloves, thinking this will protect our hands from the chemicals. While this is true, a rash can still develop on their hands. This is because of the sweat that accumulates on your hands within the rubber gloves. When you remove the gloves, the sweat evaporates and dries out your skin, which can trigger a rash. The trick is to get cotton-lined rubber gloves because the cotton lining will wick moisture away from your skin so that your hands won't dry out afterward and get irritated. If you have a cut or fissure from such a rash, a good way to seal it is to use liquid bandage, even superglue. This helps seal the crack and protects it from acidic liquids we can come into contact with. We know how much it stings if we get lemon juice on a cut!

I'm Not Hurting You, Right?

I DON'T KNOW WHEN IT STARTED, NOR DID I REALIZE I SAID IT SO OFTEN until I started really videotaping my surgeries. Perhaps I say it more now, since I know my videos on YouTube are watched on average two to four million times a day. But I'll tell you what. I have to thank this Dr. Pimple Popper phenomenon for making me a better dermatologist. Knowing that my videos are seen by millions every day certainly makes me conscious of what I say and what I do as a physician.

I'm squeezing cysts and lipomas and extracting blackheads more often than I ever imagined in my life—what is all this for, anyway? I'm not a dermatology superhero, trying to rid the world of every strange unwanted growth under the human skin! You know what really keeps me going? What really makes me love what I do? What makes this all worth it? Helping others in my field. Just recently, I was invited to speak at a dermatology conference about social media and how it can be effectively incorporated into a dermatologist's or other physician's practice.

To me, it's such a big deal that I was even asked! Of course, as expected, I freaked out only days before the big event. Normally, I'm able to speak to large nondermatologist audiences without too much anxiety, but to know that I was to speak to a room full of dermatologists really increased my blood pressure and perspiration! I can't sound like a fool, a charlatan in front of my peers. Plus, how many dermatologists actually disagree with and disapprove of what I'm doing on social media? Do they think I'm taking advantage of my patients to promote myself? Do they hate that patients who see them ask them why they don't remove a cyst or perform a surgery "like Dr. Pimple Popper does"? My lecture also wasn't wedged between really interesting topics like "Five Best Reconstructive Pearls for Repairing a Nasal Defect" or "Minimally Invasive Repair of an Aging Neck." My talk was not directly about dermatology, but instead about practice management, about incorporating social media into your medical practice. Would anyone even show up? I got there thirty minutes early to mentally prepare, and I could clearly detect the low hum of the air conditioner in the empty hotel ballroom.

My lecture was better attended than I ever imagined or hoped! Every seat was filled, and people stood lining the back wall to listen to what I was saying about my experiences growing my social media presence. I really thought many of them wouldn't be interested in what I had to say, didn't even know about this Dr. Pimple Popper phenomenon, or worse, were scoffing at me, believing what I was doing was an embarrassment to dermatology.

Then, immediately after the talk, people in the audience converged upon me. They wanted to meet me and tell me that they watched and loved my videos. The biggest compliment I got was from a dermatology resident from Chicago, who said one of the older residents in his program recommended that he watch my surgical videos before their "Lumps and Bumps" surgical session. He said he had rolled his eyes and said, "*Why* would I want to watch a pimple popper?" But he checked out my YouTube and now, he says, he is addicted. He told me that he and his fellow derm residents actually prepare to do their own surgeries and learn suture technique from watching my videos.

This, honestly, is one of the highest compliments I could ever receive. Apparently, many dermatologist residents in training follow me on Snapchat, Facebook, Instagram, and YouTube, and use my videos as a sort of master class in derm surgery and social media. As I walked around during the meeting after my lecture, dermatologists would yell out, "Hi, Dr. Lee, I *loved* your lecture!" and, wow, this surprised me as much as it made me happy. I'm so honored to possibly be inspiring a new legion of future dermatologists, and that they are entertained and educated by my work! To get support and love from your peers is a very special kind of respect. Who knew that pimple popping could lead me to such amazing things?!

There was a recent article in the most respected dermatology journal, the *Journal of the American Academy of Dermatology,* where people were asked what they thought dermatologists actually do. The responses were mainly treating acne and skin cancer, and administering cosmetics like Botox and filler. We need to change this misperception about dermatology and dermatologists. We do so much more than this.

I'm proud to be able to show what I do as a dermatologist to the world via my social media. I am proud that I'm helping to elevate the specialty. For example, most people don't know many of us dermatologists do liposuction under local anesthesia alone, that we remove facial skin cancers and perform facial surgical reconstructions and surgical repairs that are on par with the best plastic surgeons. That we are the true experts in all things concerned with the skin, the hair, and the nails. Of course, we are not the only experts; there are many other medical specialties and providers that also help people to take care of their skin. I'm proud to show people what I love about what I do, and to demonstrate to people what dermatology can be about. Thank you for letting me open a window for you into my world!

ACKNOWLEDGMENTS

MY FATHER HAS ALWAYS LOVED BOOKS AND PASSED HIS LOVE OF READING on to me. So of course I jumped at the opportunity to write a book myself and knew it would be a significant achievement in my life. It was *way* harder than I anticipated. I knew there were important things that I wanted to say, that people would find interesting, but it was really hard to actually say them! There are many people I want to thank—if it wasn't for them, I don't think I would be as proud of this achievement as I am.

Thank you to the amazing team at Dey Street Books, especially my editor, Sean Newcott, Kendra Newton, Ben Steinberg, Lynn Grady, Lauren Janiec, Heidi Richter, Paula Szafranski, and Shelby Peak. Thank you to my agent, Carol Mann, and Lydia Shamah, and Karen Kelly and Mary Ann Marshall, who helped so much to organize my thoughts and make me sound so good.

Now I need to thank the people who put up with me during this whole process: My assistant, Madisen, my two medical assistants, Kristi and Valeria, all of my staff at Skin Physicians & Surgeons, SkinPS Brands, and Dr. Pimple Popper Headquarters. My great girlfriends, especially Raquel, who has always been my cheerleader, reminding me to take care of myself, to just chill, to enjoy life. My brother, Kevin, who is helping to grow the Dr. Pimple Popper brand and my skincare line to be forces to be reckoned with. My parents, Soon and Irene, who are the best parents in the world, for so many reasons. When I grow up I want to be just. Like. Them. My kids, Chance and Stratton, who roll their eyes when I insist that I am, indeed, a YouTuber . . . thank you for being patient with me, for grounding me, and for reminding me of the good and important things in life. To my wonderful husband, Jeff: you know full well I would be living in a van down by the river if you weren't there to see the "big picture." Thank you for gently redirecting me when I go off on tangents and lose sight of the proper path. But also, thank you for letting me be me. I jokingly say you are the brains and I am the personality, and in many ways this is true—we are much bigger and better together than we are as individuals. Love you.

Oh, and I can't forget to thank all my wonderful patients and popaholics! Those of you who allowed me to film your dermatologic procedures for my social media, thank you for exposing a part of yourself to perfect strangers in the name of entertainment and education. And thank you to all of you around the world who follow me on social media and YouTube, and who are so kind, supportive, intelligent, and funny. You all remind me how much *good* there is in the world. It is because of you popaholics that I am here, writing this book, for you. I've said it many times and I'll say it again, very proudly: Popaholics Unite!

BDD AND BFRB RESOURCES

The TLC Foundation offers an entire support page here: www.bfrb.org/find-help-support

Skin Picking Support is another great resource: www.skinpickingsupport.com

The International OCD Foundation has a page dedicated to BDD: bdd.iocdf.org

The Anxiety and Depression Association of America (ADAA) has lots of helpful information about BFRB and BDD: adaa.org

They also have a YouTube video of a presentation that explains BFRB and its treatments: www.youtube.com/watch?v=THAFnbrOqhg

Get involved with the Picking Me Foundation! pickingme.org/get-involved/

NOTES

Chapter 2: Thanks for Popping In!

1. Gary W. Cole, "Freckles," MedicineNet, last modified August 14, 2017, www.medicinenet.com/freckles/page3.htm.
2. Simone Laube, "Fibrous Papule of the Face," Medscape, last modified March 10, 2017, emedicine.medscape.com/article/1057309-overview.
3. "Syringoma," Skinsight, accessed June 1, 2018, www.skinsight.com/skin-conditions/adult/syringoma.
4. Ibid.
5. "All About Rosacea," National Rosacea Society, accessed June 1, 2018, www.rosacea.org/patients/allaboutrosacea.php.
6. Kristeen Cherney, "What Causes Pilar Cysts and How Are They Treated?" Healthline, accessed June 1, 2018, www.healthline.com/health/skin-disorders/pilar-cyst.
7. Daniel Bennett and Rosalie Elenitsas, "Eruptive Vellus Hair Cyst," DermatologyAdvisor.com, accessed June 1, 2018, www.clinicaladvisor.com/dermatology/eruptive-vellus-hair-cyst/article/691571.
8. "Common Moles, Dysplastic Nevi, and Risk of Melanoma," National Cancer Institute online, accessed June 1, 2018, www.cancer.gov/types/skin/moles-fact-sheet.
9. "Actinic Keratosis," Skin Cancer Foundation, accessed June 1, 2018, www.skincancer.org/skin-cancer-information/actinic-keratosis

10. "Skin Cancer Facts & Statistics," Skin Cancer Foundation, accessed June 1, 2018, www.skincancer.org/skin-cancer-information/skin-cancer-facts.
11. "Skin Cancer," WebMD, last modified March 18, 2018, www.webmd.com/melanoma-skin-cancer/melanoma-guide/skin-cancer#1.
12. "Skin Cancer Facts & Statistics," Skin Cancer Foundation, accessed June 1, 2018, www.skincancer.org/skin-cancer-information/skin-cancer-facts.
13. Jörg Reichrath, *Sunlight, Vitamin D and Skin Cancer*, Springer Nature, 2014.
14. Dr. Colin Tidy, "Skin Cancer Types," Patient, last modified December 4, 2017, patient.info/health/skin-cancer-an-overview.

Chapter 3: Acne: An Issue for the Ages

1. "Adult Acne," American Academy of Dermatology online, accessed June 1, 2018, www.aad.org/public/diseases/acne-and-rosacea/adult-acne#sthash.P7AHDBR6.dpuf.
2. "What Is Acne?" Science of Acne, last modified March 24, 2018, thescienceofacne.com/what-is-acne.
3. "Hormonal Factors Key to Understanding Acne in Women," American Academy of Dermatology online, last modified March 13, 2012, accessed June 1, 2018, www.aad.org/media/news-releases/hormonal-factors-key-to-understanding-acne-in-women.
4. Khalid O. Abulnaja, "Oxidant/Antioxidant Status in Obese Adolescent Females with Acne Vulgaris," *Indian Journal of Dermatology* 54, no. 1 (January–March 2009): 36–40, www.ncbi.nlm.nih.gov/pmc/articles/PMC2800868.
5. "Acne: Signs and Symptoms" American Academy of Dermatology, accessed June 2, 2018, www.aad.org/public/diseases/acne-and-rosacea/acne#symptoms.
6. Catherine M. Nguyen et al., "The Psychosocial Impact of Acne, Vitiligo, and Psoriasis: A Review," *Clinical, Cosmetic and Investigational Dermatology* 9 (2016): 383–92, www.ncbi.nlm.nih.gov/pmc/articles/PMC5076546.
7. Yasin Bez et al., "High Social Phobia Frequency and Related Disability in Patients with Acne Vulgaris," *European Journal of Dermatology* 21, no. 5 (September/October 2011): 756–60, doi:10.1684/ejd.2011.1418.
8. D. A. Rapp et al., "Anger and Acne: Implications for Quality of Life, Patient Satisfaction and Clinical Care," *British Journal of Dermatology* 151, no. 1 (July 2004): 183–89, www.medscape.com/viewarticle/484747.
9. AHA, Paula's Choice online, accessed June 1, 2018, www.paulaschoice.com/cosmetic-ingredient-dictionary/definition/aha.
10. Joshua A. Zeichner, Varsha Bhatt, and Radhakrishnan Pillai, "*In Vitro* Percu-

taneous Absorption of Benzoyl Peroxide from Three Fixed Combination Acne Formulations," *Journal of Clinical and Aesthetic Dermatology* 6, no. 8 (August 2013): 19–22, www.ncbi.nlm.nih.gov/pmc/articles/PMC3760600.

11. "Azelaic Acid," Mayo Clinic, accessed June 2, 2018, www.mayoclinic.org/drugs-supplements/azelaic-acid-topical-route/description/drg-20062084
12. Amanda Oakley, "Azelaic Acid," DermNet NZ, accessed June 1, 2018, www.dermnetnz.org/topics/azelaic-acid.
13. "Acne," Mayo Clinic online, accessed June 1, 2018, www.mayoclinic.org/diseases-conditions/acne/basics/treatment/con-20020580.
14. Emmy Graber, "Hormonal Therapy for Women with Acne Vulgaris," UpToDate, www.uptodate.com/contents/hormonal-therapy-for-women-with-acne-vulgaris.
15. "Birth Control for Acne," WebMD, last modified November 28, 2017, www.webmd.com/skin-problems-and-treatments/acne/birth-control-for-acne-treatment#3–7.
16. Omudhome Ogbru, "Isotretinoin," MedicineNet.com, last modified September 8, 2016, www.medicinenet.com/isotretinoin/article.htm.
17. "Isotretinoin Capsule," WebMD, accessed June 1, 2018, www.webmd.com/drugs/2/drug-6662/isotretinoin-oral/details.
18. Alison Layton, "The Use of Isotretinoin in Acne," *Dermato-Endocrinology* 1, no. 3 (May/June 2009): 162–69, www.ncbi.nlm.nih.gov/pmc/articles/PMC2835909.
19. Philip D. Shenenfelt, "Herbal Treatment for Dermatologic Disorders," chapter 18 in *Herbal Medicine: Biomolecular and Clinical Aspects*, 2nd ed., ed. Iris F. F. Benzie and Sissi Wachtel-Galor (Boca Raton, FL: CRC Press/Taylor & Francis, 2011), www.ncbi.nlm.nih.gov/books/NBK92761.
20. Staci Brandt, "The Clinical Effects of Zinc as a Topical or Oral Agent on the Clinical Response and Pathophysiologic Mechanisms of Acne: A Systematic Review of the Literature," *Journal of Drugs in Dermatology* 12, no. 5 (May 2013): 542–45.
21. "Home Remedies: Anxiety About Acne," Mayo Clinic, accessed June 2, 2018, newsnetwork.mayoclinic.org/discussion/home-remedies-anxiety-about-acne/.
22. "Acne Scars," American Society for Dermatologic Surgery, accessed June 2, 2018, www.asds.net/Skin-Experts/Skin-Conditions/Acne-Scars.
23. "Acne Scars," American Academy of Dermatology online, www.aad.org/public/diseases/acne-and-rosacea/acne-scars#causes.

Chapter 4: Time Won't Tell

1. "Stumped by Oxidative Stress?" Weil Lifestyle online, last modified March

17, 2009, www.drweil.com/vitamins-supplements-herbs/supplements-remedies/stumped-by-oxidative-stress.

2. Samantha Williams, "Advanced Glycation End Products (AGEs)—It's Aging You Quicker," Metrin online, last modified December 13, 2016, www.metrin.com/blog/advanced-glycation-end-products-ages.
3. April Long, "Sugar and Aging: How to Fight Glycation," *Elle* online, February 1, 2012, www.elle.com/beauty/makeup-skin-care/tips/a2471/sugar-aging-how-to-fight-glycation.
4. "What Is Photoaging?" Skin Cancer Foundation, accessed June 4, 2018, www.skincancer.org/healthy-lifestyle/anti-aging/what-is-photoaging.
5. "Inflammation," DermaMedics online, www.dermamedics.com/inflammation_id55.html.
6. "Esteé Lauder Clinical Trial Finds Link Between Sleep Deprivation and Skin Aging," University Hospitals online, last modified July 17, 2013, accessed June 4, 2018, www.uhhospitals.org/about/media-news-room/current-news/2013/07/estee-lauder-clinical-trial-finds-link-between-sleep-deprivation-and-skin-aging.
7. Ibid.
8. "Is it true that smoking causes wrinkles?" Mayo Clinic, accessed June 4, 2018, www.mayoclinic.org/healthy-lifestyle/quit-smoking/expert-answers/smoking/faq-20058153.
9. David Oliver, "Survey: Stress in America Increases for the First Time in 10 Years," *U.S. News & World Report* online, last modified February 15, 2017, accessed June 4, 2018, health.usnews.com/wellness/health-buzz/articles/2017–02–15/survey-stress-in-america-increases-for-the-first-time-in-10-years.
10. Rhonda Allison, "What Causes Skin to Age?" *Dermascope* online, last modified July 14, 2004, www.dermascope.com/aging/what-causes-skin-to-age#.WPemOKKP6pA.
11. Dean Ornish et al., "Effect of Comprehensive Lifestyle Changes on Telomerase Activity and Telomere Length in Men with Biopsy-Proven Low-Risk Prostate Cancer: 5-Year Follow-up of a Descriptive Pilot Study," *Lancet Oncology* 14, no. 11 (October 2013): 1112–20, www.thelancet.com/journals/lanonc/article/PIIS1470–2045%2813%2970366–8/fulltext.
12. University of Reading, "New Research Shows Anti-Wrinkle Cream Chemical Works," news release, March 5, 2013, www.reading.ac.uk/news-and-events/releases/PR491218.aspx.

Chapter 5: Prescription for Beauty

1. "Botox Tested to Help Treat Depression and Social Anxiety," CBSNews online, last modified April 17, 2017, www.cbsnews.com/news/botox-treatment-depres sion-and-social-anxiety.
2. "Body Dysmorphic Disorder," Psychology Videos, accessed June 4, 2018, www .psychotube.net/photograph/body-dysmorphic-disorder/.
3. Jon E. Grant and Katharine A. Phillips, "Is Anorexia Nervosa a Subtype of Body Dysmorphic Disorder? Probably Not, but Read On . . . " *Harvard Review of Psychiatry*, 12, no. 2 (2004): 123–26. doi: 10.1080/10673220490447236.
4. "Body Dysmorphic Disorder," Anxiety and Depression Association of America, adaa.org/understanding-anxiety/related-illnesses/other-related-conditions /body-dysmorphic-disorder-bdd.
5. "Bullies and their victims more likely to want plastic surgery," University of Warwick, accessed June 4, 2018, warwick.ac.uk/newsandevents/pressreleases/bullies_ and_their_victims_more_likely_to_want_plastic_surgery1.

INDEX

Page numbers in *italics* indicate photos or illustrations

5-fluorouracil, 121–22
"11s" grooves (glabella), 189, 194, *194*

ABCDEs of melanoma, 43, 118, 119, 131
abscesses, 85, 90–93
acanthosis nigricans, *114*, 114–15
Accutane, 155. *See also* isotretinoin
acetylcholine (ACh), 189
acne
- adult, 134
- body acne *vs.* face acne, 246
- causes of, 142–45
- comedonal, *135,* 136–38
- and cosmetics, 243
- cystic and nodular, *135,* 139–40
- diet and, 144–45, 242
- effect on emotions, 145–46, 161–62
- embarrassment about, 134, 140
- explained, 135, *135*
- family history and, 139–40, 142
- feelings of loss of control, 133
- and hair products, 72–73
- hormones and, 142–43
- keeping dirt and oil off your face, 71–72, 246
- medication as a cause of, 144
- outbreaks, 138
- papulopustular, *135,* 138–39
- scars, 159–62
    - anetoderma (atrophic scars), *160,* 160–61, 162
    - boxcar, 161, *161,* 162
    - ice pick, 161, *161,* 162–63
    - rolling, *160,* 161, 162
    - treatments for, 162–63, *163*
- skincare products and, 144, 245
- SLMD Acne System, 72, 73, *73,* 77, 136, 140, *147,* 147–48, 245
- statistics, 133–34
- stress and, 143
- and sun exposure, 71
- and sweat, 72
- treatments
    - mechanical tools, 158–59

acne *(cont.)*
natural products, 157–58
over-the-counter medications, 148–52
prescription medications, *152,* 152–57
procedures, 157
for scars, 162–63, *163*
viewers' fascination with pimple popping, 5, 78–79
acne excoriée, *143,* 143–44
acne inversa. *See* hidradenitis suppurativa (HS)
actinic keratosis (AK), 120–23, 217
adapalene (Differin), 42, 71–72, 136, 149–50
advanced glycation end products (AGEs), 168
Afrin nasal spray, 240
age spots. *See* solar lentigos
aging and skincare
changes to the body with age, 166–67
choosing the best anti-aging products, 173–74
environmental factors affecting aging, 167
four main causes of aging skin, 167–69
intrinsic *vs.* extrinsic agers, 166–67
most effective anti-aging ingredients, 174–80
preventive measures, 169–72
research, 220–21
retinoids' anti-aging properties, 150
allergies
contact dermatitis, 34, 236, *236,* 244, *244*
hair dye, 238–39
lidocaine, 250
penicillin, 232–34
alpha hydroxy acids (AHAs), 148–49
aluminum chloride, 105
anagen phase of the hair growth cycle, *230,* 230–31
anesthesia
gate control theory, 249
techniques and instruments used, 23–24
anetoderma (atrophic scars), *160,* 160–61, 162
angiofibromas. *See* fibrous papules
angiolipomas, 100
antibacterials, topical, 152–53
antibiotics
oral, 153
risks and side effects, 153
topical, 152
antioxidants
benefits of, 174–75
coenzyme Q10, 176
green tea, 175
resveratrol, 175
vitamin C, 175–76
vitamin E, 175
apocrine glands, 115
atopic dermatitis, 33
atrophy, 22
azelaic acid, 151–52

bacteria
inflamed cyst *vs.* abscess, 85–86
Staphylococcus aureus, 91–92
basal cell carcinoma (BCC), 123–25, *126*
Beau's line, 229–30
benzoyl peroxide (BPO), 150–51
beta hydroxy acids, 149
biologics, 117
biopsy, taking a tissue, 52
biotin, 232
birth defect risks from acne medications, 153, 155–56
Birt-Hogg-Dube syndrome, 51
blackheads (open comedones)
about, 136
comedone extractors, *24,* 24–25, 75, 136
Dr. Lee's video series, 78–79
images of, 4, 70–71, 135, 137
Instagram interest in, 3–4
nose strips, 75–76
preventing, 71–74
skincare after squeezing, 76–77
solar comedones (Favre-Racouchot syndrome), 70–71, *70–71*
squeezing, 74–75
unpredictable nature of, 1, 78
bleeding
and dilated blood vessels, 63
and skin tags, 105–06
blepharitis, 58
blepharoplasty, 200, *200*
blisters
cantharidin for inducing, 108
blood vessels
treating dilated, 63
under the eyes, 198
using Afrin nasal spray to shrink, 240
body dysmorphic disorder (BDD)
about, 222
body-focused repetitive behavior (BFRB), 223–24
and bullying, 223–24

and eating disorders, 222–23
and other mental disorders, 223
raising awareness about, 224–25
statistics, 222
body-focused repetitive behavior (BFRB), 223–24
boils, 90–91
Botox, 188–90, 191, 192–97, 201, *202,* 204
boxcar scars, 161, *161,* 162
bruising (ecchymosis), 63
bulla, *21,* 21–22
bunny lines, 201
buried vertical mattress stitch, 29
B vitamins, 179

calcifying epithelioma of Malherbe. *See* pilomatricomas
cancer
basal cell carcinoma (BCC), 123–25, *126*
malignant growths, 123–21
melanoma, 43, 48, 118, 119, 123, 127–30
metastasis, 123
Mohs surgery, 125–27, *126*
precancerous growths, 120–23
squamous cell carcinoma (SCC), 120, 123–25, *126*
and sun exposure, 124–25, 130
Candida antigen, 110
cantharidin, 108
carbuncles, 90–93
catagen phase of the hair growth cycle, *230,* 230–31
cavernous sinus region of the head, 141
cellulite reduction machines, 220
ceramides, 179–80
cheeks, lifting the, 201–02
chemical peels, 42, 122, 157, 216–18
cherry angiomas, *64,* 64–65
children and skin treatments, 62
chin reshaping
Botox, 204
double chin, 204–05, *205*
Kybella, 205, *205*
liposuction, 205, *205*
weak chin, 204
chloasma, 55–56. *See also* melasma
chondrodermatitis nodularis helicis, 239
closed comedones. *See* whiteheads
CO2 laser resurfacing, 163, *163,* 218, *218*
coenzyme Q10, 176
cold sores (herpesvirus), 250
color wheel and makeup, 198–99, *199*
comedones. *See* blackheads; whiteheads
concealer, 198–99
contact dermatitis, 34, 236, *236,* 244, *244*
CoolSculpting, 212
copper peptides, 177–78
cortisone injections, 157
cosmetic injectables
Botox, 188–90, 191, 192–97, 201, *202,* 204
crow's-feet, 196–97
eyebrows, 196
forehead lines, 192–93
glabella ("11s" grooves), 189, 194, *194*
hyaluronic acid (HA) fillers, 190, 201, *201, 202,* 202–03
permanent fillers, 191–92
reversible nature of, 188
side effects of, 191
soft-tissue fillers, 163, 190
temporal atrophy, 193
temporary nature of, 188, 190
variances among products and physicians, 187
cosmetic procedures
competition among health care providers, 181–85
emotional toll of embarrassing spots, 4–5
midlevel providers (MLPs), 182–83
paying out of pocket for, 3, 185
cosmetics, 34–35, 198–99, 243, 248
crow's-feet, 196–97
crust, 22
cryosurgery. *See* cryotherapy
cryotherapy, 42, 106, 107, 121
curettage, 49, 107, 121
curette, 26, 49
cyst excisions, 26–27, 84, 88
cystic acne, *135,* 139–40
cysts. *See* epidermoid cysts; pilar cysts

dandruff (seborrheic dermatitis), *237,* 237–38
dapsone, 153
dark circles and bags under the eyes, 198–200, *200,* 241
dermabrasion/dermaplaning, 162, 219–20. *See also* microdermabrasion
dermatologists and dermatology
anesthesia, 23–24, 249
bedside manner, 7
competition for residencies, 11–12

dermatologists and dermatology *(cont.)*
  education and experience, 118
  inappropriate requests made to doctors, 6
  insurance regulations, 181–82
  job responsibilities, 1–2, 182–85, 255
  personalized treatment, 148
  and social media, 224–25, 253–55
  when to see a doctor, 43, 48, 131, 147
dermatosis papulosa nigra (DPN), 43–45, *44*
diabetes and acanthosis nigricans, 114
diet and acne, 144–45, 242
dilated blood vessels, 61–63
dilated pore of Winer (DPOW), *81–82,* 81–83, *137,* 137–38
doxycycline, 153
drinking more water for hydrating dry skin, 33
duct tape for wart removal, 111
dysplastic nevus syndrome (DNS), 117–18

ears
  chondrodermatitis nodularis helicis, 239
  earlobe reconstruction, *207,* 207–08
ecchymosis (bruising), 63
electrocautery tool, 44
electrosurgery, 60
emotional toll
  of acne, 145–46
  of acne scars, 161–62
  of benign cosmetic conditions, 4–5
  of hurtful comments, 221–22
enlarged oil glands (sebaceous hyperplasia), 65–67, *66*
environmental factors affecting aging, 167
epidermoid cysts, 83–88, *84, 86*
erbium laser resurfacing, 218
erosion, 22
eruptive syringomas, 54, *54*
eruptive vellus hair cysts (EVHCs), 93–96, *94, 95*
erythema ab igne ("laptop-on-thigh" disease), 240
erythrotelangiectatic rosacea, 57, *60*
Eskata, 49–50
excisions
  cyst, 26–27, 88
  and punch replacement grafting to treat acne scars, 162–63
  punch *vs.* standard, 25–26
  shape of, 25–26, 88
  to treat hidradenitis suppurativa (HS), 116–17
excoriation, 22
exfoliant creams and lotions, 112–13
eyebrows, 196
eye creams, 171
eyes
  blepharoplasty, 200, *200*
  crow's-feet, 196–97
  dark circles and bags, 198–200, *200,* 241
  eyelift, *209,* 209–10
  tear troughs, 200, *200*

facelift (rhytidectomy), 208
facial scrubs, 75
family history, 127–28, 130, 139–40, 142
fat, "recycling" the body's, 212
fatty acids, 179–80
Favre-Racouchot syndrome (solar comedones), 70–71, *70–71*
feeling self-conscious, 221–22
fibrous papules, *51,* 51–52
fingernail(s)
  acrylic nails as the cause of rashes, 236
  cleaning under the, 247
  fixing a split, 236–37
  health, 229–30
  onycholysis, 247
fissure, 22
Fitzpatrick, Richard, 15
Fitzpatrick Skin Type quiz, 31
flat warts, *109,* 109–11
fluid retention, 241
forehead lines, 192–93
foreign-body reaction, 86, *86*
freckles, *40,* 40–42
free radicals, 167, 172
furuncles, 90–93

gate control theory, 249
genetic factors that affect skin type, 31, 36
genital warts, 109–11
Gerri (patient), *137,* 137–38
glabella ("11s" grooves), 189, 194, *194*
glandular rosacea, 58
glycation, 168
glycolic acid, 148–49
green tea extract, 158, 175

hair
  cutting and growth rate, 228–29
  dye, allergy to, 238–39

growth cycle, *230*, 230–31
removal, laser, 214–15, *215*, 234
washing frequency and dandruff, *237*, 237–38
hair, thinning
hair transplants, 186, 231
male *vs.* female hair loss, 185–86, 231–32
minoxidil, 186
hair products, 72–73, 238–39
healing times
after lipoma removal, 102
for cosmetic treatments, 47
heat
erythema ab igne ("laptop-on-thigh" disease), 240
heat-based acne therapies, 157
herpesvirus (cold sores), 250
hexapeptides (Argireline), 178
hidradenitis suppurativa (HS), *115*, 115–17
hidrocystomas, *5*
home remedies, scarring from, 55, *55*
hormones and skin conditions
acanthosis nigricans, 114
acne, 142–43, 154–55
melasma and chloasma, 55–56
oral contraceptives, 154
polycystic ovarian syndrome (PCOS), 154–55
spironolactone, 154–55
human papillomavirus (HPV), 109
hyaluronic acid (HA)
benefits of, 178
fillers, 190, 201, *201*, *202*, 202–03
low molecular weight hyaluronic acid, 178
sodium hyaluronate, 179
hydrocortisone cream, 113
hydroquinone, 41–42, 56
hypopigmentation, 50

ice pick scars, 161, *161*, 162–63
imiquimod, 110, 122
immune system's response to warts, 109–10
incision and drainage (I&D), 86, 92–93
inflammation, *86*, 86–88, 139, 158, 159–60, 169
inflammatory cells, *86*, 86–88
instruments and techniques used
11 blade, 24, *24*
15 blade, 24, *24*
30-gauge needle, 23
buried vertical mattress stitch, 29
comedone extractors, *24*, 24–25, 75, 80, 136
curette, 26, 49
electrocautery tool, 44
electrosurgery, 60
incision and drainage (I&D), 86, 92–93
interrupted stitch, *29*, 29–30
laser treatments, 42, 44–45
liquid nitrogen, 42, 45, 106, 107
numbing medication, 23–24
punch biopsy tool, 25–26, 162–63
running subcuticular stitch, *29*, 30
shave removal, 50
suspension stitch, 29, *29*
insurance regulations, 181–82
intense pulsed light (IPL) treatments, 42
interrupted stitch, *29*, 29–30
intuition, trusting your, 67
iPLEDGE program, 156
irritants, common skin, 34, 173
isotretinoin (oral retinoid), 155–56, *155–56*
isthmus-catagen cyst. *See* pilar cysts

jawline, softening the, 205–06
Jenner, Kylie, 203
Jolie, Angelina, 203
jowling, improving, 201–02

keratin, 84, 89, 111–12
keratosis pilaris (KP), 111–13, *112*
Koebnerization, 108, *109*
Kybella, 205, *205*

laser treatments
for acne, 157
for acne scars, 163
CO2 laser resurfacing, 163, *163*, 218, *218*
for dermatosis papulosa nigra (DPN), 44–45
for dilated blood vessels, 63
erbium laser resurfacing, 218
false advertisements regarding, 63
for freckles, 42
for hair removal, 214–15, *215*, 234
nonablative laser resurfacing, 218–19
for tattoo removal, *215*, 215–16, 234
for warts, warning against, 110
layers of the skin, 168
Lee, Sandra ("Dr. Pimple Popper")
adolescence, 221
atopic dermatitis, 33, 241

Lee, Sandra ("Dr. Pimple Popper") *(cont.)*
- dermatology residency and early career, 12–16
- education and medical school experiences, 9–13, 184–85
- family life, 7–9, *8–10,* 15–16
- friendships, 228, *228*
- Instagram presence, 2
- personal Botox experiences, 193, 195, 197
- practice specialties and exclusions, 184–85, 187
- shaking hands of, 249
- SLMD Acne System, 72, 73, *73,* 77, 136, 140, *147,* 147–48, 245
- social media popularity, 3–4
- Southern Illinois University training, 13–14, *14*
- as a TV personality, *6*
- on YouTube and social media, 1–4, 78–79, 249, 253–55

lesion terminology, 20–22
lichenification, 22
lidocaine, 23, 250
lipidosis, 52–53
lipids, 179
lipomas
- composition of, 100
- healing and recovery from, 102
- images of, *101, 103*
- treatment of, 101
- *vs.* angiolipomas, 100
- *vs.* keloids, 102
- watching the removal of, 100–01, 103

liposuction
- alternatives to, 212
- of the chin and neck, 205, *205*
- effects on future weight gain, 213, 247–78
- ideal candidates for, 210–11, 248
- true tumescent, *210,* 211–12

lips
- celebrities envied for their, 203
- changes due to aging, 202
- cultural differences, 203
- full lips trend, 202–03
- hyaluronic acid (HA) fillers, *202,* 202–03
- improving a gummy smile, 204
- lip balm, 246
- perleche, 233, *233*

liquid nitrogen, 42, 45, 106, 107
liver spots. *See* solar lentigos
macule, 20, *20*
the Masked Man (patient), 70, *70*
mechanical tools for fighting acne
- brushes, 159
- cleansing cloths, 159
- scrubs, 75, 159

medical school
- author's experiences, 10–12
- clinical rotations, 11
- competition for residencies, 11–12
- gross anatomy courses, 10
- Match Day, 12

medication to treat acne
- over-the-counter, 148–52
- prescription, *152,* 152–57

melanin, 128
melanocytes, 106, 128
melanoma
- ABCDEs of, 43, 118, 119, 131
- about, 127–30
- images of, *128*
- and metastasis, 123
- risk factors of, 129–30
- when to see a doctor, 43, 48

melasma, 55–57, *56, 57. See also* chloasma
metastasis, 123
microdermabrasion, 219. *See also* dermabrasion/dermaplaning
midlevel providers (MLPs), 182–83
milia, *5, 68,* 68–70, 80–81
minimally invasive procedures. *See also* surgical procedures
- cellulite reduction machines, 220
- chemical peel, 42, 122, 157, 216–18
- CO2 laser resurfacing, 163, *163,* 218, *218*
- dermabrasion/dermaplaning, 162, 219–20
- erbium laser resurfacing, 218
- laser hair removal, 214–15, *215,* 234
- microdermabrasion, 219
- nonablative laser resurfacing, 218–19
- tattoo removal, *215,* 215–16, 234
- tissue tightening, 220

minocycline, 153
minoxidil, 186
Mirvaso, 59
Mohs surgery, 125–27, *126*
moisturizer, 171, 173, 241–42, 247
moles (nevi)
- atypical (dysplastic) nevi, 117–18, 129
- common, 117, 128–29
- dysplastic nevus syndrome (DNS), 117–18
- giant congenital nevus, 117

images of, *117*
removing and evaluating, 119
shave biopsy, 119, 120
molluscum contagiosum, *106,* 106–08
Momma Squishy (patient), *97,* 97–98
Mr. and Mrs. Gold (patients), 28, *28*
Mr. Wilson (patient), *58, 78,* 78–79
myths about skin, nails, and hair
acne and washing, 246
base tans, 242–43
body acne *vs.* face acne, 246
bumps on the edges of the ear, 239
cold sores (herpesvirus), 250
cosmetics and acne, 243
cosmetics that contain sunscreen, 248
diet and acne, 144–45, 242
fragranced moisturizers and cleansers, 247
hair dye allergy after years of use, 238–39
hair-washing frequency and dandruff, *237,* 237–38
"laptop-on-thigh" disease (erythema ab igne), 240
lidocaine allergies, 250
lip balm, 246
liposuction, 247–48
moisturizer application after bathing, 241–42
oil-based cleansers, 245
penicillin allergies, 232–34
permanent laser hair removal, 234
rashes around the eyes, 34, 236
rate of hair growth, 228–29
spider bites, 249
sudden hair loss, 230–32
sunscreen and acne, 243–44
universal product effectiveness, 238
vitamin D from sun exposure, 235
waiting after sunscreen application, 235
wearing rubber gloves to prevent a rash, 251

nail(s)
acrylic nails as the cause of rashes, 236
cleaning under the, 247
fixing a split, 236–37
health, 229–30
onycholysis, 247
natural products to treat acne
green tea extract, 158
tea tree oil, 158
zinc, 158
neck
cervicoplasty, 209
cosmetic procedures, 206
neck lift, 209, *209*
platysmaplasty, 209
neuromodulators
Botox, 188–90, 191, 192–97, 201, *202,* 204
neurotic excoriations, *143,* 143–44
nevi (moles)
atypical (dysplastic), 117–18, 129
common, 117, 128–29
dysplastic nevus syndrome (DNS), 117–18
giant congenital nevus, 117
images of, *117*
removing and evaluating, 119
shave biopsy, 119, 120
nevus araneus, *62. See also* dilated blood vessels
niacinamide (vitamin B3), 179
nodules, 20–21, *21*
nodulocystic acne, *135,* 139–40
nonablative laser resurfacing, 218–19
nose
bunny lines, 201
reshaping using hyaluronic acid (HA) filler, 201, *201*
nose strips, 75–76
numbing medication, 23–24

obsessive-compulsive disorder (OCD), 143
ochronosis, *41,* 41–42
odor
of cyst excisions, 27, 84
fragranced moisturizers and cleansers, 247
oil glands, enlarged (sebaceous hyperplasia), 65–67, *66*
onycholysis, 247
open comedones. *See* blackheads
oral contraceptives for treating acne, 154
oxymetazoline, 240

papules, 20, *20, 135,* 138–39
papulopustular rosacea, 57
parentheses lines, 201–02
patch, 20, *20*
patient stories
Gerri, *137,* 137–38
the Masked Man, 70, *70*
Momma Squishy, *97,* 97–98

patient stories *(cont.)*
Mr. and Mrs. Gold, 28, *28*
Mr. Wilson, *58, 78,* 78–79
Pops, 1–4, *3*
penicillin allergies, 232–34
pentapeptides (Matrixyl), 177
peptides
benefits of, 176–77
copper peptides, 177–78
hexapeptides (Argireline), 178
limitations of, 177
pentapeptides (Matrixyl), 177
perleche, 233, *233*
permanent fillers, 191–92
phytophotodermatitis, 245
pigmentation, 45, 50, 106, 198
pilar cysts, 88–90, *89*
pilomatricomas, *98,* 98–100
pimple popping, viewers' fascination with, 5, 78–79
pimples. *See* acne
plantar warts, 109–11
plaque, 20, *20*
polycystic ovarian syndrome (PCOS), 154–55
Pops (patient), 1–4, *3*
pore size, 36, 76–77
postinflammatory hyperpigmentation, 45
precancerous growths
actinic keratosis (AK), 120–23, 217
product
effectiveness, myth of universal, 238
labels, importance of reading, 173–74
psoriasis, 20, *21,* 237, *238*
ptosis, 194, *194*
punch biopsy tool, 25–26, 162–63
punctum, 84
pus, 91
pustules, *21,* 22, *135,* 138–39

rash
after taking penicillin, 232–34
from allergic contact dermatitis, 34, 236, *236,* 244, *244*
from sweat inside rubber gloves, 251
Rebish, Jeff, *10,* 10–13, 15–16
resveratrol, 175
retinoids, 42, 95, 113, 136, 149–50, 152, 176
retinol, 67, 69, 136, 149–50, 176
rhinophyma, 58, *58,* 59–60, *60, 78,* 78–79
Rhofade, 59
"rodent ulcers" (squamous cell carcinoma), 124
rolling scars, *160,* 161, 162
rosacea
incidence of, 57–58
misconceptions regarding, 58
rhinophyma, 58, *58,* 59–60, *60, 78,* 78–79
symptoms, 61
topical treatments for, 59
treatment of, 58–60
types of, 57–58
running subcuticular stitch, *29,* 30

salicylic acid, 72, 73, 77, 111, 149
scale, 22
scalp
hair-washing frequency and dandruff, *237,* 237–38
pilar cysts, 88–90, *89*
psoriasis, 237, *238*
scarring
from acne inflammation, 139–40, 159–62
from home remedies, 55, *55*
treatment for acne scars, 162–63, *163*
scrubs, facial, 75, 159
"sebaceous cysts," 89
sebaceous hyperplasia (enlarged oil glands), 65–67, *66*
seborrheic dermatitis (dandruff), *237,* 237–38
seborrheic keratoses (SK), 48–50, *49*
sebum, 36, 135–36, 154–55, 158
sensitivity to skin products, 35
sexually transmitted diseases (STDs)
cold sores (herpesvirus), 250
molluscum contagiosum, *106,* 106–08
shadow cells, *98,* 99
shave biopsy, 119, 120
shave removal, 50
skin cancer. *See* cancer
skincare
combination skin, 36
dry skin, 34
normal skin, 32
oily skin, 37
sensitive skin, 35
skin color
and melanoma, 127
phytophotodermatitis, 245
skin-lightening creams, 41–42
skin tags, *104,* 104–06
skin type
combination, 35–36
dry, 33–34, 112–13

as a factor is treating acne, 30–31
Fitzpatrick quiz, 31
genetic factors that affect, 31
normal, 32
oily, 36–37
and pore size, 76–77
sensitive, 34–35
sleep's effect on skin health, 170–71, 242
SLMD Acne System, 72, 73, *73,* 77, 136, 140, *147,* 147–48, 245
smell
of cyst excisions, 27, 84
fragranced moisturizers and cleansers, 247
smile, improving your, 204
smoking
and skin health, 171–72
and smoker's lines around the lips, 203
soap
antibacterial, 32
moisturizing, 32
vs. cleansers and washes, 32
soft-tissue fillers, 163, 190
solar keratosis, 120–23
solar lentigos, 45–48, *46*
spider angioma. *See* dilated blood vessels
spider bites, 249
spironolactone, 154–55
spray tans, 48
squamous cell carcinoma (SCC), 120, 123–25, *126*
squeezing
blackheads (open comedones), 74–75
unsuccessful, 80–81
whiteheads (closed comedones), 79–81
Staphylococcus aureus bacteria, 91–92
steatocystomas, 94–95, *95, 97,* 97–98
steroid injections, 157
stitches
buried vertical mattress, 29
interrupted stitch, *29,* 29–30
running subcuticular stitch, *29,* 30
suspension, 29, *29*
suture removal guidelines, 96
stress
and acne, 143
and aging, 172
and hair loss, 232
and nail health, 229–30
sulfur, 150, 151
sun exposure
and acne, 71
after a chemical peel, 216–18
and aging, 168–69
base tan, dangers of a, 242–43
and melasma, 55–56
phytophotodermatitis, 245
and rosacea, 59, 60
and skin cancer, 124–25, 128, 130, 168–69
and solar lentigos, 45–47
and vitamin D, 235
sunscreen
chemical *vs.* physical, 243–44
to combat photoaging, 169–70
cosmetics containing, 248
to prevent freckles, 43
to prevent melanoma, 130
to prevent postinflammatory hyperpigmentation, 45
recommendations, 170, 173
usage guidelines, 130
waiting time after application, 235
surgical procedures. *See also* minimally invasive procedures
earlobe reconstruction, *207,* 207–08
eyelift, *209,* 209–10
facelift (rhytidectomy), 208
liposuction, *211–13*
neck lift, 209, *209*
screening for bullying before providing, 223–24
true tumescent liposuction, *210,* 211–12
suspension stitch, 29, *29*
sweat, 72
syringoma, 53–55, *54*

tanning
base tans, 242–43
spray tans, 48
tattoo removal, *215,* 215–16, 234
tazarotene (Tazorac), 42, 152
tear troughs, 200, *200*
tea tree oil, 158
techniques and instruments used
11 blade, 24, *24*
15 blade, 24, *24*
30-gauge needle, 23
buried vertical mattress stitch, 29
comedone extractors, *24,* 24–25, 75, 80, 136
curette, 26, 49
electrocautery tool, 44

techniques and instruments used *(cont.)*
electrosurgery, 60
incision and drainage (I&D), 86, 92–93
interrupted stitch, *29,* 29–30
laser treatments, 42, 44–45
liquid nitrogen, 42, 45, 106, 107
numbing medication, 23–24
punch biopsy tool, 25–26, 162–63
running subcuticular stitch, *29,* 30
shave removal, 50
suspension stitch, 29, *29*
telangiectasias. *See* dilated blood vessels
telogen phase of the hair growth cycle, *230,* 230–31
temporal atrophy, 193
terminology, 20–22
tetracyclines, 153
tissue tightening procedures, 220
tools for dermatology. *See* instruments and techniques used
tretinoin (Retin-A), 42, 136, 152, 176
"triangle of death," 141
trichilemmal cyst. *See* pilar cysts
trichloracetic (TCA) acid, 217
tuberous sclerosis, 51
tumescent liposuction, *210,* 211–12
tumors, 22, 84
Tyndall effect, 191
T-zone, 35

ulceration, 22
ultraviolet (UV) rays, 40–41, 124–25, 130, 168–70, 235

vellus hair, 93–94, *94*
vesicle, 21, *21*
viral infections
molluscum contagiosum, *106,* 106–08
warts, *109,* 109–11
vitamin B3 (niacinamide), 179
vitamin B5 (panthenol), 179
vitamin B7 (biotin), 179
vitamin C, 175–76
vitamin D, 235
vitamin E, 175

warts, *109,* 109–11
weight gain after liposuction, 213
wen. *See* pilar cysts
whiteheads (closed comedones)
about, 136
comedone extractors, 80, 136
images of, *70, 135*
preventing, 71–74
similarity to other skin conditions, 80
squeezing, 79–81
vs. pustules, 71
wrinkles
eliminating, 178, 190
preventing, 171–72, 189, 242

xanthelasma, 52–53, *53*

zinc, 158, 169

ABOUT THE AUTHOR

Sandra Lee, MD, is a board-certified dermatologist and a member of the American Academy of Dermatology, the American Academy of Cosmetic Surgery, the American Society for Dermatologic Surgery, and the American Society for Mohs Surgery. Dr. Lee specializes in cosmetic and surgical dermatology in Southern California and has become a global YouTube and social media sensation. She is the star of the TLC television series *Dr. Pimple Popper* and the founder of SLMD Skincare. She lives in Southern California with her husband, also a board-certified dermatologist, and their two sons.